AF752419

SUGAR COATED

CALIFORNIA STUDIES IN FOOD AND CULTURE

Darra Goldstein, Editor

SUGAR COATED

Unboxing the Hidden Forces Shaping America's Favorite Breakfast Food

Marion Nestle and
Lisa Sutherland

UNIVERSITY OF CALIFORNIA PRESS

The publisher gratefully acknowledges the generous support of the Literati Circle of the University of California Press Foundation, whose members are the Melony and Adam Lewis Advised Fund at Aspen Community Foundation, Harriett Gold, Richard Greene in memory of Lorrie Greene, and The Dido Fund at the East Bay Community Foundation.

The publisher and the University of California Press Foundation also gratefully acknowledge the generous support of Jessica Lipnack and Peter Booth Wiley in making this book possible.

UNIVERSITY OF CALIFORNIA PRESS
Oakland, California

©2026 by Marion Nestle and Lisa Sutherland

All rights reserved.

Cataloging-in-Publication data is on file
at the Library of Congress

ISBN 978-0-520-42127-1 (cloth : alk. paper)
ISBN 978-0-520-42128-8 (ebook)

Text design by Kevin Barrett Kane

Manufactured in the United States of America

GPSR AUTHORIZED REPRESENTATIVE:
Easy Access System Europe,
Mustamäe tee 50, 10621 Tallinn,
Estonia, gpsr.requests@easproject.com

35 34 33 32 31 30 29 28 27 26
10 9 8 7 6 5 4 3 2 1

DEDICATION

To cereal lovers, now and future

CONTENTS

PART III. MARKETING

INTRODUCTION

This book is about how the food industry, publicly and behind the scenes, sells products and entices people to eat junk food, regardless of its health consequences—as illustrated by breakfast cereals. Cereals are perfect for telling this story. Their boxes are much more than packages for selling processed grains; they are a wide-open window into American popular culture and the politics of food. Because of their size, cereal boxes are unique vehicles for food marketing. And because their designs are updated frequently, they can immediately respond to new regulations and take advantage of dietary fads, holidays, and celebrity popularity. Every word and illustration on a cereal box has one of two purposes: to comply with regulatory requirements or to promote sales. In this book, we explain each design element, why it is there, what inspired it, what it means, and for a surprisingly large number, how it was contested. But before getting into all that, we need to tell you why we wanted to write this book and how our collaboration got started.

In Marion Nestle's words

I first noticed how cereal boxes reflect current events when I was working as senior nutrition policy advisor for the Reagan administration's Department of Health and Human Services in the late 1980s. My job was managing the editorial production of *The Surgeon General's Report on Nutrition and Health*. This 727-page report was intended to settle nutrition controversies by giving the public up-to-date, evidence-based advice about how to eat healthfully. Its recommendations were much the same as dietary guidelines then and now: balance calories; reduce saturated fat, salt, and sugar; drink alcohol only in moderation; and eat more vegetables, fruits, and whole grains. The report was published in July 1988. Within just a few months, General Mills used it to market Total cereal as we show in Figure 1—a revelation about how cereal marketing works.

Once I moved to New York University (NYU), where I have been ever since, I started to collect an occasional cereal box whenever I spotted one responding to some new food fad or regulation. I made slides of them to illustrate teaching points about health claims, food labeling rules, or over-the-top marketing. Sometime in the early 2000s, I met Lisa Sutherland through her work developing the Guiding Stars front-of-package labeling system for Hannaford supermarkets, and I later ran into her at meetings she organized while consulting for Walmart.

In spring 2010, Kellogg's senior vice president for nutrition, Celeste Clark, asked me to consult with her and another official about some product they had in mind. To avoid conflicts of interest, I do not accept funds from food companies. But I did ask for a favor: Would it be possible for me to look through Kellogg's archives to examine cereal box labels issued before Congress passed the Nutrition Labeling and Education Act in 1990 that still governs their details? I could not remember what the old labels looked like and had not been able to find suitable examples online. Celeste said they would try.

Weeks went by with no response. But at the end of June, Lisa wrote that she had just started a job as vice president of nutrition for Kellogg. After wishing her well, I asked if she could please get me into Kellogg's files. Some months later, she told me the company had agreed to my visit, and I flew out to Battle Creek.

When I arrived, Lisa and Celeste asked which I wanted first: the good news or the bad. I asked for the bad news and got it. Kellogg's lawyers were not going to let me anywhere near the archives. But the good news could not have been better. They handed me three flat cartons, each containing a set of color scans of the cereal boxes for every consecutive year since they were first introduced: one for All-Bran since 1919, another for Rice Krispies since 1928, and the third for Froot Loops since 1963.

Their significance was instantly evident. Paging through them, we could see how the designs changed year by year in response to new regulations

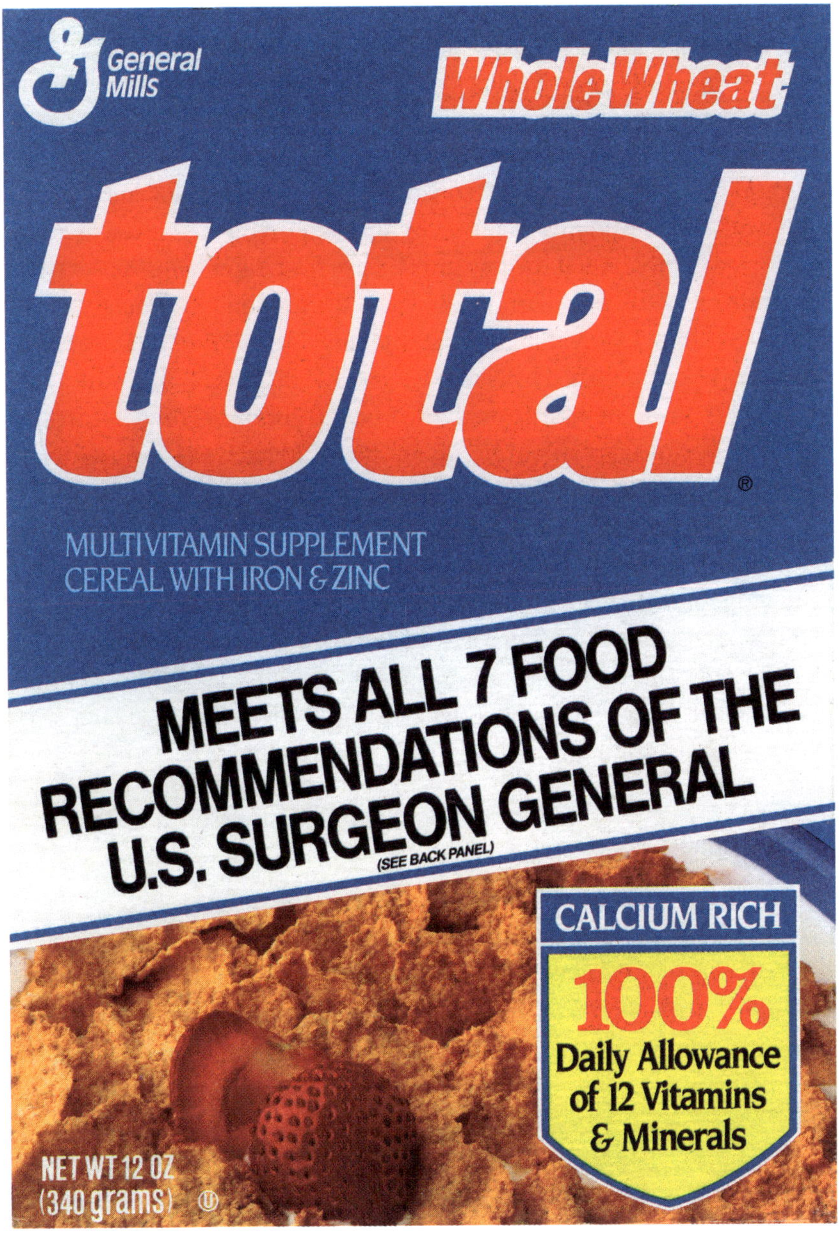

FIGURE 1 In 1989, shortly after publication of *The Surgeon General's Report on Nutrition and Health*, General Mills advertised Total cereal as a way to meet all of the report's food recommendations.

and cultural trends. Cereal boxes illustrate the contemporary history of food policy and American culture. And they sit on millions of breakfast tables across America, engaging children and adults. We knew right away there was a book in this.

But busy with other career matters, we did not pursue the idea. In 2015, Lisa and I met in New York and corresponded about the book idea, and we each went so far as to investigate copyright requirements for use of cereal box images (lawyers tell us they are fair use for academic purposes). But the timing was still not right. We dropped the idea and lost touch.

Late in 2023, I turned in the draft manuscript of *What to Eat Now*, my 700-page book published by North Point Press in 2025. While waiting for its editor to work his way through the manuscript, I had time to consider what the next project might be. In February 2024, I was amazed to see supermarket shelves loaded with heart-shaped Honey Nut Cheerios in multiple versions for individual family members (mom, dad, grandparents, grandkids, dogs, cats), some in Spanish (*mamá, familia, abuelo*). These reminded me of the cereal book project. I could put my box collection to good use. But I remembered my discussions with Lisa and thought I needed to make sure she would not mind if I did this. It took a full morning of internet searching to track her down, but I did and wrote to tell her what I had in mind. “I'm doing this with you,” she wrote back.

Lisa Sutherland's version

While Marion was building her academic career and place in food policy history, I was acquiring my own expertise in breakfast cereals. As a kid of the '70s, I ate cereal for breakfast, for snacks, and often for supper on Sunday nights. I watched Saturday morning cartoons laden with cereal commercials, memorized the catchy jingles, loved the mascots, and couldn't wait to dig out the toys and prizes from the bottom of the sugary sweet cereal boxes. Our home always had three to four cereals in our cupboards, typically Sugar Corn Pops, Cocoa Puffs, Frosted Flakes, and Lucky Charms. Cereal was inexpensive, was convenient, and never went to waste. I was the core cereal consumer, a captive fan of all its marketing and advertising gimmicks. Nutrition was not something I thought much about—until years later.

As a student of nutrition and food policy at the University of North Carolina, how could I not know who Dr. Marion Nestle was. Her first book, *Food Politics*, was published the year I received my PhD. I spent the next few years studying product placement, advertising to kids in popular media, and teaching food policy before embarking on a 20-year corporate career.

With my doctorate in hand and considerable experience consulting in the corporate food sector, including advising the Walmart food team, I became Kellogg's vice president of nutrition, overseeing strategy development and implementation for nutrition labeling and regulatory policy, marketing, and communication. One of my first calls after setting up shop there was to Marion. I can't remember what we were working on, but I wanted her counsel. She would come—but only if we gave her access to our archives. Marion knew what I didn't; Kellogg has one of the best packaging and historical libraries in the food industry.

Over the next several weeks, I met with our "morning foods" (breakfast cereal) leadership, company lawyers, and CEO David Mackay to discuss Marion's request. She had written a few times about Kellogg for her blog (foodpolitics.com), not always in the most positive light. Kellogg's missteps landed them in trouble with the Federal Trade Commission (FTC) over advertising that Marion considered to be anything but "truthful and not misleading." Despite the published criticisms, our executive team agreed to the visit. I promised to make sure Marion was accompanied at all times and that she would not run off with trade secrets. As a compromise to unlimited access to the archives, our librarian made copies of three complete packaging sets from the cereals' inceptions through Marion's visit in 2010. I was surprised we agreed to let Marion keep them; we even mailed them to her after the visit.

I was thrilled when she contacted me. For years, I wanted to do this book. Marion was reluctant to have an unfamiliar co-author, but we agreed that if we could make it through the writing of the proposal without issue, we'd make a go of it. We did, and this book is the result.

Our collaboration

Our combined expertise in food and nutrition policy (Marion) and corporate background in the cereal industry (Lisa) and, most important, our joint appreciation and love of cereal boxes and what they signify, made this book a perfect project for us. Right from the start, we knew we were onto something. We are not alone in our quasi-fanatical interest in cereals. Nearly 300 million Americans eat breakfast cereals at least occasionally, many with intense attachments to particular brands. Whenever we talk to people about this project, they immediately recount childhood memories. Collectors—there are lots of them—seem willing to spend fortunes on rare vintage items; in 2024, we saw a 1951 Stan Muṣial Wheaties box for sale on Etsy for $5,000. Collectible, fan club, YouTube, and social media sites are devoted to cereals. In 2025, a Reddit thread, "What is/was your favorite breakfast cereal," had 46 million followers. Search for "cereal" on TikTok, and you can watch thousands of posts. The hashtag #cereal has 2.4 million posts on Instagram. You can even celebrate National Cereal Day on March 7.

In this book, we use cereal boxes to describe and analyze the history and present status of food, nutrition, and health in the United States, as well as to investigate examples of heavily researched and highly sophisticated food marketing. This is by no means the first book about cereals (see our Bibliography), although it uniquely focuses on how the packaging of these products exploits regulatory and cultural trends.

We approached our writing by examining a particular element on a particular box and analyzing what it was and why it was there. We were fortunate to have so many boxes to choose from, and not only from Marion's collection of about 200 (1989 to the present) and the Kellogg facsimiles (1919 to 2010). Unexpectedly, the NYU library houses the David Pollack collection of 300 boxes from 1976 to 2017. And because so many people collect cereal boxes, we were able to borrow or buy the ones we wanted online.

This book's themes

This book highlights several overarching themes worth noting. The chapters demonstrate how these themes developed over time, illustrated by box designs, marketing strategies, and legal challenges.

Nostalgia sells. The emotional attachment of American adults to the cereal brands they loved as children emerges as a constant, underlying theme throughout this book.

Sugar sells. Cereals may have started out as simple, highly nutritious grain foods for the health conscious, but they ended up as candy and cookies for breakfast for adults as well as kids.

Vitamins sell. Cereal companies struggled for decades to convince a reluctant Food and Drug Administration (FDA) to permit them to add nutrients to fortify cereals; many of today's cereals are no more than sugary one-a-day nutrient supplements.

Health sells. Cereal marketers have pushed the FDA to allow them to extol the benefits of their products for heart health, cancer prevention, and promotion of immunity, bone health, weight loss, and more, however poorly backed up by research.

Consolidation sells. Historically, four companies—the Big Four—thoroughly dominated the US cereal market: General Mills, Kellogg Company (now split into companies owned by Mars and Ferrero), Post Consumer Brands, and The Quaker Oats Company (owned by PepsiCo).

Marketing sells. Besides the required elements, everything on a cereal box, no matter how seemingly trivial, is designed to promote sales.

Marketing to children sells. The most heavily sweetened cereals, in brightly colored boxes illustrated with cartoon mascots, are aimed at children.

The Big Four vs. the FDA and FTC. This book records the historic—and still ongoing—struggle between cereal companies and the FDA and FTC over what the boxes are allowed to claim or advertise about what cereals do for health.

The Big Four vs. consumer advocates. For decades, consumer groups and child-health advocates have petitioned the FDA—or have sued cereal companies—to remove unhealthful ingredients and misleading statements from the boxes. This, too, is an ongoing struggle.

An overview

We begin this book with a brief recounting of the history of the development and production of cereals and of the industry that produces them (Chapter 1). This is not a history book, but we do provide the historical context for what is in cereals and how they are marketed. We then move on to explain the structure of a cereal box (Chapter 2). The rest of the chapters are organized into three parts: ingredients, claims, and marketing. In Part I, we discuss the principal ingredients that comprise ready-to-eat cold cereals. Although these products naturally and most prominently contain grains and fiber, we begin with their most controversial ingredient: sugars (Chapter 3). Chapter 4 covers grains and fiber, and Chapters 5 and 6 deal with the other common ingredient additions—flavors, colors, and nutrients.

Part II deals with claims for health benefits. Once Kellogg tricked the FDA into allowing health claims on food products, companies could market cereals as helping to prevent cancer and heart disease (Chapters 7 and 8). Later, companies could use more poorly substantiated claims such as those permitted for dietary supplements (Chapter 9). Chapter 10 covers the small icons—which we call widgets—that appear on boxes to signal cereals as especially healthy. Chapter 11 deals with cereal box claims about specific diets: weight loss, gluten-free, and keto. In Chapter 12, we focus on claims about how the cereals were produced—naturally, organically, or not genetically modified—often interpreted as implying that the products are healthier.

In Part III, we describe the tactics used to market cereal to kids (Chapter 13); adults and families (Chapter 14); and consumer groups included under the heading of diversity, equity, and inclusion (Chapter 15). In Chapter 16, we explain how companies use philanthropy (feel-good marketing) to sell cereals. Chapter 17 analyzes how the Big Four sell cereals internationally. In the conclusion, we discuss what all this means for American culture and food systems.

A few points about some of this book's idiosyncrasies: The majority of cereal brand names and many components on the boxes are trademarked, but we think the ™ or the ® symbols are distracting and left them out. We know that boxes cannot talk, but using "the box says" is so much easier than saying "the text on the back of the box includes this statement." We hope you will forgive us for the imprecision.

As for the box illustrations, we wrote every part of the book with a particular box in mind, selecting each for historical, aesthetic, or sentimental reasons to illustrate the points under discussion. Each illustrated box is dated by its year of production. Since the early 1970s, a best-used-by date is stamped on the box top; this is one full year after the cereal was produced (for production dates, we subtracted a year from the sell-by dates).

One final observation: As a result of consumer advocacy and actions by the FDA and FTC, the cereal aisles of supermarkets are much less fun to investigate than they used to be. Whereas the boxes used to display outrageous or ridiculous health claims (as in the examples we include), hardly any do that now. Even so, we love looking at the new boxes when they arrive in supermarkets. We hope this book will encourage you to view cereal boxes as fascinating objects, historical treasures, indicators of food regulation, and works of pop art—and as profoundly serious but thoroughly enjoyable examples of food industry marketing, as we do.

Marion Nestle and Lisa Sutherland
MARCH 2026

CHAPTER 1

BREAKFAST CEREALS

THE BASICS

TO CEREAL MAKERS, grains are more than just food. They are the core of civilization. Grains shape human history in many ways, ranging from how they are planted (agriculture), stored (societal stability), exchanged and traded (economics), cooked (techniques), harvested, and prayed over (religion). Though it might seem a stretch, cereal staples—mainly wheat, rice, corn, oats, barley, and sorghum—have been and continue to be principal sources of calories and nutrients in the diets of all populations. For millennia, people have eaten grains as porridges or ground them into flour to make breads.[1] But ready-to-eat breakfast cereals? These are a far more recent invention.

The invention of these products has been recounted in riveting detail in books we recommend highly (see our Bibliography). This chapter draws on these and other sources to provide a brief overview of the development of ready-to-eat breakfast cereals, describe trends in cereal sales and consumption, and introduce the companies, brands, and marketing that drive this multibillion-dollar global food category.

As recounted by scholars, the history of cereals is entertaining—and weird—as it involves a succession of religiously influenced health-food faddists and fanatics. To get a feeling for the weirdness, we suggest taking a look at *The Road to Wellville*, the 1994 film based on the novel by T. C. Boyle, a fictional, but not all that far off, reenactment of Dr. John Harvey Kellogg's experiments with corn flakes.

Breakfast cereal: A bizarre start

The early inventors of cereal held in common a firm belief that most major illnesses derived from dyspepsia, the term then used to describe disorders of digestion and elimination resulting from poor diets, but also from the effects of sexual sins, particularly masturbation.[2] Their solution? An abstemious and thoroughly bland diet based on cereal grains. In such beliefs, they established a now century-long tradition of considering breakfast cereals the cure-all for everything that ails you.

Credit for the first breakfast cereal goes to Dr. James Caleb Jackson, who ran a sanitorium health resort in upstate New York. In 1863, he invented Granula, a cereal of bran-rich graham flour, so difficult to chew that it had to be soaked overnight.[3] One of his patients was Ellen White, who co-founded the Seventh-day Adventist Church; she claimed to have received the word of God to promote grain-based vegetarian diets and to establish an institute for wellness in Battle Creek, Michigan.

Next came the Kellogg brothers. Dr. John Harvey, a physician, and his younger brother, William Keith (W. K.). John Harvey visited Jackson's sanitorium, began working for Ellen White, adopted her religious and vegetarian views, and founded her wished-for sanitorium, "The San," in 1866, which eventually evolved into "the Vatican of the Seventh Day Adventist church." In 1880, he hired W. K. to run the San's publishing and food businesses. Together, the Kellogg brothers promoted health reform and created grain-based cereals, reflecting their dietary ideology but also less attractive beliefs in eugenics and racial superiority.[4]

John Harvey experimented with his versions of Granula, but when Jackson filed a lawsuit, he renamed it granola. After accidentally pressing wheat grains into flakes, he applied the same process to corn, creating corn flakes in 1898.[5]

W. K. Kellogg worked at the sanitorium for many years, but eventually the two split over issues of ownership of the Kellogg name—and sugar. W. K. thought sugar essential for improving the taste of the flakes and making them more appealing to a mass audience, whereas John Harvey viewed sugar as poison (shades of Robert F. Kennedy Jr. in 2025).[6] W. K. bought the cereal recipe from John Harvey in the early 1900s, added a little sugar, and created the Battle Creek Toasted Corn Flake Company in 1906, which became the Kellogg Company in 1922. Remarkably, Kellogg's Corn Flakes grace supermarket shelves to this day, virtually unchanged.

At this point, meet a third founder, Charles William (C. W.) Post, a patient at John Harvey's sanitorium. Short of money to pay for his stay, he worked in the kitchen, where he watched how granola was made, "borrowed" the techniques, created the Postum Company, and in 1897 invented wheat-and-barley-based Grape-Nuts. This cereal, he proclaimed, "makes and rebuilds the soft gray matter in the Brain, in the Solar Plexus and in the many Nerve Centres all over the body." He promised that eating Grape-Nuts with every meal "will put you safely on the Road to Wellville."[7]

Post also bought the rights to one of W. K. Kellogg's cereal-making machines. With the right equipment, cereals were easy to make, and many competitors copied the techniques. By 1906, Battle Creek—nicknamed Cereal City—housed more than 100 cereal companies marketing and selling to anyone who would buy them; today, only two remain (Kellogg and Post). The cereals had immediate wide appeal. They did, in fact, help with digestion, and they were convenient, inexpensive, and so easy to use that even children could grab a box, pour out the cereal, and add milk (and sugar) on their own.[8]

Manufacturing breakfast cereal

At first, cereal inventors had to solve some formidable technical problems. Except for sweet corn, cereal grains are too tough to be digested. They have to be soaked for hours to be edible as porridge or mush. That is why most cereals are extruded, shredded, flaked, or puffed. In 1893, Henry Perky invented the first machine with grooved rollers to do this; it allowed wheat to be extruded and shredded, then layered into biscuits, creating shredded wheat.

These inventions solved the indigestibility problem. The grains were cooked, dried, rolled, and toasted to make flaked cereals. When puffing guns were introduced in 1904, they allowed cooked whole-grain rice or wheat to be loaded and, under intense pressure, puffed and shot out to make puffed wheat. For making O-shaped circles (as in Cheerios and Froot Loops), the grains are cooked, forced through a die to make tubes, sliced into small O's, and subjected to pressure and its quick release. A similar technique is used to make balls (Kix and Trix). Later, other dies were invented to make more interesting shapes, and new equipment and manufacturing techniques allowed the addition of sugars and fortifying nutrients. Companies also introduced methods for packaging the finished cereals to preserve their shape and crispness.[9]

In making cereals, an important botanical consideration is that wheat, corn, oats, and rice seeds are composed of three layers: the bran (the outer, nutrient-rich fibrous layer), the inner endosperm (starch and protein), and the germ (the embryo). Because whole grains are difficult to form into shapes, and because the germ contains easily oxidized oils, manufacturers mill off most of the germ and bran, a process that extends shelf life but unfortunately removes most of the nutrients. Cereals that are 100% whole grain retain all three components of the original seed and all its nutrients. For the more-processed US cereals, a few nutrients (thiamine, niacin, riboflavin, folic acid, iron) must be added back; other nutrients may also be added voluntarily as "fortification." Later chapters discuss these additions in more detail.

Breakfast trends

The first challenge for the early cereal makers was to convince Americans to replace cooked breakfasts with ready-to-eat cold cereals. They did this by extolling breakfast as the most important meal of the day, and equating breakfast with cereal. No other product could do a better job of providing taste, convenience, and health, all in one box, and for pennies on the dollar, they said, arguments still used today. As Kellogg puts it, "A large body of international research supports the key role of breakfast in achieving nutrition recommendations, staying mentally alert, reaching peak physical performance, and maintaining a healthy body weight," and "breakfast and cereal are too important to miss." Ready-to-eat cereals, Kellogg says, rank as top choices for their grain, fiber, and nutrients—and you don't need to worry about the sugars; cereals have less sugar than either orange juice or flavored yogurts.[10]

Kellogg avoids mentioning that it and other cereal companies paid for much of that "large body of international research."[11] Independently funded research tends to conclude that for adults, at least, whether you eat breakfast or not is up to you; what matters for nutrient intake and health is what you eat, not when you eat it. For children and adolescents, eating breakfast of *any* kind has been shown to result in healthier diets and better academic performance.[12]

For decades, the idea that breakfast means cereals succeeded and endured, but the effectiveness of this message appears to be waning. In the early 1900s, the American food supply included about 300 pounds of cereal grains per year—nearly a pound per day—for every man, woman, and child in the country (those pounds went for bread, pasta, and porridge as well as cold cereal). The amount fluctuated but remained relatively constant until the 1960s, when demand began to decline. Today, the food supply offers approximately 170 pounds of grains per capita per year.[13] Hence, less cereal.

Not everyone eats breakfast cereals, but an estimated 300 million Americans say they do at some time during the year. The peak year for cereal buying was 1994; except for a slight uptick during the COVID-19 pandemic, sales have stagnated or declined ever since. In the early 2000s, about 25% of American children were reported to eat breakfast cereals, and so were 15% to 30% of adults, depending on age; older adults consume more cereals than younger adults. But by the early 2020s, the percentages had dropped by a few points in all age categories.[14]

Multiple trends, social as well as demographic, explain the decline in buying ready-to-eat cereals: skipping breakfast, more meals consumed outside the home, higher demand for portable breakfast foods (shakes and bars), the increasing popularity of the protein fad (yogurt, eggs, bars), and more focus on what's in our food (sugars, color additives). The declining birth rate is also a factor; it means fewer kid customers.[15]

Pouring cereal into a bowl, adding milk to it, and eating it is so quick and easy that even children can do it, but the process is apparently not easy or quick enough for today's busy individuals and families. Bagels, Pop-Tarts, and anything portable that can be eaten on the go give breakfast cereals stiff competition. The downward trend is also explained by increasing dietary preferences for whole-grain, natural, organic, and non-GMO foods (which most cereals are not) as well as for products that have minimal sugar but plenty of protein and for keto- and paleo-friendly foods (which leaves out all but niche cereals).[16] Even so, the best-selling cereals—mostly sugary and artificially colored—remain highly popular and continue to occupy substantial space on supermarket shelves.

The cereal industry: A consolidated global powerhouse

By one account (others differ, sometimes substantially), breakfast cereals were projected to generate $88 billion in revenues in 2025, $23 billion from the United States alone, with the next-largest cereal-purchasing populations in China, France, India, and Russia, in that order. China houses more than 600 cereal manufacturers, and India more than 500. But the global market is controlled largely by the two biggest producers, General Mills and Kellogg, which together account for 60% of cold cereal sales worldwide.[17]

Although more than 80 cereal makers are now located in the United States, only four companies—the Big Four (as we refer to them)—controlled 80% of the US cereal market through 2024 (the year after Kellogg split into two companies): General Mills (31%), Kellogg (26%), Post Consumer Brands (18%), and PepsiCo/Quaker (5%). The rest of the market was and is distributed among the smaller, niche brands (11%) and store brands (9%). Corporate concentration has major effects on consumers' food choices. It enables the industry to set prices, determine the market, and influence food policy through lobbying and other means—all of which the Big Four cereal companies do.[18]

For these reasons, cereal companies have been targets of antitrust action. In the early 1970s, the Federal Trade Commission (FTC) filed an antitrust suit against Kellogg, General Mills, and General Foods (which owned Post cereals at the time). Quaker was initially included in the suit but was later removed. Even then, the remaining three companies collectively held 80% of the cereal market. After a 10-year battle, the FTC dismissed the case "with prejudice," which meant it could not be appealed. Kellogg's chief attorney said this decision put him "in a state of happiness."[19] We bet it did. If the companies had lost the case, they would have been required to be split into any number of smaller companies.

In 1992, RJR Nabisco (Nabisco had been acquired by R. J. Reynolds Tobacco in 1985) attempted to sell its cereal business to General Mills, but that deal failed during antitrust investigations. Instead, Nabisco was acquired by Philip Morris/Kraft General Foods. The New York attorney general challenged the sale's reduction of competition in the cereal category, but that case also was dismissed. In 1995, two US representatives called for an antitrust investigation into the Big Four. New York Representative Charles Schumer said of the cereal industry, "We are paying caviar prices for corn flakes quality." Although he urged the US attorney general to open a pricing investigation, his plea went nowhere.[20] Control of the cereal industry remains highly concentrated.

The cereal industry is also highly differentiated. Cereals are distinguished by brands—such as Frosted Flakes and Cheerios—and ingredients, as well as by marketing through advertising, cartoon mascots, packaging, coupons, licensing deals, and special offers. Because the industry is so consolidated, Big Four cereals do not differ much by price; the average cost for a box of cereal in 2024 was $4.64 from General Mills, $4.59 from Kellogg, $4.76 from Post, and $4.63 from Quaker Oats. In contrast, organic and niche brands averaged $6.60 per box, whereas store brands were at the low end at $2.98.[21]

The Big Four non-price competition shows up in the constant introduction and repackaging of tried-and-true brands to introduce "new" products with slightly different shapes or flavors—"line extensions." Cheerios and Special K are examples of brands that are constantly reinvented to keep consumer interest, dominate cereal aisle shelf space, and boost sales. Overall, business analysts view the cereal industry as highly regulated, mature, capital intensive, innovative, and competitive. One key point: its profit margins are exceptionally high, ranging in 2024 from 13% (Kellogg) to 19% (General Mills).[22]

The Big Four

In business jargon, "mature" refers to market share, but all of the Big Four cereal companies are venerable; they originated in the late 1800s or early 1900s. Over the years, all have been involved in mergers or acquisitions that expanded their product offerings beyond cereals. But to focus on cereals, here are the leading companies and brands in 2025:

The Kellogg Company was founded by W. K. Kellogg in 1906. His Battle Creek company lasted until 2023, when declining sales led to its split into two distinct independent entities: the WK Kellogg Co, which retained distribution and marketing of cereals in the US, Caribbean, and Canada, and a new company, Kellanova, with snacks, frozen foods, and international cereals. This division would have left WK Kellogg Co as the only remaining company selling its cereals exclusively in the United States. But once launched, the split companies became vulnerable to takeover. In 2025, Mars bought Kellanova, and the WK Kellogg Co was acquired by Ferrero, the global candy and confection company that makes Nutella. WK Kellogg/Mars cereals included these brands: All-Bran, Apple Jacks, Bear Naked, Corn Flakes, Corn Pops, Cracklin' Oat Bran, Crispix, Extra, Froot Loops, Frosted Flakes, Frosted Mini-Wheats, Honey Smacks, Kashi, Krave, Mueslix, Raisin Bran, Rice Krispies, and Special K.

General Mills dates to the Washburn-Crosby Company flour mill of the late 1860s but was not established formally until 1928, when it merged with three other mills. It makes many other products besides cereals. In the United States, its mainstream cereals are sold under the Big G banner—the G stands for Goodness. To sell cereals internationally, General Mills partnered with Nestlé in 1990 to form Cereal Partners Worldwide, a joint venture that makes and distributes more than 100 cereals in 130 countries. General Mills owned these brands in 2025: Annie's, Basic 4, Cascadian Farm, Cheerios, Chex Cereal, Cinnamon Toast Crunch, Cocoa Puffs, Cookie Crisp, Fiber One, Golden Grahams, Kix, Lucky Charms, Monster Cereals, Nature Valley, Oatmeal Crisp, Raisin Nut Bran, Reese's Puffs, Total, Trix, and Wheaties (of these, all are considered Big G except for the health-food brands—Annie's, Cascadian Farm, and Nature Valley).

Post Consumer Brands was founded by C. W. Post in 1895. It soon began acquiring other food companies, and in 1929, it bought General Foods and adopted that name. Beginning in 1985, the company went through a head-spinning series of mergers and acquisitions:

1895: C. W. Post founds the Postum Cereal Company.

1929: Postum buys and merges with General Foods.

1985: Philip Morris acquires General Foods.

1989: Philip Morris acquires Kraft Foods; merges General Foods and Kraft into Kraft Foods (which includes Post Foods).

2007: Philip Morris sells Kraft/Post to Ralcorp Holdings.
2012: Ralcorp spins off Post Foods.
2014: Michael Foods acquires Post Foods.
2015: Post buys Malt-O-Meal (MOM) brands; they merge into Post Consumer Brands.

In 2025, Post's cereals included Barbara's, Bran Flakes, Chips Ahoy!, Golden Crisp, Grape-Nuts, Honey Bunches of Oats, Honey-Comb, Malt-O-Meal, Mom's Best, Oreo O's, Oreo Puffs, Pebbles (Fruity and Cocoa), Puffins, Raisin Bran, Shredded Wheat, and Weetabix.

The Quaker Oats Company started out as Quaker Mill in 1877. It introduced the Quaker man, meant to project values of honesty, integrity, purity, and strength, in the early 1900s. In 1983, Quaker bought Stokely-Van Camp, which made Gatorade. To acquire Gatorade, PepsiCo bought Quaker in 2001. Quaker cereals are now part of the PepsiCo empire, worth $91 billion in 2025, and include, in addition to hot oat cereals, Cap'n Crunch, Life, Oatmeal Squares, Puffed Granola, and Simply Granola.

In addition to selling cereals, these companies are political entities. They have stayed in business and flourished for so long not only as a result of brilliant marketing, but also because of their unceasing efforts to influence federal and state policy on product contents (ingredients and nutrition), labeling, and health claims. They also pay lobbyists to make sure cereals are well represented in federal food assistance programs, school meals, and dietary guidelines. In 2024, the WK Kellogg company spent $350,000 on lobbyists and lobbying, while Kellanova and General Mills each spent more than $1.1 million for such purposes. PepsiCo's lobbying expenditures are even greater, but not all of them focus on cereals.[23]

Cereals as marketing billboards

As noted, most Americans eat breakfast cereals at least sometimes during the year, and sales of these products are staggering. For example, General Mills reportedly sold 1,400 boxes of cereal every *minute* in the United States in 2024. That year, Kellogg sold 121 million boxes of Frosted Flakes,

77 million of Froot Loops, and 51 million of Frosted Mini-Wheats. General Mills sold 138 million boxes of Honey Nut Cheerios, 107 million of Cinnamon Toast Crunch, and 78 million of original Cheerios. Post sold 103 million boxes of Honey Bunches of Oats and 62 million of Fruity Pebbles. Quaker's Oatmeal hot cereals sell more than 250 million boxes a year. Collectively, private label brands such as those from Walmart and Wegmans accounted for more than 345 million boxes sold that year. Note that while cereal companies market products to people of all ages, about a third particularly target children.[24]

Cereal brands are in constant competition for sales, with boxes as prime vehicles for marketing. While marketing channels have evolved over the years (think social media), the Big Four's proven strategies for using cereal boxes as advertising vehicles have lasted decades. The aim of marketing is to create demand for products, whether needed or not. For cereal companies, marketing isn't just about selling a convenient, nutritious breakfast food; it's about capturing customers by shaping early preferences and creating lifetime brand loyalty, which is why so many are aimed at children. The Big Four employ consumer-insight teams to study all aspects of the demographics, lifestyle, and cultural preferences, purchasing behaviors, and values of every consumer group.[25] This information enables them to "speak" directly to targeted market segments (as companies refer to their consumers).

Marketing and *advertising* are often used interchangeably, but marketing is specifically about building brand awareness and loyalty, whereas advertising aims to drive sales. These distinctions matter to advertising executives and academics, but we use *marketing* to refer to all of the ways cereal companies work to build brands and sell products: in-store promotions, social media campaigns, TV advertising, endorsements, and sponsorships, but also behind-the-scenes lobbying and paying for research studies.

Marketing methods, which often draw on the use of celebrities, pop culture, or holidays, are visible on the boxes—the core of cereal brand-building and sales promotion. The boxes establish the basis for the nostalgia many people feel about the look and taste of cereals and the childhood memories they evoke. Consider, for example, the drawing by illustrator J. C. Leyendecker shown in Figure 2. This illustration is one of several used by Kellogg in kids' cereal advertisements in the early 20th century.[26] Kellogg is invoking nostalgia to celebrate the 60th anniversary of Rice

Krispies' introduction, recalling simpler times and the cereal's humble beginnings.

We think of cereal boxes as billboards displaying marketing messages on supermarket shelves and breakfast tables across America. The marketing of every cereal, especially those for kids, begins by giving it a memorable brand name: Lucky Charms, Froot Loops, Cap'n Crunch's Crunch Berries. The mere mention of the name conjures up images of the box's color, design, mascot, and even what is in the box: green clover marshmallows, multicolored rings, and round pink balls. Academics as we are, we classify cereal names in three broad categories: grains, sugar, and fruit. Others may be named for healthy ingredients like protein or fiber, but grains, sugar, and fruit apply to most cereals on supermarket shelves.

What they are called within those categories can make or break a product. Kellogg knew this as early as 1949, stating: "If you had an Aladdin's Lamp or a magic mill that could grind out your commands, what would you ask for? . . . John Q. Public doesn't buy just any product. He wants one with a good NAME. . . . But what gives a name such magical power? The magic is advertising."[27]

Grain names came first. Companies named the earliest cereals after their main ingredient: Corn Flakes, All-Bran, Cheerioats, Rice Krispies, Shredded Wheat. Those cereals contained just a few ingredients and were promoted for their wholesomeness. A century later, cereals are still named for grains—Rice, Corn, and Wheat Chex, for example.

Many original grain-based cereal names have remained unchanged for decades. Cheerioats, what we now know as Cheerios, is a rare exception, as the result of a legal dispute. In 1938, Quaker Oats attempted to register "OATIES" as a trademark with the United States Patent Office. General Mills objected on the grounds of interference with its own registered trademarks for Wheaties and two other cereals that were never marketed, Kornies and Maizies. Quaker, in turn, filed a trademark infringement lawsuit against General Mills for using "oats" in Cheerioats.[28] It makes no sense to us that "oats" should belong to only one company, but lawyers had other ideas. Rather than engaging in a drawn-out, costly legal battle, General Mills renamed the cereal Cheerios in 1945. Its marketers brilliantly incorporated the O-shaped oat rings into the name and, in the end, had the last laugh. The court ruled that "OATIES" could not be trademarked.

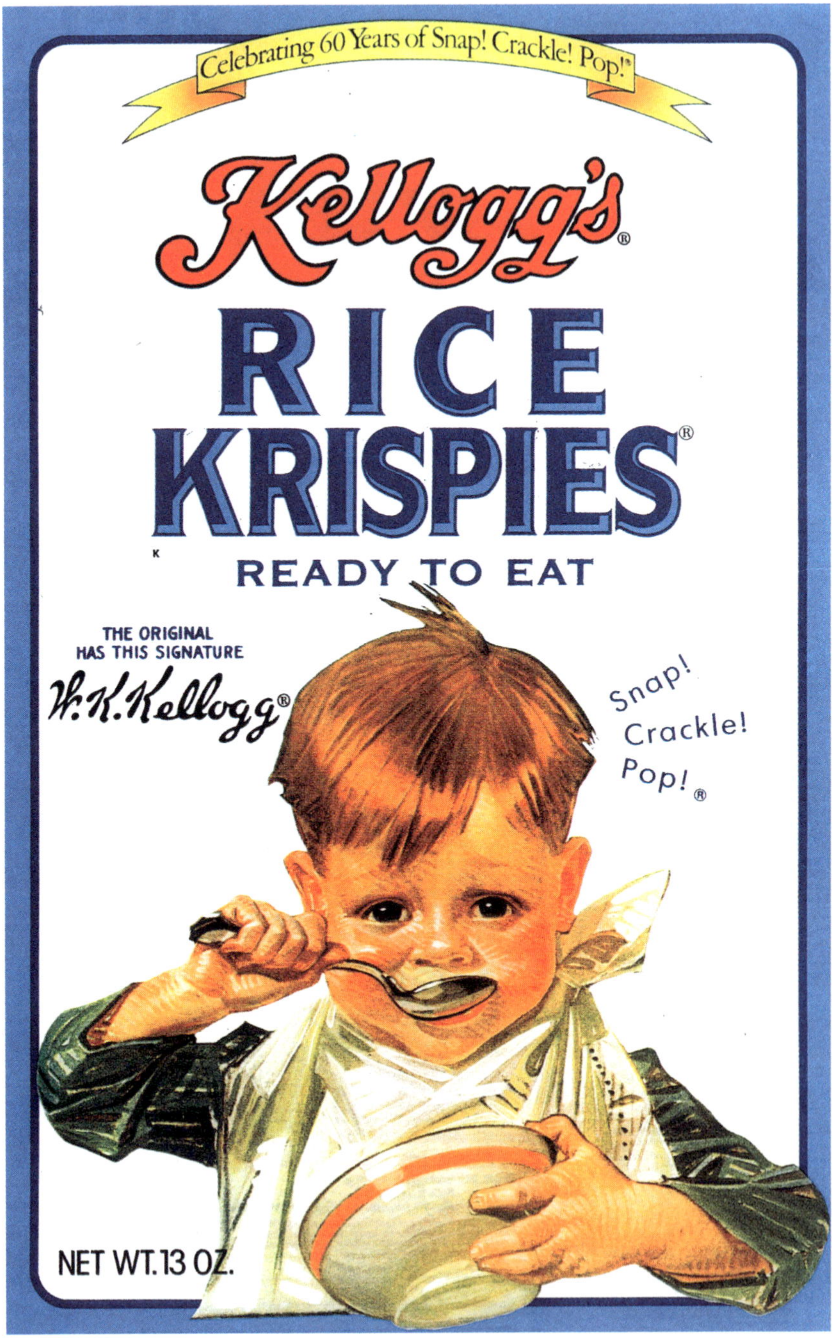

FIGURE 2 This nostalgia-inducing box from 1990 is a throwback to early 20th-century cereal advertisements by the famous illustrator J. C. Leyendecker. Kellogg reproduced the drawing to celebrate the 60th anniversary of Rice Krispies' 1928 introduction.

It disappeared as a brand, leaving the original Cheerios in its iconic yellow box as an all-time best seller. When General Mills issued a retro Cheerioats box in 2021 to celebrate its humble oats beginnings and 80th birthday, Quaker neither objected nor sued.

By the 1950s, companies had introduced cereals with "sugar" in the name, followed by brands referring to fruit. When consumers were asked in 2024 whether they knew cereals by name, more than 92% recognized Froot Loops.[29]

With this brief introduction, we take a look next at what a cereal box is required to display. In subsequent chapters, we discuss how companies use the boxes to compete for sales and market share.

CHAPTER 2

THE CEREAL BOX

AN OVERVIEW

YOU MIGHT THINK of cereal boxes as containers for something to eat for breakfast, but we have come to view them as billboards—valuable real estate for marketing. Because the major cereal manufacturers redesign them several times a year, cereal boxes, more than any other food packaging, reveal trends in nutrition fads, labeling regulations, ingredients, popular culture, and political history. They are a window (a box!) into the past and often foreshadow the future. Each word and image on a cereal box has a specific purpose.

In this book, we examine how the Big Four cereal companies use what's on the boxes to entice you to buy their products or get kids to beg for them. The boxes aimed at kids often display brightly colored, vivid food images and lively cartoons, but all boxes provide nutrition and other information and marketing messages targeting a wide range of potential buyers. Nevertheless, a surprisingly large amount of the box is devoted to elements required by labeling laws as interpreted by the Food and Drug Administration (FDA), such as the manufacturer's name and address and nutrition information, as well as elements required by retailers (barcodes).[1] In this overview of the box, we focus on the *obligatory* design elements relevant to the themes of this book. We use the contemporary box in Figure 3 as our starting point for this discussion.

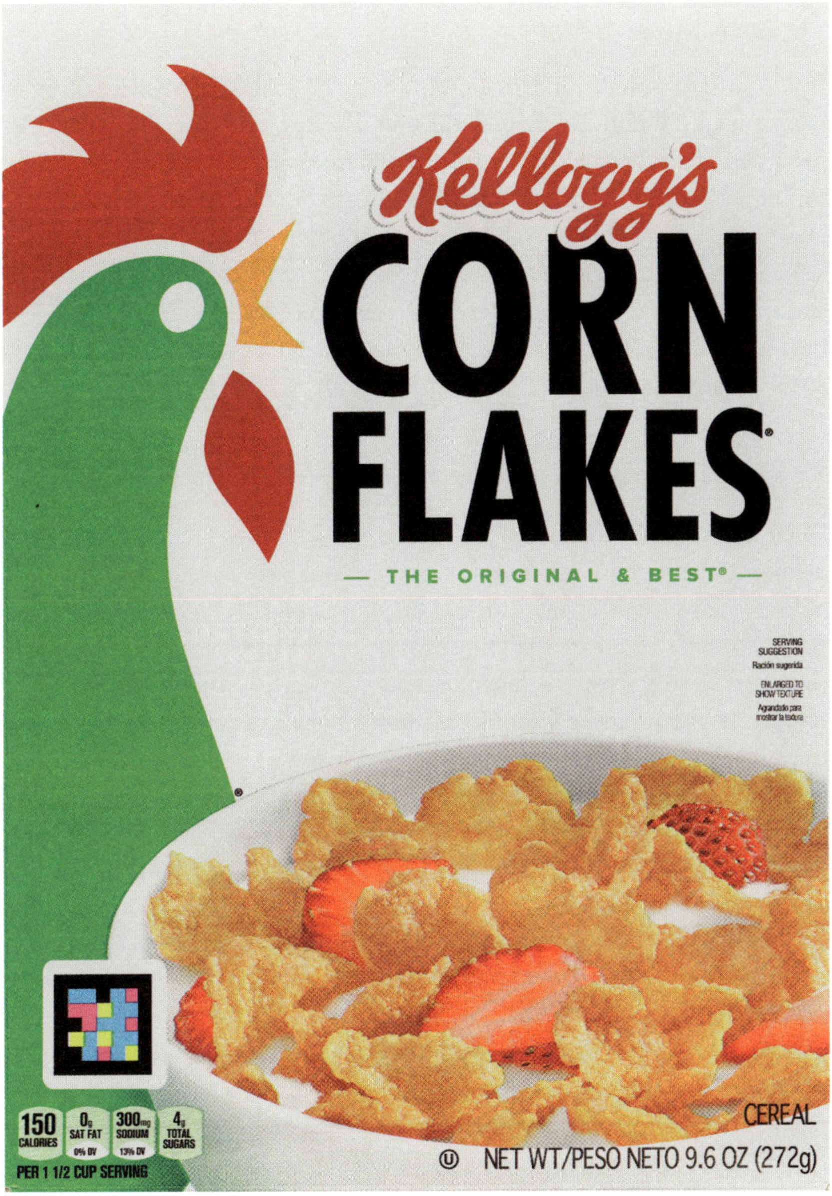

FIGURE 3 A typical cereal box in 2025. Every word and design element on this Kellogg box has a purpose, either for marketing or to comply with federal labeling regulations and retailers' requirements.

The best-if-used-by date

It is standard practice in the food industry to voluntarily use a sell-by or best-if-used-by date that gives the month, day, and year by which the product should be sold or consumed. These dates usually appear on the top flap of cereal boxes and merely indicate how long the manufacturer guarantees the optimal product quality. Ready-to-eat cereals are dry and sealed in airtight bags; they are safe to eat long past the marked date. The stamped dates are one year after the cereals were boxed at the factory. The best-if-used-by date on the box in Figure 3 is 2025; it was manufactured a year earlier in 2024.

FDA-regulated elements

What amazes us is the level of codification involved for each FDA-required element. The details are so specific that some are assigned names and abbreviations, such as the principal display panel (PDP). FDA regulations cover not only where everything must go on the box but also in what size font and how far letters must be spaced apart. Cereal companies are obliged to follow these tedious and mind-boggling rules. If they do not, the FDA can force the products to be recalled.

The FDA's labeling requirements, for example, divide the box into two sections: the principal display panel and the information panel. *PDP* is for the front of the box, or front of package. The information panel is the side of the box, or side panel.

The principal display panel

The PDP is the most prominent and valuable cereal box real estate; it is the first thing a shopper sees. The front of the box is where the marketing begins, although it continues onto the sides and back of the box. Much of this book is devoted to analyzing how this marketing works and has evolved over time. Here, we consider the FDA's labeling requirements. For starters, the FDA requires the PDP to include two elements:

Statement of identity. This is the legal name of the cereal product (examples: Froot Loops, Raisin Bran, Cocoa Pebbles, or, as shown in Figure 3,

Corn Flakes). The box must display this name in a font height not less than half that of the largest font on the package (we are not making this up).

Net quantity of contents. This is the weight of cereal in the package, which must appear in the bottom third of the PDP in a specific font size determined by the available area in a style that is "prominent, conspicuous, and easy to read." The quantity must be stated in both metric (grams) and the US customary system (ounces).

The FDA does not require the manufacturer's name—Kellogg or General Mills, for example—to appear on the PDP, though it can. Kellogg puts *Kellogg's* before most of its cereal names (Kellogg's Corn Flakes), and General Mills uses its blue *G* logo in the upper left corner of its PDPs. For Big Four cereals, the manufacturer's name is often on the PDP, but the FDA allows it to be placed in other locations, such as a side panel, along with the required company address or optional contact information.

Everything else on the PDP is voluntary and left up to manufacturers as long as they abide by whatever other rules the FDA has set for such matters as illustrations, health claims, nutrient content claims, marketing statements, content statements, icons or symbols ("widgets"), endorsements, games, announcements, and everything else we examine throughout this book. Occasionally, cereal companies land in trouble for taking advantage of loopholes in FDA regulations, giving us plenty of fodder for discussion.

The information panel

This brings us to the information panel, or side panel. This, the FDA specifies, is "that part of the label immediately contiguous and to the right of the principal display panel as observed by an individual facing the principal display panel."[2] What's in that panel is laid out in excruciating detail. It contains three major elements: nutrition facts, ingredient statement, and allergens declaration.

Nutrition Facts panel. The items and fonts in this panel are derived from the Nutrition Labeling and Education Act (NLEA) of 1990 and the hundreds of pages of regulatory descriptions in the final rule published in the *Federal Register* in 1993, and as later amended. The FDA required this design as of 1994 and has kept it much the same since then, with a few subsequent modifications, most notably to require the inclusion of added sugars in 2016 (this rule went into effect on January 1, 2020).[3] The FDA specifies which nutrients must be included in the panel, the order in which they must be listed, how they are presented, when to include a Daily Value (DV), how to calculate the DV, and much more. There are precise "rounding rules" for each nutrient—for example, any amount under 0.5 grams of total sugars per serving can be labeled as 0 grams. The FDA requires vitamin D, calcium, iron, and potassium to be included in the Nutrition Facts panel; all other vitamins and minerals are optional, unless they are added to the cereal or if a statement is made about them on the PDP. Most cereal boxes list many more than the required four.

Serving size. The first items listed on the Nutrition Facts panel are the number of servings in a box and serving size by household measure (in cups, pieces, etc.), followed by weight (in grams). The FDA bases the serving size on what it calls the RACC, the Reference Amount Customarily Consumed, which is derived from what people self-report eating in one sitting. The RACC for cereals is defined by weight per cup. It is 15 grams for puffed cereals weighing less than 20 grams per cup, 40 grams for cereals weighing between 20 and 43 grams per cup, and 60 grams for those weighing more than 43 grams per cup.[4]

One result is that cereal serving sizes are all over the place: 1 cup (16 grams) for Nature's Path Wheat Puffs, 1 cup (36 grams) for Lucky Charms, 1⅓ cup (60 grams) for Post Shredded Wheat, and 1½ cup (40 grams) for Rice Krispies. Wegmans Bite-Size Shredded Wheat says 25 biscuits (60 grams) is one serving. We guess you are supposed to count them.

The RACC is not a recommendation; it has nothing to do with what anyone *should* eat; it is based on what people *say* they eat. This distinction is crucial. The RACC underestimates actual amounts of cereal consumed. When researchers asked volunteers to pour the amount of cereal they would typically eat into bowls of different sizes, all amounts exceeded standard serving sizes; the bigger the bowl and the denser the cereal, the more the amount poured exceeded the standard serving size.[5] Double the serving size, and you double the ingredients—including the sugar and calories.

Daily Value. The DV is of particular importance—and is particularly confusing—because it refers to two different goals, both based on a 2,000-calories-a-day diet. For the positive ("eat more") nutrients—vitamins, minerals, and fiber—it refers to the recommended amount that *should* be consumed in a day. But for the negative ("eat less") nutrients—fats, sodium, and sugars—it is the suggested upper limit, the amount you *should not* eat more of in a day.[6] If a cereal's DV for added sugars is 25%, one serving makes up one-quarter of the upper limit for one day. If a DV for iron is 10%, then 90% of a day's iron must come from other foods. The FDA says 5% of the DV is low and 20% is high; these standards apply to *both* the positive (eat more of) and negative (eat less of) nutrients. Got that?

The ingredients list. Prior to the NLEA, nutrition labeling was much more haphazard. Our collection of facsimiles of Rice Krispies boxes begins in 1928, the year Kellogg first produced this "delicious cereal made from choice rice, cooked, puffed, and toasted." In 1933, the front of the box listed its ingredients as "Deliciously flavored with malt, sugar and salt." It said nothing about other nutrients until World War II, when it noted, "Rice Krispies are restored to the whole-grain nutritive values of natural brown rice by the addition of thiamine (vitamin B_1), niacin, and iron" and started listing calories and the amounts of several nutrients per cup, with and without milk. The advertised nutrients varied over the years, but as a result of congressional hearings promoting cereal fortification in 1972 (see Chapter 6), the FDA specified that the order of ingredients must be listed by descending weight on the panel. By the time the NLEA passed, cereal companies were already listing ingredients as they do today.

The NLEA required lists of ingredients to begin with the one most prevalent by weight and to continue in order of decreasing weight. In 1994, all cereal boxes put these lists on their right-side panels. The law allowed one exception to listing by descending weight: the statement that a cereal "contains X% or less of _____," where the X% is 2% or, sometimes, less (but never below 0.5%). Each of the ingredients following this statement must make up less than that percent of the total product recipe, but they do not have to be in any specific order. The box shown in Figure 3 lists "Milled Corn, Sugar, Malt Flavor," but then "Contains 2% or Less of Salt and

Vitamins and Minerals." Using the statement is voluntary, and companies list ingredients after the less-than-statement in any order they please.

The rules also specify how certain ingredients are to be labeled. For example, certified synthetic colors must be listed using the additive name—FD&C Blue 1 or just Blue 1, for example. But colors from natural sources like vegetables and spices can be listed by their common names (beet or turmeric) or simply as "color added." Vitamins and minerals must use both the common or usual name (vitamin B_6, iron) and the technical name (pyridoxine hydrochloride, ferric phosphate). Some companies use bolded common names to explain the chemical terms; no rule says they can't. Multiple terms make for particularly long ingredient statements, especially when printed in all-capital letters in a color barely distinguishable from the box background, an all-too-common obscuring practice. Sometimes these nutrients are listed in a separate line as "Vitamins and Minerals," which makes the overall list of ingredients appear shorter.

The allergen declaration. Congress passed the Food Allergen Labeling and Consumer Protection Act (FALCPA) in 2004; it went into effect in 2006. This law requires that foods containing one or more of the nine most common food allergens specified by that act—milk, eggs, fish, shellfish, tree nuts, peanuts, soybeans, sesame, and wheat—must "declare" those allergens and clearly label the packages. The allergens can be identified in either of two ways. The box can list the common name of its source in parentheses after the ingredient, as in "whey (milk)." Or it can use the method most common on cereal boxes: a "contains" statement near the ingredient list, such as "Contains Wheat."[7]

Almost everything on the Nutrition Facts side panel is required by one law or another, and companies must follow the intricate and often bewildering rules to the letter. Everything else on the box is marketing. And what varied, flagrant, and complicated marketing it is! Read on.

PART I

INGREDIENTS

CHAPTER 3

SUGARS

INGREDIENT #1 OR #2

"As a cereal, it's dandy; for snacks, it's so handy; or eat it like candy." This cheerful Post jingle tells you cereals are about sugar, the ingredient we all love—and love to hate. In 2023, the global cereal industry used more than 800 *million* pounds of sugar. If sugar is not the first cereal ingredient, it is usually second; this happens because of a labeling trick. By the 1990s, cereal companies hit on a clever strategy. If they used multiple sugar types, they could list grains first but sprinkle sugars throughout the list. This makes cereal appear healthier.

Sugars have no nutrients beyond calories, which is why their calories are considered "empty." Sugars are carbohydrates. The simplest are one-sugar monosaccharides: glucose and fructose. Sucrose, common table sugar, is a two-sugar disaccharide of glucose and fructose. In cereals, "sugar" means sucrose, but sugars, plural, include many other types appearing on ingredient lists, such as brown sugar (and syrup), honey, maple syrup, fructose, dextrose, corn syrup, agave nectar, fruit juice concentrate, and high-fructose corn syrup.

Nearly all ready-to-eat breakfast cereals are presweetened. The addition of sugars has a vital marketing purpose: it entices kids to love specific brands, solidifies the place of those brands on breakfast tables across

America, and induces nostalgia among adults for the brands they ate as children. How sugar came to dominate the cereal aisle has a century-long history involving feuding brothers, company sugar wars, shunned sugars, litigation, and policy showdowns. This complicated and not always sweet history is worth recounting.

"Eat it like candy"

In the early 1900s, some companies sweetened their cereals with barley malt syrup (sugar) to make them taste better. But Dr. John Harvey Kellogg had banned sugar from the diets prescribed to patients at his Battle Creek Sanitarium. He viewed the American population as suffering from sugar overload, blaming it for nutrient deficiencies, anemia, lack of muscle tone, weak bones, and tooth decay, among other illnesses. Far ahead of his time, he spent decades calling for diets with less sugar.[1] Add sugar to cereals? Out of the question.

His brother, W. K. Kellogg, did not share this view. He envisioned cereals as changing what families across America ate for breakfast—and making him a fortune. But corn flakes tasted bland. To reach more customers than his brother's health-faddist followers, he added cane sugar to the first commercially produced Sanitas Toasted Corn Flakes in 1906. Renamed Kellogg's Corn Flakes the following year, the package said: "Deliciously flavored with malt, sugar, and salt." We do not know how much sugar was in this cereal (such details were not required until much later). What we do know is that the addition of sugar contributed to the legendary rift between the Kellogg brothers that lasted until John Harvey died in 1943. Only then could sugar be added to cereals with abandon.

The presweetening of America

The earliest cereals were sweetened, but not excessively; today's Kellogg's Corn Flakes contain a modest 4 grams per serving. Sugar's tripling or quadrupling in cereals has been attributed to a single person, Jim Rex, a heating equipment salesman in Pennsylvania. As the story goes, he was appalled by the spoonfuls of sugar his kids added to their breakfast cereals. He set out to create a version that would not induce kids to do this. His brilliant contribution: a glossy honey coating on puffed wheat, a cereal he named Ranger Joe Wheat Honnies in 1939. This was sold locally, and sold well, but had logistical problems, and Rex sold off the brand. Nabisco acquired it in 1954, but Wheat Honnies was soon discontinued.

Rex kicked off the great sugar rush. By 1949, Post had launched Sugar Crisp, a cereal targeting children, using three little bears, Dandy, Handy, and Candy, matching the catchy tagline quoted earlier. As shown in Figure 4, when Sugar Bear offered a bear-shaped bicycle reflector, no kid could resist.

With John Harvey out of the way, Kellogg could introduce Sugar Pops in 1951, Sugar Frosted Flakes in 1952, and Sugar Smacks in 1953, each among the company's all-time best sellers. General Mills jumped in with Sugar Smiles in 1953, later renamed Sugar Jets, complete with an endorsement by the trusted homemaker Betty Crocker. The company had introduced Kix in 1937 with minimal sugar, but it later added more sugar and artificial colors to create Trix, in 1954, and added chocolate, in 1958, to make Cocoa Puffs—still on supermarket shelves.

In the 1950s, presweetened cereals accounted for just 5% of all cereal sales, but they increased to 20% in the 1960s. By the mid-1970s, kids' sugary varieties were 38% of all cereals sold. The great irony: Jim Rex's efforts to reduce his kids' sugar intake led to this dubious distinction: cereals are among the top sources of sugar in the diets of American children.[2]

Sugar: The "s-word"

Pressures to reduce the sugars in breakfast cereals came to public attention in the early 1970s when Congress held hearings to highlight their inadequate nutritional quality. Witnesses testified that nearly all leading cereal brands ranged from 30% to 45% sugar by weight and were programming children to demand sweetness in every food.[3]

Cereal companies objected, arguing, correctly, that grains are nutritious. But they also responded by trying to make their products appear less sugary, beginning by removing the "s-word" from cereal names. General Mills discontinued Sugar Jets in 1974. Kellogg dropped the *Sugar* from Sugar Frosted Flakes in 1984 and rebranded Sugar Pops as Corn Pops in 1985. Post dropped the *Sugar* from Sugar Crisp, changing its name several times

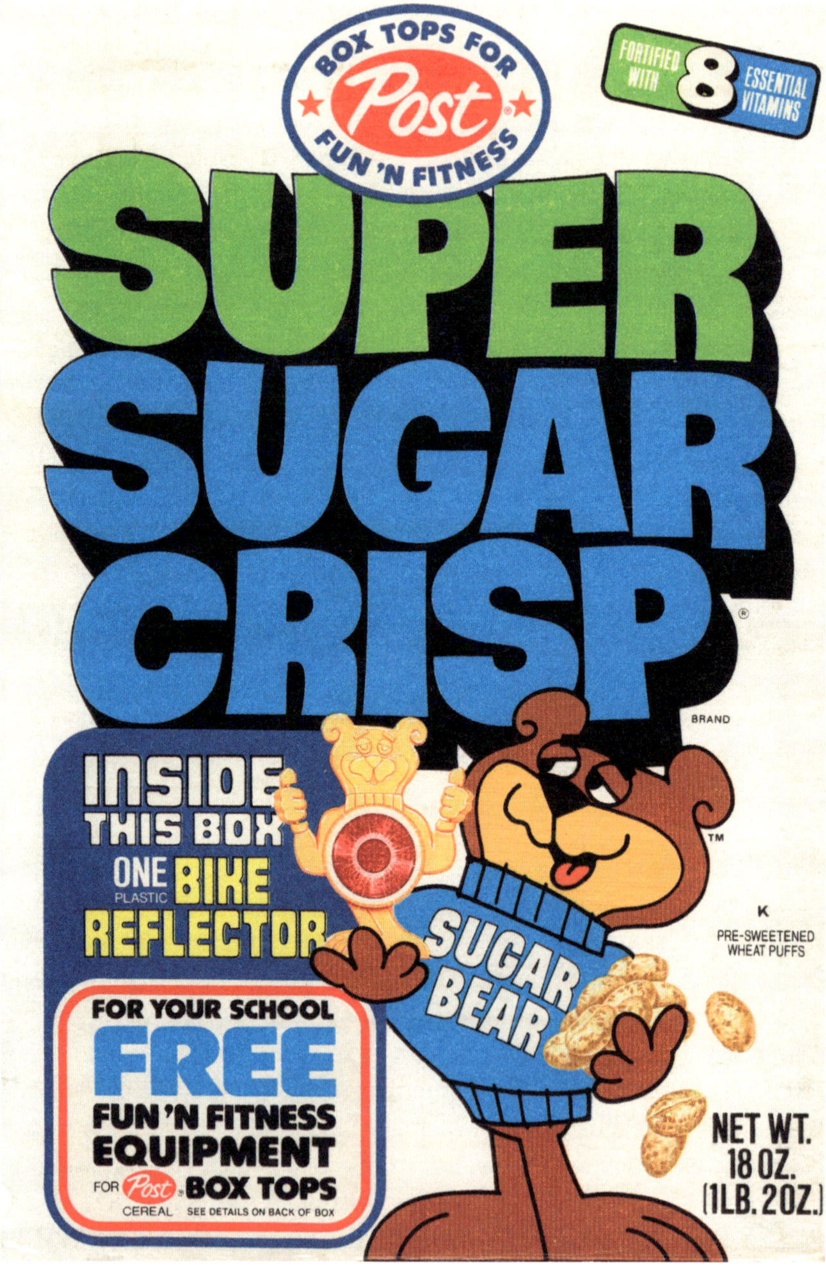

FIGURE 4 This 1976 Post Super Sugar Crisp box from General Foods lists sugar as the first ingredient and corn syrup as the third; sugars comprise half of the cereal's weight and calories.

before ending up with Golden Crisp in 1985.[4] Fun fact: It is still sold as Sugar Crisp in Canada.

Another trick was to substitute honey for sugar, on the theory that people perceive honey as more wholesome and nutritious (alas, honey contains glucose and fructose just like table sugar). Kellogg changed Sugar Smacks to Honey Smacks in the 1980s, dropped *Honey* leaving it as Smacks in the 1990s, but reverted to Honey Smacks in 2004.[5] Today, three kinds of sugars in this cereal (sugar, glucose syrup, and honey) make up 55% of its calories.

Over the years, the sugar in breakfast cereals has ranged from zero to as high as 88% by weight (Lieber's Cocoa Frosted Flakes holds this distinction), and many had more than 50%. In 2014, the Environmental Working Group analyzed more than 1,500 cereals, nearly 200 of them aimed at children, and estimated that kids could consume 10 pounds of sugar a year from cereals alone.[6] No exaggeration. The 2025 Post Golden Crisp (formerly Sugar Crisp) lists 21 grams of sugars per 38-gram (1 cup) serving. Sugar is the first ingredient, followed by corn syrup (#3) and honey (#5); combined, they account for more than 40% of the daily upper limit for added sugars.

Under pressure from consumer and public health advocacy groups, cereal companies removed *sugar* from their brand names. Instead, they use euphemisms:

Frosted: Frosted Flakes, Frosted Mini-Wheats, Frosted Cheerios
Honey: Honey Nut Chex, Honey-Comb, Honey Bunches of Oats
Chocolate: Cocoa Puffs, Chocolate Chex, Cocoa Pebbles
Cinnamon: Cinnamon Toast Crunch, Cinnamon Life
Cookies: Oreo O's, Cookie Crisp, Chips Ahoy!
Candy: KitKat, Reese's Puffs, Jolly Rancher

Sugar may have disappeared from the names of cereals, but it still tops ingredient lists.

Cookies, candy, and cake for breakfast

The cereal aisle is full of products bearing the names of cookie, candy, and snack cake brands, all promoting sugar. This is co-branding; cereal companies purchase or otherwise obtain the right to use the brand names of other foods in the naming and marketing of their products.

Cookies for breakfast started with Ralston Purina Cookie Crisp in 1977, a cereal now owned by General Mills. But the Oreo O's box shown in Figure 5 illustrates how cereals contract with popular cookie brands to sell new products. When Post launched Oreo O's in 1998, Post belonged to Kraft (then owned by Philip Morris—yes, the tobacco company), and Kraft owned Nabisco, maker of Oreo cookies. Co-branding was inevitable. The box celebrated the crème-coated, chocolatey, crunchy, O-shaped cereal as tasting like cookies dipped in milk. What could be better?

Oreo O's got caught up in a 2007 corporate merger when Kraft sold Post to Ralcorp Holdings (formerly Ralston Purina). Kraft still owned Nabisco and the Oreo brand, but Post/Ralcorp owned the cereal business, ending the licensing deal and Oreo O's cereal. Ten years later, Kraft sold Nabisco to Mondelēz International, allowing the partnership to revive and relaunch Oreo O's. Post discontinued the cereal late in 2024, replacing it with the more trendy Oreo Puffs, with crème-flavored marshmallows: "For those who love dunking their Oreo cookies in milk, Oreo Puffs cereal is a brand-new, delicious way to enjoy the taste of the iconic Oreo cookie—during breakfast time!"[7]

Co-branding of candy, cookie, and snack cake brands expanded in the late 2000s despite calls for eating less sugar. Cereal sales had fallen almost 20% over the past decade, and companies were desperate to compensate for the lost revenue.[8] The solution: new cereals with nostalgic sugary brands people knew and loved.

General Mills extended its licensing deal with Hershey in order to deliver cereals like Hershey's Kisses, Jolly Rancher (we can't even imagine), KitKat, and Reese's Puffs Big Puffs, a cereal first launched in 1994 as Reese's Peanut Butter Cups. In 2021, Reese's Puffs sold over 35 million boxes. Post partnered with Hostess Brands to use Honey Bun and Twinkies brand names, creating cereal versions of the popular snack cakes. Although 72% of surveyed consumers reported avoiding sugar, they viewed sugary cereals as a "permissible indulgence." As always, the sweeter the better; sales increased.[9] Thanks to the cereal companies, kids can finally have their candy, cookies, and cake, and eat them for breakfast too.

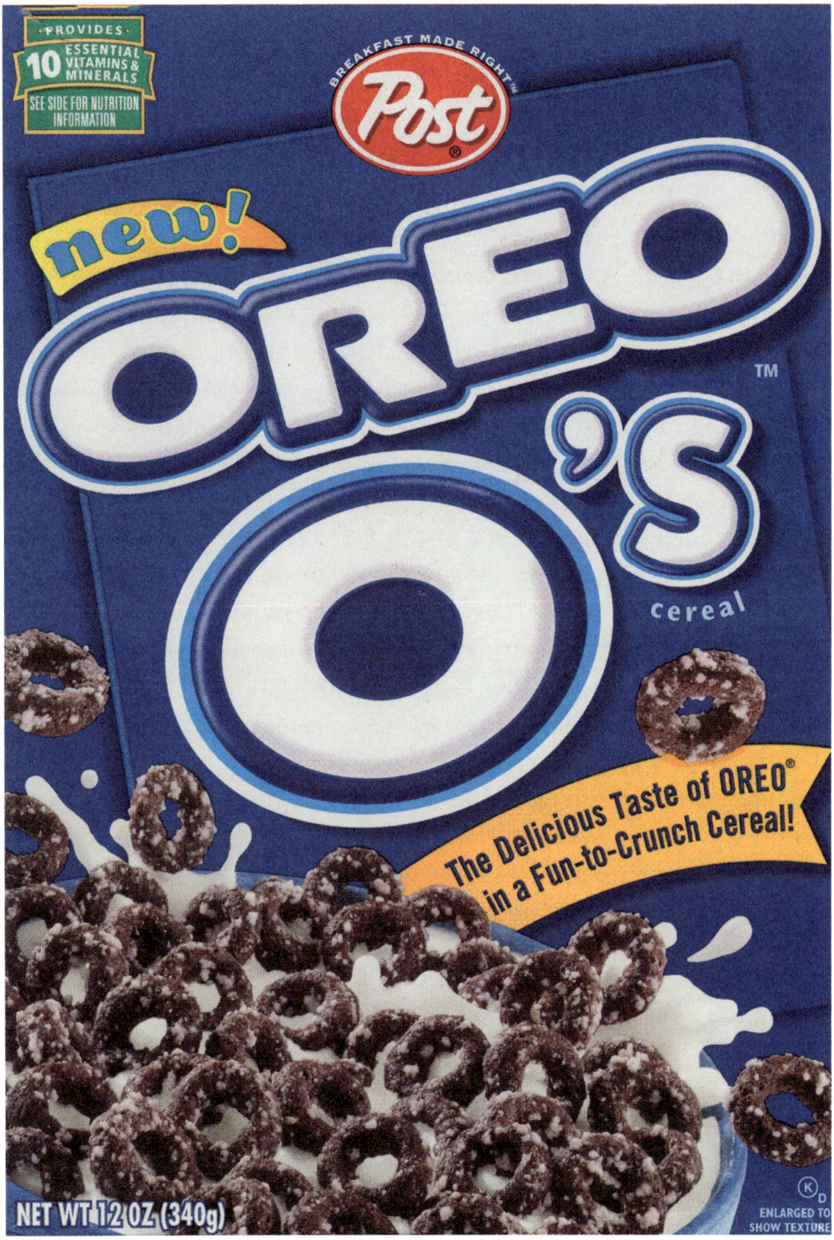

FIGURE 5 This 1998 box of new Post Oreo O's cereal (then owned by Kraft Foods) advertised "The Delicious Taste of OREO in a Fun-to-Crunch Cereal!"—Oreo cookies for breakfast.

Sugar wars: Minimizing sugar

Advocates for children's health have long complained about the high sugar content of breakfast cereals. Eventually, their "eat less sugar" complaints gained traction. Whereas the 1970s and 1980s were the heyday of presweetened kids' cereals, the 2000s marked a decade of effort—and competition—to reduce the sugar.

In 2003, Kraft Foods, which then owned Post cereals, announced its intention to reformulate some of its products to make them healthier. Cereals were an obvious place to begin. At the time, Alpha-Bits contained typical amounts of sugar; we have seen boxes from 1982 with 11 grams per serving, and from 1998 with 13 grams. Kraft intended Alpha-Bits for parents concerned about education (eat your letters), but also health. It first reformulated the cereal to contain 3 grams of fiber from whole grains per serving (similar to Cheerios) and fortified it with 14 vitamins and minerals. It produced the no-sugar version shown in Figure 6 in 2005. But removing the sugar had unfortunate consequences. Zero-sugar Alpha-Bits had "letter-integrity" issues; the extruded letters got soggy in milk, did not hold their shape, and, to some critics, tasted like "wet cardboard."[10] As you might guess, this cereal did not sell and soon disappeared. Post tried introducing the zero-sugar version again later but by 2013 had settled on 6 grams per serving, and kept it there until discontinuing the brand in 2021.

Post was not alone in confronting pressures to reduce sugar. In 2008, *Consumer Reports* compared the sugars in 27 breakfast cereals, noting that many were still 50% sugar by weight, and some, like Kellogg's Honey Smacks, contained at least as much sugar as a glazed Dunkin' Donut.[11] This required a response.

General Mills led the way. A year earlier, without saying anything publicly, it began reducing the sugars in its kids' cereals by an average of 14%.[12] But on December 10, 2009, this company made the loudest possible public announcement, pledging to reduce sugar in its most popular kids' cereals to single digits, this at a time when most had at least 12 grams per serving. As stated in its full-page ad in *The New York Times*, "our commitment to further lower sugar levels is among the most aggressive goals in the food industry." Its pledge would apply to ten cereals, including some of its most popular, such as Lucky Charms and Cocoa Puffs.

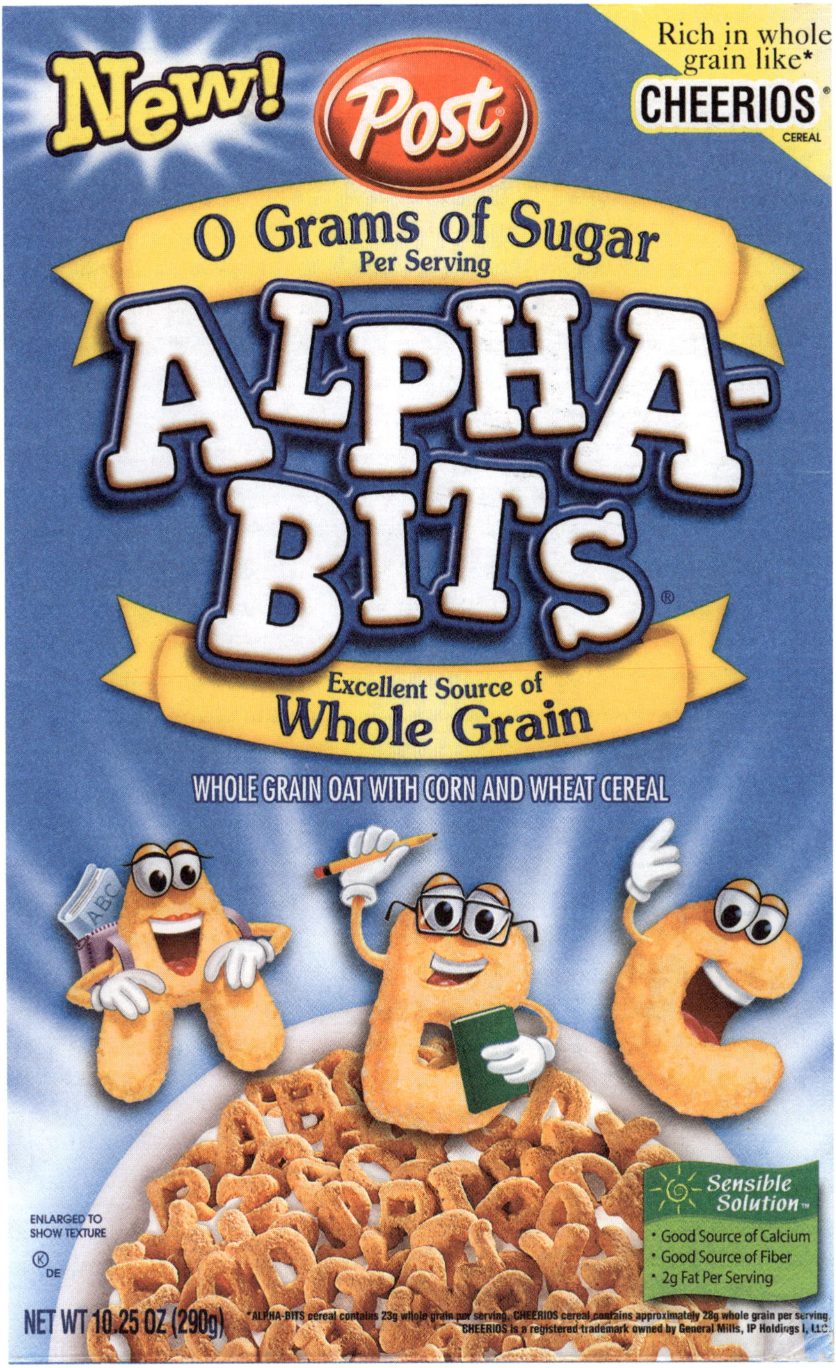

FIGURE 6 In 2005, Post (then owned by Kraft Foods) introduced a version of Alpha-Bits with 0 grams of sugar. It flopped. Later, Post reintroduced it with 6 grams of sugar per serving but discontinued the brand in 2021.

The company's bold promise was in part a response to rumors that federal agencies were working to set nutrition standards for foods advertised on television programs aimed at children under the age of 12 (see Chapter 13). General Mills said, "Ready-to-eat cereals, including presweetened cereals, account for only five percent of the sugar in children's diets. . . . Still, some consumers would prefer to see cereals that are even lower in sugar, especially children's cereals."[13] Although Kellogg interpreted this announcement as direct competition, it did not have an immediate response, and the company continued to insist that it offered consumers choice and that cereal makes many nutritious contributions to the diet.

A year later, General Mills reaffirmed its commitment to single-digit sugar content: "As of December 31 [2010], all shipments of the company's 11 cereals advertised to children will have 10 grams or less"—not exactly a single digit, but close. But a year later, the single-digit promises were history. In the company's taste tests, kids said they did not like cereals with less than 10 grams of sugar per serving. Worse, reducing the sugars caused cereals to lose their shapes, become soggier, and fail to float in milk for 3 minutes—the essential test criterion for acceptance, apparently.[14] The result: declining sales.

But General Mills did reach the single-digit goal for Cinnamon Toast Crunch, Honey Nut Cheerios, Reese's Puffs, and Cookie Crisp. Some of this success was due to a trick: decreased serving size. Whereas in 1999 a serving of Cookie Crisp was 1 cup (29 g) with 12 grams of sugar, in 2011 it was ¾ cup (26 grams) with only 9 grams of sugar. The best General Mills could do for Lucky Charms was 10 grams of sugar per ¾ cup serving—the minimum sweet spot for kids' acceptance.

Was the single-digit sugar goal a publicity stunt? Perhaps. It did keep the company's sugary cereals in the news. But the attempt encountered a harsh reality: kids like sugar, sugar is structurally important to kids' cereals, and companies remove it at their peril.

Shunning sugar: No high-fructose corn syrup

Cereal boxes reveal how ingredients come in and out of favor. Take high-fructose corn syrup (HFCS), a corn-derived sweetener not much different from table sugar (sucrose); it has the same 4 calories per gram and nearly identical glucose and fructose content. HFCS is made by adding enzymes to corn syrup to convert some of its glucose to fructose. Whereas sucrose is 50% glucose and 50% fructose, the HFCS used in cereal is 42% glucose and 55% fructose (the rest of the sugar is in small glucose chains). Despite its biochemical similarity to sucrose, HFCS became a symbol of cheap junk food in the 2000s. It is now a marker of an "ultra-processed food." This pejorative term is used to describe industrially produced foods that are high in added sugars and industrial additives, designed to be irresistibly attractive and profitable, and linked to poor health.[15] The term applies to many breakfast cereals, especially those marketed to children.

HFCS use expanded in the 1980s because it was cheaper than sucrose (US farmers grow a lot of corn). HFCS-containing foods and drinks proliferated in the food supply, in parallel with a sharp rise in the prevalence of obesity. A 2004 study associated HFCS consumption with that increase. In 2010, investigators reported that rats fed HFCS gained more weight than those fed sucrose, even with similar caloric intake.[16] We had our doubts about these results, but the study received widespread attention.

When a report from President George W. Bush's Cancer Panel said that HFCS and sugar might affect the body differently (which we also doubt), the idea was criticized by unlikely allies: the advocacy group Center for Science in the Public Interest (CSPI) and the trade group representing makers of HFCS, the Corn Refiners Association. In a joint letter, these groups correctly argued that correlation does not equal causation and the idea that HFCS differs from sugar "diverges from science in its unfair effort to identify high fructose corn syrup as a uniquely important contributor to obesity."[17] Too late. HFCS had already been demonized.

By 2010, one in 50 new products carried a "No HFCS" claim, and 35% of consumers said they looked for that claim when shopping. To get around the demonization, the Corn Refiners Association petitioned the Food and Drug Administration (FDA) to allow HFCS to be labeled "corn sugar." When the FDA denied the petition in 2012, the Sugar Association (which represents producers of cane and beet sucrose) declared this decision a "victory for American consumers." At the time, one of us (MN) pointed out that "this was nothing more than a fight between two trade associations about market share."[18]

Companies began claiming "No HFCS" to market their cereals, and lawsuits followed: "General Mills has capitalized on consumer aversion toward high fructose corn syrup by frequently touting the absence of that ingredient, deceptively suggesting that its products are healthier because HFCS is absent." The deception? The no-HFCS claim was on cereals with up to 40% of their calories from sugars. After 3 years of litigation, General Mills won this case. The judge noted that the company had fully disclosed its ingredients and said consumers could decide for themselves what to choose. Post cereals were named in a similar suit, but after a 5-year battle, that company agreed to pay out $15 million and discontinue the "No-HFCS" claim.[19]

This battle continues. Although the use of HFCS has declined and most cereals no longer contain it, a Florida legislator introduced the Stop Spoonfuls of Fake Sugar Act in 2024, a bill to classify foods containing HFCS as adulterated (and, therefore, illegal to sell in interstate commerce). In 2025, newly appointed Secretary of Health and Human Services Robert F. Kennedy Jr. declared "war on corn syrup" as part of his campaign to Make America Healthy Again. HFCS, he said, "is just a formula for making you obese and diabetic."[20] But cereals without HFCS still have plenty of other sugars.

"Lightly" litigated

At the low end of sugar content, Post Shredded Wheat has 0 grams; Kellogg's Corn Flakes and Rice Krispies have just 4, and General Mills' Wheaties has 5. The original Cheerios has only 2 grams per serving, but most of its other varieties have the usual 12.

For cereals, claiming low sugar is a hard sell. One way to avoid that problem is to use *lightly sweetened*, as on Honey Kix (7 grams) and Berry Berry Kix (8 grams). But some cereals using this claim have up to 12 grams. "Lightly" is about marketing and not the amount of sugar, as litigious consumers would soon point out.

Beginning in 2016, "lightly" became litigated, most notably in Hadley v. Kellogg. The plaintiff alleged that *lightly sweetened* implied "that Defendant's products [Smart Start and Frosted Mini-Wheats varieties] are lower in sugar when they actually are composed of 18% to 40% added sugar." The case settled in 2021 when Kellogg, maintaining it did nothing wrong, agreed to establish a $13 million fund to pay administrative costs, attorneys' fees, and claims by class action members.[21]

The settlement prohibited Kellogg from using "lightly sweetened" on any cereal containing sugars at more than 10% of calories—for at least 3 years (it did not specify what was to happen after that). In 2025, we do not see the claim on any Kellogg boxes, although its website describes Smart Start as "lightly sweetened, toasted multi-grain flakes and crunchy oat clusters." In the same year, Kellogg announced via X (the former social media site Twitter) that the cereal was discontinued because "it didn't have enough fans."

General Mills faced a similar 2016 lawsuit against Honey Kix and several Cheerios and Fiber One varieties. Plaintiffs argued that it was deceptive to advertise Multi Grain Cheerios, for example, as "5 lightly sweetened whole grains in every serving" when sugar comprised nearly 22% of its calories.[22] General Mills must have better lawyers. A judge dismissed the case in 2019, and the company continues to use that description.

The WIC sugar cap

Sugar is not just a consumer concern; it is also a matter of government nutrition policy. The federal Supplemental Nutrition Program for Women, Infants, and Children (WIC) provides low-income participants with services and benefits, including vouchers for free foods—all of which must meet the program's nutrition standards. Managed by the US Department of Agriculture (USDA), WIC is implemented locally by states. In 2024, it served more than 6.7 million women and children each month at an annual cost of more than $7 billion.[23] WIC is a lucrative business for cereal companies that can supply products that meet the program's sugar standard.

Since the 1980s, WIC has limited the sugars in cereals to 6 grams per ounce, half the amount in typical cereals aimed at kids. This limit has induced cereal companies to take two actions: petition to exclude the sugar naturally present in fruit (like raisins) from the cap, and formulate new cereals with less sugar specifically for the WIC market. In 2006, for example, General Mills introduced a new kid-targeted cereal—Dora the Explorer, "lightly sweetened cinnamon corn puffs," based on the Nickelodeon kids' television show and Latina character. The star-shaped cereal had 6 grams of sugar per 27-gram serving, precisely the amount permitted by the WIC standards.

WIC did not always limit sugar. The program began in the 1960s, when physicians reported shockingly poor nutrition among pregnant women and young children. This led Congress to establish WIC as a 2-year pilot program in 1972 and as a permanent program in 1975.[24] The WIC food package included a defined list of nutrient-rich foods, including cereals fortified with iron (at a minimum of 45% of the Daily Value).

To the dismay of advocates, the initial nutrition standards said nothing about sugar. Revisions to the food package in 1977 acknowledged this dismay: "A number of comments were received objecting to the high sugar content of the cereals and flavored milk allowed in the food packages." But Congress did not set a sugar limit; instead, it told states if they were worried about high-sugar cereals, they could exclude such products from lists of eligible foods.[25] Not helpful.

In the late 1970s, the only scientific concern about sugars and health was tooth decay. When the USDA asked for public input on sugars in the WIC package, it received 230 comments, almost all supporting limits on the sugar in WIC-eligible cereals. Comments opposing a sugar cap came from the Sugar Association and "two cereal companies" (we can guess which). Ultimately, the USDA agreed with supporters of a sugar cap and, in 1980, proposed the 6-gram limit.[26] The Big Four cereal companies objected that the science was uncertain and the limit was "arbitrary and capricious." Nevertheless, the 6-gram rule went into effect in 1982.

Kellogg immediately objected. Its Bran Flakes met the WIC standards, but Raisin Bran did not; it contained 12 grams of sugar, 7 from the raisins. The company needed a cereal that could compete with General Mills' "cash cow"—Cheerios, the best-selling WIC cereal; in 1991, WIC participants spent $200 million of their benefits on cereal, two-thirds of that on Cheerios. As *The Washington Post* put it on August 22, 1991, "Kellogg's Raisin' a Fuss." Kellogg argued that raisins are healthy, and WIC was encouraging women to add raisins to increase their iron intake, which it was. Raisin Bran, the company insisted, had more iron than Cheerios and was less expensive.

We view these points as valid, but General Mills did not; it opposed allowing Kellogg's Raisin Bran in WIC, ostensibly because it would open up the program to more sugary products, but its real reason was competition. As a former Kellogg lobbyist put it, Cheerios is "found money." All

General Mills needed to do was to make sure the cereal was "placed on a store shelf and WIC participants pick up the familiar yellow Cheerios box."[27]

As it happened, General Mills' opposition to raisins got support from some vocal public health advocates such as CSPI and the Food Research & Action Center (an antihunger group promoting food assistance). These groups worried that allowing Raisin Bran would open the floodgates to loosening WIC's strict nutrition criteria. Despite Kellogg's persistent efforts, the USDA did not budge.

But times change. In 2024, the USDA issued its third update to the WIC food package since 1975. The agency retained the 6-gram limit but specified that it applied only to *added*, not total, sugars. It said the policy change was justified to align with listing "added sugars" on food labels and with the Dietary Guidelines for Americans, and to create a "more permissive standard for products containing naturally occurring sugars."[28] After nearly 40 years of trying, Kellogg's Raisin Bran finally achieved WIC eligibility.

As for what is at stake, cereals make up the second-largest share of all WIC purchases (milk and milk alternatives come first). The USDA sets the nutrition criteria, but states decide which WIC cereals to include on their lists based on cost, availability, and popularity. In May 2024, for example, New York State's list of approved cereals included 575 options differing in brands, flavors, and sizes. Big Four cereals make up 35% of those options, but the majority come from lower-cost private brands, with Walmart's Great Value leading the way. WIC participants, however, prefer the more expensive Big Four cereals and are willing to use their WIC benefits to pay for them.[29] This explains why Cheerios, Kix, and Corn Flakes, all below 6 grams of sugar per ounce, are on the lists of more than 40 states.

One last observation about General Mills' WIC-inspired Dora the Explorer cereal. Only 12 states adopted it, mainly those with large Hispanic/Latino WIC-eligible populations. But that wasn't enough. In 2018, the Texas WIC office told local state agencies it was discontinuing Dora due to "low distribution nationally."[30] A WIC agency in Virginia posted on social media, "Adios Dora." Cereal company concerns about sugar are not really about health; they are about market share.

CHAPTER 4

GRAINS AND FIBER

THE WHOLE POINT

BREAKFAST CEREALS USUALLY LIST a grain as the first ingredient (unless sugar takes that spot). Grains are the edible seeds of the Poaceae family of grasses, which includes oats, wheat, corn, and rice—90% of all cereals. Quaker Oats has been oat based since its start. General Mills relies largely on wheat (Wheaties), oats (Cheerios), and corn (Kix). Kellogg started out with wheat and corn cereals, then added rice (Rice Krispies). Post often combines grains, such as corn and oats, in Honey-Comb and Oreo O's. Boring as they might seem, grains are the focus of intense competition. Witness the grain wars: General Mills' focus on whole grains versus Kellogg's on fiber.

General Mills: Whole Grain Nation

Whole grains are demonstrably good for health. Because of their nutrients and fiber, they are strongly associated with a reduced risk of premature death from all causes, including coronary heart disease.[1] You might think whole grains would be an obvious way to sell cereals, but most breakfast grains are so highly processed that hardly any fiber or nutrients remain. For cereal manufacturers, using whole grains poses challenges in processing, texture, and taste. Intact or minimally processed whole grains are hard to eat and digest. Nearly everybody prefers the taste and texture of refined-grain foods—white bread as opposed to whole wheat.

Turning seeds into easily digestible cereals with broad consumer appeal requires grinding, crushing, and further processing ("refining") to remove most of the bran and germ. Refining, unfortunately, removes most of the fiber and nutrients, which is why some are added back through fortification (see Chapter 6). Thus, General Mills refines whole oats into oat flour and sends it to manufacturing facilities to produce Cheerios, which has few nutrients except those added back through fortification.

General Mills' use and promotion of whole grains dates back to some of its first cereals: Washburn's Whole Wheat Flakes, now Wheaties (1921), and whole-grain oat Cheerios (1941). Over the next five decades, the company introduced highly refined sugary cereals such as Trix, Lucky Charms, Cocoa Puffs, and Cinnamon Toast Crunch, none a particularly healthy or obvious way to consume whole grains. Although General Mills experienced decades of record growth for its Big G cereals, sales slowed by the mid-1990s.[2] The company needed to innovate. Whole grains seemed like a good way to attract health-conscious consumers, especially the aging baby boomer population.

General Mills' first attempt to push whole grains followed the Food and Drug Administration (FDA) Modernization Act of 1997, which allowed companies to use health claims backed up by reports from federal agencies or the National Academy of Sciences (NAS). Companies merely had to notify the FDA when they wanted to use a claim; they could use it if the agency did not object within 120 days. In 1999, General Mills petitioned the FDA for a claim that whole-grain foods could reduce the risk of heart disease and certain cancers, based on the NAS's 1989 report *Diet and Health: Implications for Reducing Chronic Disease Risk*. The FDA consulted with the NAS but chose to take no action. As soon as the 120 days were up, General Mills exulted: "The FDA agrees that eating whole-grain foods like Cheerios, Wheaties, and Total . . . may reduce your risk of heart disease and some cancers."[3] The FDA's nonaction launched two decades of intense whole-grain marketing. By 2000, General Mills led the cereal category for the first time with a 33% share and touted its "healthy innovation" as a primary reason for its reinvigorated growth.[4]

In 2003, General Mills became a founding member of the Whole Grains Council, an entity managed by Oldways Preservation and Exchange Trust, a group founded in 1990 as a think tank on food issues. The council was, and is, supported by food industry members.[5] It ran an education campaign to encourage increased whole-grain consumption.

Shortly after joining the council, General Mills announced that it would soon convert all its Big G cereals, including sugary kids' cereals made mostly from refined grains, to "good" or "excellent" sources of whole grains.[6] Its boxes stated the whole-grain promise, "ALL General Mills Cereals Are Made With WHOLE GRAIN!" We show an example in Figure 7. These boxes also displayed "goodness corners" with icons promoting a variety of nutrition qualities; one showed a wheat shaft and stated whether the cereal was a "good" or "excellent" source of whole grain.

One problem: although the FDA had defined the meaning of *good* and *excellent* for nutrients, it had not done so for whole grains—a food ingredient. To solve that problem, General Mills petitioned the FDA to define the claim. It suggested its own cut points: "excellent" (16 grams whole grains per serving), "good" (8 grams), and "made with." When the FDA rejected the petition, citing the absence of a defined Daily Value (DV) for whole-grain consumption, the company had to remove the whole-grain icon and the unauthorized claims.[7] But it continued to relentlessly promote whole grains.

The workaround: The Whole Grain Stamp

At about that time, the Whole Grains Council created a bright-gold Whole Grain Stamp as an "aid for busy shoppers" (see Figure 22a). The first stamps followed General Mills' lead. They defined a "good source" as at least 8 grams per serving and an "excellent source" as 16 grams, and they added a third category, "100% excellent" (all grains whole and at least 16 grams). An advertising campaign promoted "Trust the Stamp" on television, in magazines, and in newspapers. The first products displaying the stamp appeared in supermarkets in 2005. General Mills put the stamp on many of its cereals, including kids' cereals like Cocoa Puffs and Lucky Charms, despite their 12 grams of sugar and only 1 gram of fiber. Within a year, nearly 50 companies were using the stamp on more than 550 products.

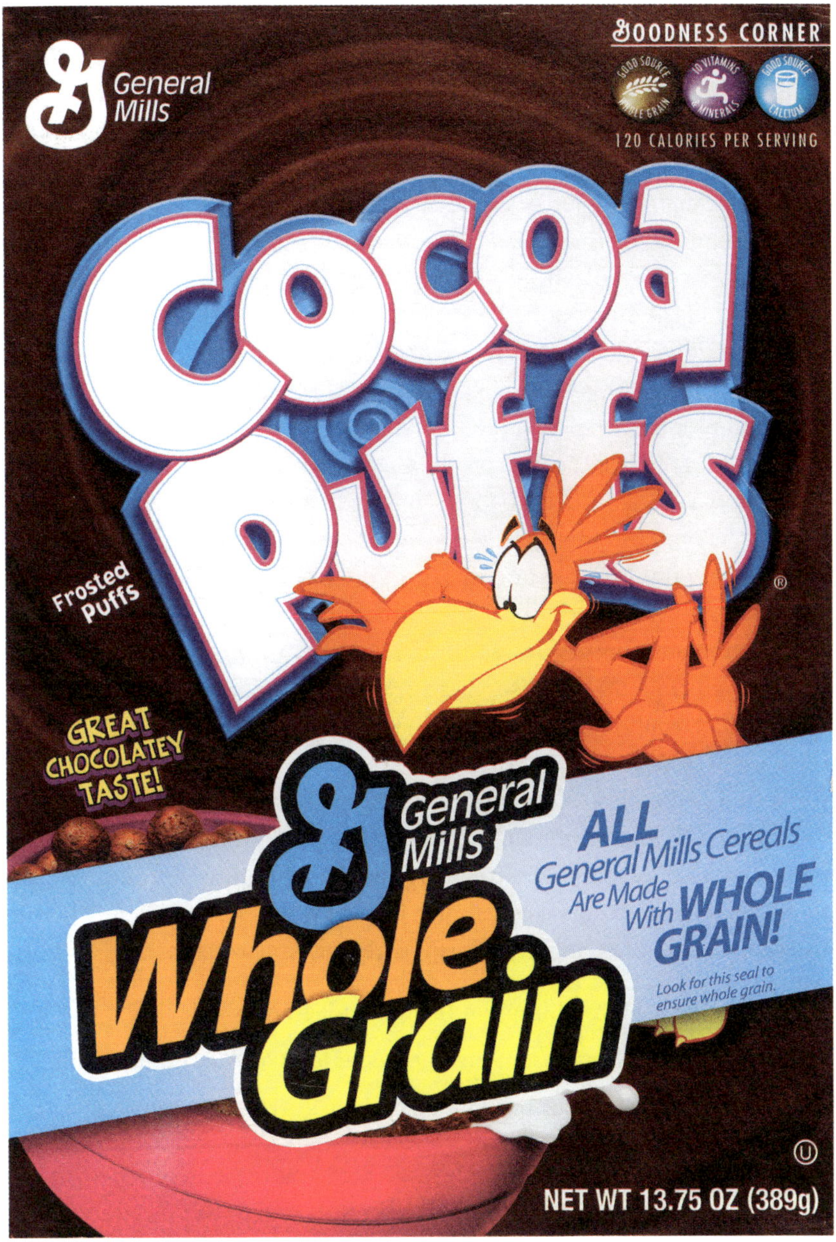

FIGURE 7 This 2005 box displays General Mills' promise to make all its cereals with whole grains. The GOODNESS CORNER highlights this cereal as a "GOOD SOURCE" of whole grain, a designation the FDA had not—and still has not—defined.

So where was the FDA? It immediately objected, since it still had not defined "good" or "excellent" sources of whole grains. Under pressure from companies and consumer groups, the FDA developed *Whole Grain Guidance for Industry* in 2006, which was voluntary and not enforceable. This suggested that label statements should not imply comparative levels of whole grains (like good or excellent), as such comparisons would be false and misleading. Instead, the FDA suggested companies use factual statements like "xx% whole grain" or "xx grams of whole grain."[8]

The Whole Grains Council complained that "the FDA's nonbinding recommendations, released today, are a guidance document, which does 'not establish legally enforceable responsibilities.'" True. But it had to comply.

The Center for Science in the Public Interest (CSPI) disapproved of the Whole Grain Stamp. It called on the FDA to focus resources on "the most common type of deceptive labeling—misleading whole grain claims."[9] CSPI argued that without identifying the actual percentage of whole grains, the stamp could not help anyone interpret dietary advice to make half your grains whole. It also could mislead consumers into eating more refined grains, since it allowed claims for products containing only 8 grams of whole grains in a 30-gram serving (27% whole grain but 73% *not* whole grain). Most troubling, the stamps appeared on sugary kids' cereals, making them seem healthier. CSPI urged the FDA to insist that the stamps include the actual percentage of whole grain and the number of grams.

Despite CSPI's objections, the FDA has issued no further guidance or regulations for labeling whole grains, and General Mills continues to use the Whole Grain Stamp on cereals like Cocoa Puffs, Trix, and Lucky Charms. In 2025, the Whole Grain Stamp appeared in three versions:

- 100% whole grain: minimum 16 grams, all grains whole
- 50%+ whole grain: minimum 8 grams, at least half the grains whole
- Basic: at least 8 grams but contains primarily refined grain

A basic stamp might say "Whole grain 8 g or more per serving," with the admonition "Eat 48 g or more of whole grains daily." The program is voluntary. Companies self-determine whether their products qualify for the stamp; the program runs on the honor system. They pay to use the stamps through membership fees to the Whole Grains Council. In 2024, these ranged from $525 per year for small companies with sales up to $500,000, to $15,750 per year for companies with sales exceeding $1 billion. The Whole Grains Council says it represents more than 350 companies, and its stamps appear on more than 13,000 products in 64 countries.

Whole grains in dietary guidance

General Mills repeatedly petitioned the FDA to allow it to market whole-grain cereals as nutritionally superior despite their sugar content. It also lobbied for dietary guidelines that called for consumption of whole grains (and, therefore, General Mills' cereals). For the first time, the 2005 Dietary Guidelines did just that: "In general at least half the grains should come from whole grains." The guidelines advised Americans to eat three or more "ounce-equivalent servings of whole grains per day," meaning 16 grams each, for a total of 48 grams per day.

General Mills declared victory and launched its Whole Grain Nation marketing campaign, which included TV and print ads and a dedicated website (now gone).[10] When the US Department of Agriculture (USDA) issued a new Food Guide Pyramid to accompany the 2005 guidelines, General Mills put a banner on the Frosted Cheerios box we show in Figure 8: "New Pyramid Recommends More WHOLE GRAIN!" It followed this statement with "For more info go to MyPyramid.gov," implying government endorsement. The back of the box said, "9 out of 10 Americans don't get enough whole grain" and "Aim for at least 3 servings of whole grain each day." The eat-more-cereal message could not have been more explicit.

Whole Grain Guaranteed: The struggles

General Mills was nothing if not persistent in its attempts to market its cereals as packed with healthy whole grains. When the FDA objected to the "goodness corner," the company replaced it with a blue banner and a trademarked white check mark, "With Whole Grain Guaranteed." It continued to try to position whole grains as essential to dietary guidance. Company officials submitted recommendations to the 2010 Dietary Guidelines Advisory Committee to tell the public to look for products with "whole" or "whole grain" ingredients (e.g., "whole grain corn"), and

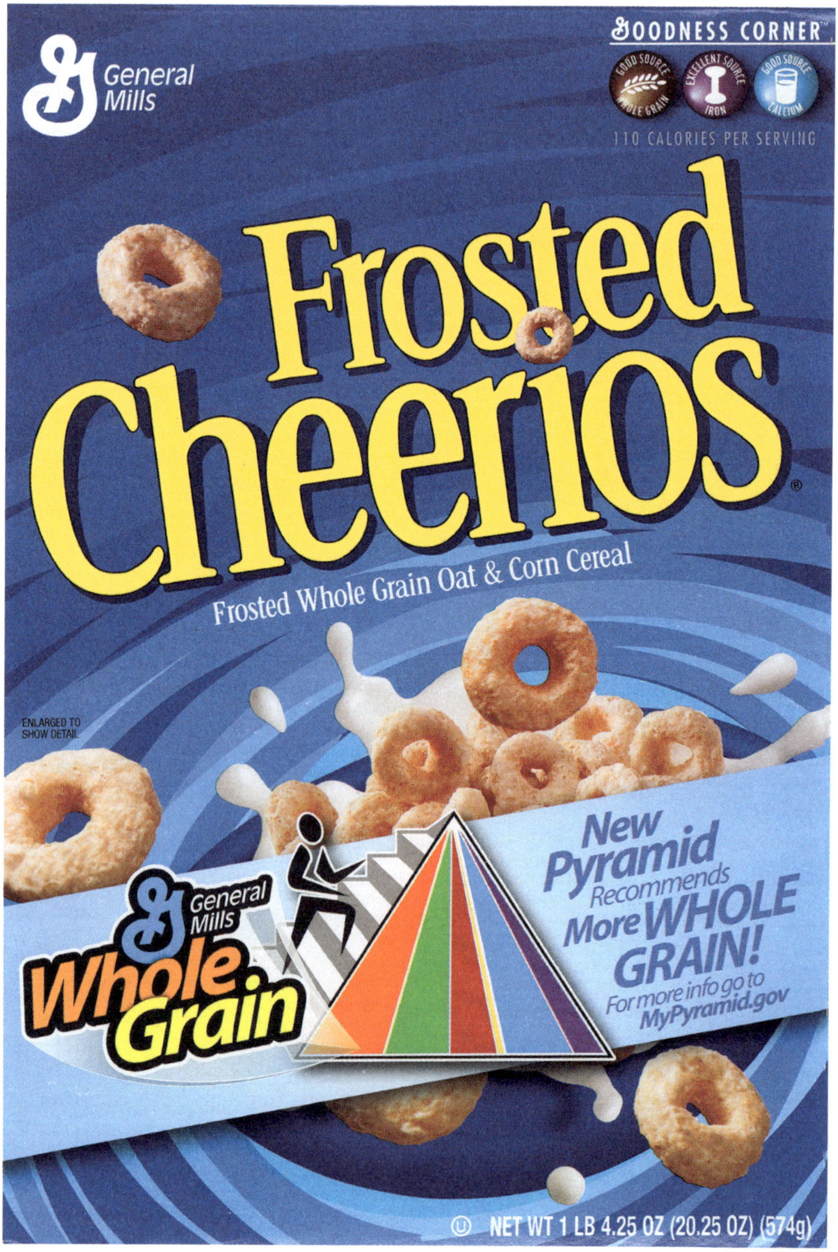

FIGURE 8 The USDA revised the Food Guide Pyramid soon after releasing the 2005 Dietary Guidelines. In 2006, General Mills used the new pyramid's recommendation of whole grains to promote sugary Frosted Cheerios.

for whole grain to be listed as the first ingredient.[11] The 2010 Dietary Guidelines did both.

But CSPI complained that General Mills' Whole Grain Guaranteed banner was deceptive, as it led consumers to believe that even kids' cereals were 100% whole grain and healthier than other kids' cereals.[12] When CSPI threatened to sue, General Mills agreed to update the banner to read "with Whole Grains xx grams," but instead it revised the banner to say "With First Ingredient Whole Grain," the 2010 guidance it had lobbied for. CSPI again objected, this time to "whole grain" appearing in a much larger print than other text; it said nobody would understand the "first ingredient" qualifier. General Mills responded by adding a second banner to the middle of its boxes: "More WHOLE GRAIN than any other ingredient!*" The asterisk led to the small print on the side panel: "as compared to any other single ingredient."

In 2011, General Mills put yet another banner on cereals like Chocolate Cheerios and Cookie Crisp: "Big G Cereals are America's #1 Source of Whole Grain at Breakfast." When the company increased its advertising spending on whole-grain cereals that year to $245 million, the Public Health Advocacy Institute accused it of using the campaign to distract from the sugar content.[13] Eventually, the complaints led General Mills to abandon the banner and wheat check mark and replace both with the FDA-suggested factual statement: "16 g whole grain per serving." In 2025, we saw this statement on Cocoa Puffs, raising the question, Is a sugary cereal with whole grains meaningfully healthier? We don't think so. Cocoa Puffs provides only 2 grams of fiber per serving, but 12 grams of sugar.

Has the Whole Grains Council achieved its goal of increasing the intake of whole-grain foods? The USDA reported a negligible 0.05-ounce equivalent increase per 1,000 calories for whole grains between 1994 and 2018, but the increase in consumption of refined grains was seven times higher.[14] Are customers really cuckoo for whole grains in Cocoa Puffs? Maybe, if they think whole grains make sugary cereals healthier. Truly whole-grain, high-fiber cereals such as Post Shredded Wheat (49 grams of whole grains, 8 grams of fiber per serving) do not sell nearly as well.

Kellogg's fiber "big bet"

The alternative to marketing whole grains is to market a cereal's fiber content. Kellogg proudly claims that it brought the first two high-fiber cereals to market, with Bran Flakes in 1915 and All-Bran in 1919. But when Kellogg began introducing sugary kids' cereals in the 1950s, its focus on fiber waned. By 2008, Kellogg's long-standing US market lead was declining; it had a 33% share, but General Mills was closing in at 30%.[15] What to do?

Kellogg's kids' cereals are best sellers, but most have little or no fiber. In 2009, Kellogg promised that 80% of its kids' cereals would provide at least 3 grams of fiber per serving, the amount qualifying as a "good" source (the DV for fiber is 28 grams; a "good" source is 10% of that).[16] The new fiber campaign began with two kids' favorites, Apple Jacks and Froot Loops, and later, Corn Pops. The fiber-reformulated cereals displayed large banners: "NOW PROVIDES FIBER. A GREAT WAY TO KEEP KIDS HEALTHY" (see Figure 23). By 2011, a green banner across the top of Froot Loops said, "Good Source of Fiber," despite a third of its calories coming from sugars.

Upping the fiber made good marketing sense. Kellogg had promoted the benefits of fiber for digestive health since its start, and public pressures to make kids' foods healthier were increasing during the Obama administration. By May 2009, 6.5% of all new food products sported fiber claims, and the food industry was "embracing fiber-fortified products at warp speed." Kellogg's CEO said, "The fiber additions in a number of kids products are all about trying to strengthen and differentiate our foods"—an admission that fiber really was about marketing, not health.[17]

Fiber, indigestible by us but food for our gut microbiome, naturally occurs in food plants—fruits, vegetables, beans, nuts, and whole grains. It is "intrinsic" or "intact" in these foods and in unrefined corn, wheat, and oats. But Kellogg boosted the fiber to 3 grams per serving by adding *isolated* oat fiber, corn fiber, or soluble corn fiber. The FDA allows these and other kinds of extracted substances—guar gum, cellulose, psyllium, pectin, and inulin—to be considered dietary fiber, and to count toward source claims as "good" or "excellent."[18] Fibers may not be created equal, but the FDA views them as equal for labeling purposes.

Despite Kellogg's aggressive fiber campaign, General Mills' whole-grain strategy was succeeding; the company reported record financial results in 2010, with sales of Big G cereals increasing by 5% that year. By 2011, it was spending 20% more on whole-grain advertising to make sure customers knew that "General Mills' Cereals are America's number one source of whole grain at breakfast."[19] The marketing positions—whole grains for General Mills and fiber for Kellogg—were in direct competition.

Kellogg was losing out. Needing a better way to compete, it moved right in on General Mills' approach. By 2012, the front banners of Kellogg's kids' cereals said, "Good source of fiber & made with whole grain." The ampersand (&) was the key. The company could now say it "offers more cereals with at least a 'good' source (3 grams) of fiber *and* 8 grams of whole grains than any other U.S. food company."[20] Customers would not have to decide between fiber and whole grains; Kellogg's kids' cereals delivered both.

Did lovers of Froot Loops, Apple Jacks, or Corn Pops care? Probably not. By 2025, these cereals no longer claimed fiber or whole grains on the box. Instead, the marketing messages were "Sweet crispy crunch" (Corn Pops) and "Cinnalicious" (Apple Jacks). Froot Loops even came with marshmallows. The fiber content of these cereals is zero; their sugars are half the weight and at least 40% of the calories. In today's market, sugar is what sells—not fiber, and not whole grains.

But in January 2026, the Trump administration's Departments of Health and Human Services and of Agriculture issued the *Dietary Guidelines for Americans* for 2025–2030. These advised severe restrictions on sugars along with a guideline to "focus on whole grains" and advice to "prioritize fiber-rich whole grains." But their overall message about grains was inconsistent. A new food guide, an inverted pyramid, placed whole grains at the bottom tip, suggesting that intake should be minimized in comparison to the more prominently displayed protein, dairy, healthy fats, vegetables, and fruits. How cereal companies would respond to these messages remained to be seen. The companies were already dealing with the departments' pressures to eliminate petroleum-based artificial food dyes, as we discuss in the next chapter.

CHAPTER 5

FLAVORS AND COLORS

NATURAL AND ARTIFICIAL

WITH SUGARS AND GRAINS as the main ingredients in most breakfast cereals, companies struggle to differentiate their brands. Flavor innovations are an easy way to create line extensions, increase supermarket shelf space, and expand sales. Cheerios, with more than 20 varieties (e.g., honey, chocolate, peanut butter, cinnamon, and fruit flavors), is today's most prominent example; its boxes occupy major portions of supermarket cereal aisles.

The cereal aisle is hardly a place where you would expect to find fruit, but here we find Froot Loops, Fruity Pebbles, Cap'n Crunch's Crunch Berries, Blueberry Toast Crunch, and Strawberry Krispies, all grains and sugars, but fruit flavored and brightly colored. We concede that Kellogg's Apple Jacks does have some fruit. Of its 22 ingredients (not counting the vitamins and minerals), dried apples constitute ingredient #10, appearing under the "Contains less than 2%" statement.

"Natural" flavors

Ingredient #14 in Apple Jacks is "natural flavor." And what, pray tell, is that? The Food and Drug Administration (FDA) has rules about such things; these refer to how companies can use, label, and market natural and artificial flavors. We love the FDA's definitions. "Natural flavors" are

> the essential oil, oleoresin, essence or extractive, protein hydrolysate, distillate, or any product of roasting, heating or enzymolysis, which contains the flavoring constituents derived from a spice, fruit or fruit juice, vegetable or vegetable juice, edible yeast, herb, bark, bud, root, leaf or similar plant material, meat, seafood, poultry, eggs, dairy products, or fermentation products thereof, whose significant function in food is flavoring rather than nutritional.[1]

Simply put, natural flavors are extracted from plant or animal sources. In contrast, artificial flavors are chemicals originating in a lab. But natural flavors are not what anyone might consider natural. By the time they are added to cereals, they may contain as many as 250 different chemicals, some of which are artificial and synthetic.[2] This is why both natural and synthetic flavors are considered markers of ultra-processed foods.

The FDA also regulates how flavors appear in ingredient statements or on box fronts. Most kids' cereals use a combination of natural and artificial flavors. Sometimes, boxes will say "With other natural flavors" (WONFs in regulation-speak). *WONF* means that some flavor comes from a natural ingredient, like the dried apples or apple juice concentrate (ingredient #11) in Apple Jacks, but the "other natural flavor" boosts it, creating a more intense apple flavor.

When first introduced, Froot Loops promised fruit flavors as shown in Figure 9. By the 1980s, its boxes said "All natural flavors: orange, lemon, cherry" and, in tiny print, "and other flavors." Its mascot Toucan Sam sings, "Follow my nose, wherever it goes, to the flavor of fruit." The cereal still only contains natural flavors, but fun fact: the different artificially colored loops all taste the same.

The FDA says companies can use fruit names and images to describe a flavor, but the Federal Trade Commission requires the advertising on a cereal box to be "truthful and not misleading." Thus, the use of fruit in cereal names and images occasionally landed the companies in trouble with regulatory agencies and consumer advocates.

Again, consider Froot Loops. Urban lore has it that Kellogg first wanted to name its brightly colored rings "Fruit Loops" but was quickly threatened

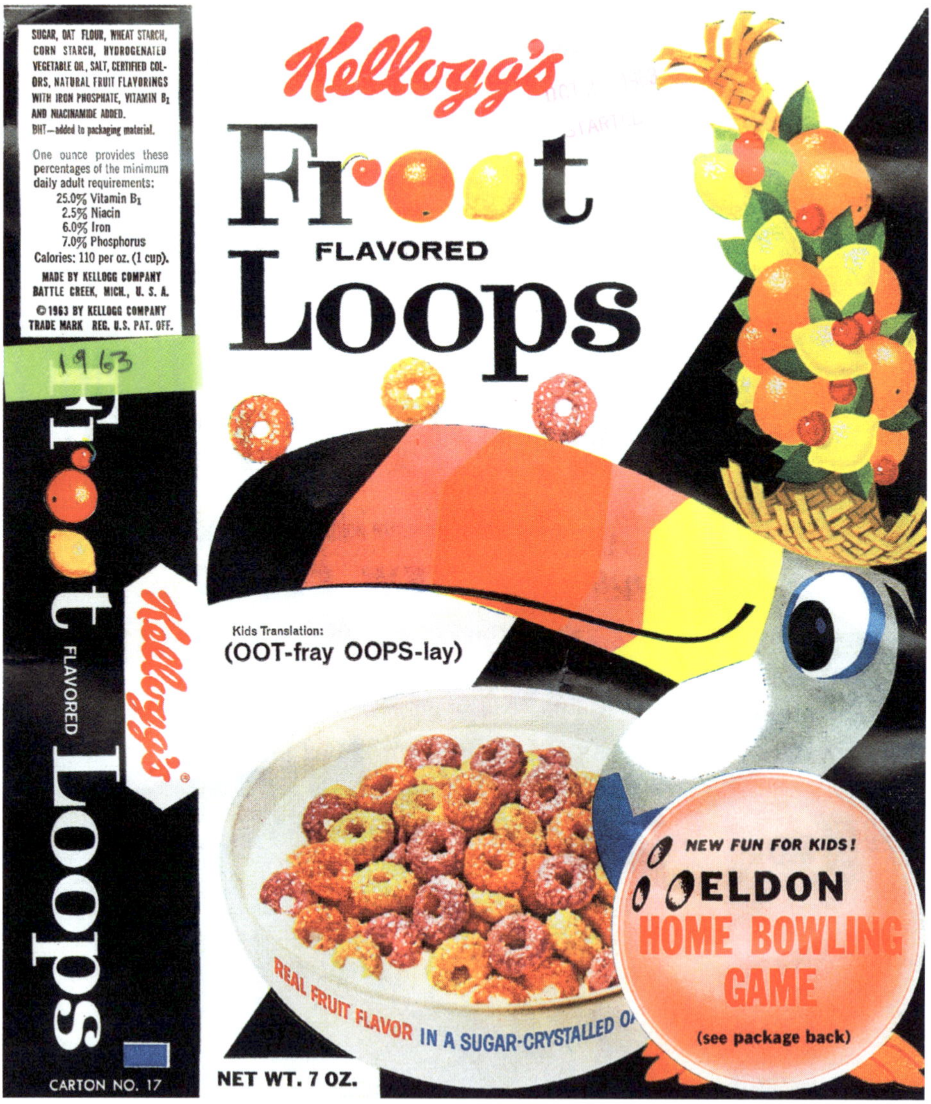

FIGURE 9 In 1963, Kellogg introduced Froot Loops "(Kids Translation: OOT-fray OOPS-lay)" with "REAL FRUIT FLAVOR" and "certified colors," but not a trace of real fruit.

with a lawsuit. We cannot confirm this legend, but we think it plausible. By the time Kellogg introduced Froot Loops as a "sugar-crystalled oat cereal in a puffed crisp form" with "real fruit flavor" in 1963, it knew enough not to use *fruit* in the name of a product that had none. "Froot Loops" also could be trademarked, preventing others from copying it—but not protecting it from litigation.

At least four lawsuits have been filed against Kellogg over Froot Loops, none of them successful. Each argued that Froot Loops misled consumers into thinking the cereal contained real fruit. Federal judges disagreed; they said no reasonable person would interpret "froot" as suggesting real fruit; a box of Froot Loops "truthfully depicts that cereal in the shape of multi-colored rings that do not resemble any known fruit" and "the fanciful use of a nonsensical word cannot reasonably be interpreted to imply that the Product contains or is made from actual fruit." In 2009, a similar complaint was filed against Quaker's Cap'n Crunch's Crunch Berries. In that case, the judge said, "Any reasonable consumer would know that 'Crunchberries' were not berries."[3] Count these decisions as wins for cereal companies.

Still, the lawsuits over fruit names continue. In the mid-2000s, blueberries were marketed as a superfood, and they turned up in the names of cereals. The result: "Blueberry-Gate." When General Mills introduced "naturally and artificially flavored" Total Blueberry Pomegranate cereal in 2009, plaintiffs filed the usual lawsuit: "Where's the fruit?" In dismissing the case, the judge said, "If you look at the ingredients table, blueberry and pomegranate aren't there. So I don't understand how a reasonable consumer is somehow tricked into thinking it contains blueberry and pomegranate."[4]

Around that same time, Kellogg introduced Frosted Mini-Wheats Blueberry, also "naturally and artificially flavored." The box shows "Mini," its wheat biscuit mascot, juggling blueberries, but not one blueberry turns up in the cereal. To avoid further trouble, Kellogg changed the cereal's name to Frosted Mini-Wheats Blueberry Muffin. Blueberries? Not a chance. The moral: "froot" is not fruit. If you want fruit, add blueberries or whatever other kinds you like to your cereal.

Spicing up the cereal aisle

While cereals with sugar and fruity flavors are mostly targeted to kids, those with seasonal flavors such as apple pie, chai, or gingerbread target adults. But none is more popular than pumpkin spice, the gateway flavor to the fall season. Pumpkin spice flavor took off as a trend—a craze—after Starbucks introduced the Pumpkin Spice Latte in 2003. By fall 2020, the Big Four filled cereal aisles with limited-edition, orange, pumpkin-illustrated boxes.

Kellogg, for example, introduced Frosted Mini-Wheats Pumpkin Spice in 2015, and added Special K Pumpkin Spice to its fall lineup in 2016. General Mills also launched Pumpkin Spice Cheerios that year. Pumpkin spice also shows up in Post's Life cereal and Quaker Instant Oatmeal. Although the boxes say "Naturally flavored" or "With natural flavors," the flavor does not come from pumpkin. Instead, it comes from the spices commonly used with pumpkin, like cinnamon, nutmeg, allspice, or ginger, along with the usual "natural flavor."[5]

This was not always the case. When General Mills first introduced Pumpkin Spice Cheerios, pumpkin puree was one of its ingredients, and the sugars were only 8 grams per serving. Today, the puree is gone, and the sugars are 11 grams. Pumpkin-flavored products, including cereals, accounted for more than $800 million in sales in 2023.[6] Pumpkin spice may sell, but in cereals, it's more sugar than spice.

Eating the rainbow: Artificial colors

Kellogg's Froot Loops is the poster child for bright colors in cereals (see Figures 23 and 29). Alas, its colors—FD&C Red 40, Blue 1, and Yellow 5 and 6—are artificial, synthesized originally from coal tar and now from petroleum by-products. Throughout 2024, investor and consumer activists protested Kellogg's failure to fulfill its 2015 promise to eliminate these dyes from kids' cereals. In October 2024, activist shareholders staged a demonstration at the WK Kellogg Co's Battle Creek headquarters to demand the removal of these and other artificial dyes.[7] Also in Battle Creek that week was the food industry critic Vani Hari (the "Food Babe"), who delivered a petition with 400,000 signatures making the same demand: get rid of the artificial colors. Kellogg officials refused to meet with her.

The petition particularly noted the dyes in Baby Shark, the cereal aimed at toddlers (see Figure 28). Although Baby Shark cereal was no longer available in 2024, the petition pointed out that Kellogg does not use these dyes in many other countries: "Kellogg's, we deserve the safer cereals other countries get!" It compared the ingredient lists for American Froot Loops (16 ingredients in addition to vitamins and minerals) to the Australian version (7 ingredients). Hari said, "This is a moral issue. . . . American food companies are knowingly using ingredients here in this country that they removed abroad due to stricter regulations and to avoid warning labels. This is unethical, and it needs to stop."[8]

Even more astonishing, the artificial colors in cereals got caught up in the electoral politics of 2024. Hari was invited to testify before a Senate roundtable alongside former presidential hopeful and then Trump supporter Robert F. Kennedy Jr., who incorporated her demands in his campaign to Make America Healthy Again (MAHA). Kennedy, who would soon be confirmed as the secretary of Health and Human Services (HHS) in the Trump administration, said, "The first thing I'd do isn't going to cost you anything because I'm just gonna tell the cereal companies, take all the dyes out of their food."[9] He called for revisiting pesticide and other chemical-use standards, noting that some chemicals allowed in American foods are banned in the European Union.

In April 2025, the FDA, which is part of HHS, announced its intention to phase out the dyes, and in May, the MAHA Commission increased the urgency of such action by suggesting links between food dyes and mental disorders, hyperactivity, and autism in children. We can hardly believe that the colors of Froot Loops and Apple Jacks could elicit demonstrations, petitions, congressional testimony, campaign promises, and White House action, but they most certainly did. As to why Kellogg did not respond to the Food Babe, the answer is obvious: artificial food dyes are *essential* to kids' cereals. People much prefer intensely colored foods, are more likely to buy them, and perceive them as tasting better. General Mills learned this early; it attributed a 13% growth in sales of Lucky Charms in 1996 to the incorporation of "brighter colored marshmallows." That year, it also gave Trix a makeover with enhanced colors—drivers of the brand's growth.[10]

Regulating food colors

The FDA categorizes colors added to food as either certified or exempt from certification. The original 1963 Froot Loops label listed "certified colors," of which there seemed to be just three, none as bright as in current versions. Exempt colors are extracted from natural sources like vegetables, spices, and minerals. Other countries use exempt colors such as beet juice (red), annatto (yellow), and grape skin extract (purple) to color kids' cereals. But certified colors are artificial or synthetic; they are made in laboratories.

When Congress passed the Pure Food and Drug Act of 1906, which prohibited "poisonous or deleterious colors in confectionery and the coloring or staining of food to conceal damage or inferiority," it reduced the number of permitted colors from more than 700 to 7 considered safe for use in food: Blue 2, Green 3, Red 1, 2, and 3, Yellow 1, and Orange 1.[11]

The 1938 Food, Drug, and Cosmetic Act established a premarket approval process for new synthetic colors. In 1960, Congress passed the Color Additives Amendment in response to a tragedy; children got sick after eating Halloween candy made with Orange 1 (subsequently delisted for food). The amendment defined *color additive* and set conditions for safe use and labeling.

Since then, the FDA reviewed the safety of colors in use and delisted all of those it found harmful, and it now requires all synthetic colors to be tested and certified before use. Colors can be used in food as long as they follow "good manufacturing practices," a rather subjective criterion. In 2024, the FDA reported that more than 23 million pounds of the seven permitted colors—Blue 1 and 2, Green 3, Red 3 and 40, and Yellow 5 and 6—had been certified for use in US food products. Of these, Red 40, Yellow 5, and Yellow 6 made up 86% of all colors used that year.[12]

Health implications

The effects of artificial food colors on health have been debated, and safety arguments continue to this day. Synthetic colors may be bright and attractive, but some have been shown in animal studies to damage the immune system, disrupt endocrine function, and cause cancer. Collectively, they also have been linked to hyperactivity and other disruptive behaviors in children, especially through the work of the Feingold Association. "Linked" does not necessarily imply causation. Even the MAHA Commission admits that research on the harm of food colors is not definitive.

Studying the effects of food colors is inherently difficult because they are consumed in such small amounts. One of the earliest placebo-controlled trials of synthetic food dyes, for example, showed no effect on hyperactivity except in one of six children studied.[13] Such results are typical, but hard to interpret.

Thus, the FDA says, "Because of inherent limitations of science, the FDA can never be absolutely certain of the absence of any risk from the use of any substance." It considers synthetic colors safe at current levels of intake. But in 2008, the Center for Science in the Public Interest (CSPI) called for settling this matter when it petitioned the FDA to ban artificial colors linked to hyperactivity and other behavioral problems in children; it published a scientific report on food dye hazards in 2010. The FDA responded by asking its Food Advisory Committee to consider whether science supported a causal link between synthetic colors and hyperactivity. The committee said no, but it called for more research. CSPI published yet another scientific report on color additives in 2016. In 2019, the FDA asked its Science Board to review that science. Again, the board found no link, and again it called for more research. On this basis, the FDA continued to maintain that synthetic colors are safe.[14] In 2025, under pressure from the MAHA movement, the FDA appeared to be changing its stance.

All of this makes life difficult for the makers of kids' cereals. Eliminating synthetic dyes is bad for business; the dyes from natural sources cost more, their colors are less vivid and less stable, and people perceive the foods as less tasty than those more brightly colored. The FDA's rules do not help, as it considers all color additives, vegetable and synthetic, to be artificial when added to breakfast cereals, and it does not allow claims for "natural color" or "no artificial colors" on these brightly colored cereals. In 2026, the FDA reversed its stance and allowed the claim for natural colors.[15] We do see "no artificial colors" on uncolored cereals—another marketing strategy, apparently.

Companies pledge to replace dyes

In 2015, under mounting pressure to eliminate or replace the synthetic dyes, cereal companies pledged to reduce their use. General Mills promised that 90% of its cereals would be free of artificial colors within a year, up from its then-current level of 60%. Kellogg said 75% of its North American cereals were already made without artificial colors, but it would eliminate the dyes completely by 2018. Business analysts viewed these pledges as efforts to overcome flagging cereal sales.[16]

Attempts to meet those promises did not go well. In 2016, General Mills said 75%—not 90%—of its cereals were free of artificial colors. In 2017, it reformulated and repackaged Trix, marketing it as containing "NO high fructose corn syrup, NO colors from artificial sources, and NO artificial flavors." But the reformulated Trix cereal looked nothing like the original; its colors had gone from technicolor reds, blues, and yellows to autumnal yellowish and brownish shades. Sales declined. By the end of 2017, General Mills had reinstalled the artificial colors in Trix; in 2021, 15% of its cereals still contained artificial colors.[17]

States force action

But in 2021, California's Environmental Protection Agency assessed studies of the effects of synthetic food dyes on children's behavior. Its conclusion differed from that of the FDA: "The body of evidence from human studies indicates that synthetic food dyes are associated with adverse neurobehavioral outcomes in children, and that children vary in their sensitivity to synthetic food dyes." The report elicited immediate criticism from the International Association of Color Manufacturers, which argued that evidence was insufficient to establish a causal relationship. Nevertheless, in 2023, California banned some commonly used food additives, including Red 3, and 10 other states soon introduced similar legislation.[18]

A year earlier, CSPI had invoked the Delaney amendment to the Food, Drug, and Cosmetic Act in calling on the FDA to revoke authorization for the use of Red 3 (erythrosine) in foods and drugs. The Delaney clause prohibits additives found to induce cancer in humans or animals. Red 3 had been found to cause cancer in male rats under certain circumstances, and in 1990, the FDA had banned it from cosmetics, but not foods. Red 3 is not used in breakfast cereals, but the writing was on the wall. In 2025, the FDA revoked authorization for Red 3 and announced that it would soon take action to phase out the remaining petroleum-based food dyes.[19] Cereal companies would have to respond.

In 2024, General Mills had announced it would stop making Trix, Cocoa Puffs, and Reese's Puffs with artificial colors and flavors by the end of that year. Activists pressed General Mills to act on this commitment. Kellogg made no such commitment, however, bringing on the wrath of investor as well as consumer activists.[20]

In October 2024, California's governor signed a bill banning synthetic food dyes from its public schools (they have until the end of 2027 to comply). West Virginia's governor soon did the same. Other states soon followed. By that time, General Mills was already supplying schools with a version of Trix made without synthetic dyes or flavors. HHS Secretary Kennedy was calling for the voluntary elimination of the dyes within months. A newly formed consumer group, The People's Union, calling General Mills "a symbol of unchecked corporate power," called for a boycott of the company's products, and in 2025 the Texas attorney general launched an investigation into General Mills' promotion of its cereals as healthy when in fact they contained petroleum-based dyes "linked to a host of health issues, including hyperactivity disorders, endocrine disruption, and obesity."[21]

Farewell to artificial colors?

In July 2025, we made supermarket field trips to assess the state of synthetic colors in cereals. Kids' cereals from Kellogg, but also General Mills (e.g., Lucky Charms), Post (Fruity Pebbles), and Quaker (Cap'n Crunch), all contained artificial colors, as did house brands for Walmart (Magic Treasures) and Wegmans (Berry Corn Crunch). But we suspect cereal makers will have to get rid of the dyes soon under pressure from schools, states, and the federal government. Kellogg said "85% of its cereals contain no artificial colors" and it is "removing synthetic colors from those sold in schools."[22] In June 2025, General Mills said it would remove all synthetic food dyes from its cereals sold in schools by summer 2026 and from all of its cereals and other products by the end of 2027. WK Kellogg, two weeks after agreeing to be acquired by candymaker Ferrero, conceded it too would eliminate artificial colors by 2027, which appeared to be a move to help gain federal approval for its sale deal. As one commentator warned the food industry, "When MAHA comes for your rainbow, no brand is safe."[23]

In early January 2026, the Trump administration issued the 2025–2030 *Dietary Guidelines for Americans*, which included a specific admonition to limit highly processed foods with petroleum-based dyes.[24] Despite all this, plenty of artificially colored kids' cereals were still widely available in stores and online. Early in 2026, the retail chain Target delivered another blow. It announced that by the end of May, its nearly 2,000 stores would stop selling cereals with artificial dyes.

While waiting for the Big Four to meet their promises and deal with these threats, you can buy kids' cereals free of artificial colors in health food stores. The organic, whole-grain Cascadian Farm makes its cereals with natural colors and flavors. Can major cereals really eliminate artificial colors? Of course they can. They have done so in Europe, Australia, and New Zealand (see Chapter 17). General Mills has removed them from cereals sold in schools, and that company has owned Cascadian Farm since 2000. It looks to us as though it's not a matter of "if" anymore; it's a matter of "when." And that should be soon.

CHAPTER 6

NUTRIENTS

THE MORE, THE BETTER

ONCE CEREAL MARKETERS figured out how to use sugars, grains, and fiber to encourage sales, they looked for more ways to differentiate and market their products. Nutrients were an obvious strategy. In 1952, Kellogg bragged that each cereal box "tells a story . . . what vitamins and food values it contains, and tells it plainly to an increasingly nutrition-conscious people."[1] By then, companies well understood that nutrients sell cereals.

Breakfast cereals now contain as many as 16 added vitamins and minerals and display banners touting 100% of the Daily Value (DV) for whatever nutrient is trending. In the early 20th century, scientists identified nutrients essential for human nutrition (those our bodies cannot make), the first, vitamin A, in 1913 and the last, vitamin B_{12}, in 1948. They were still discovering the physiological roles of essential trace minerals, those needed in milligram rather than gram amounts, up through the early 1970s.[2]

Adding nutrients to cereals would surely boost sales, but the Food and Drug Administration (FDA) opposed that idea. In this chapter, we discuss how the Big Four convinced the FDA to allow them to add vitamins, minerals, antioxidants, omega-3 fats, protein, and powdered vegetables, of all things, to their best-selling breakfast cereals.

Vitamins and minerals

Almost as soon as each nutrient was discovered, companies began advertising its availability in cereals. Kellogg led the way. In 1933, boxes of All-Bran promoted fiber, vitamin B, and iron: "Iron is necessary for red blood, and vitamin B is necessary for the best intestinal tone." Wheat bran naturally contains these nutrients, but once vitamins were chemically synthesized in the 1930s, they could be cheaply added to cereal. Kellogg again was first; it added "Sunshine Vitamin D and Energy Vitamin B_1" to PEP whole wheat flakes in 1938.[3]

Let's now distinguish between *enrichment*, the restoration of nutrients at levels equivalent to those of the natural, unmilled whole grains, and *fortification*, the addition of nutrients not present in whole grains or added at higher-than-restoration levels. Vitamin B_1 in PEP was enriched (restored); vitamin D was fortified (cereal grains do not naturally have any).

All-Bran boxes in 1938 promoted the cereal as "A good source [as yet undefined] of the important vitamin B_1"—meaning thiamine, which had been synthesized 2 years earlier. All-Bran boasted that its B_1 content was equal to that in bread, twice the level in spinach, and four times the level in lettuce, and it had twice the iron of liver and six times that of spinach.

Cereal companies wanted to add even more nutrients to cereals, and at higher-than-enrichment levels. But they faced a formidable barrier: FDA opposition. The FDA agreed that replacing nutrients lost in grain processing was useful, but it disapproved of "indiscriminate" (scientifically unjustified) nutrient additions purely to sell products. Vitamins are required in small amounts; consuming more does not make healthy people healthier.

The FDA's opposition dated back to 1941, when the US entered World War II, when many men drafted into the military appeared malnourished. Needing to recruit healthy soldiers, President Roosevelt called for nutritional help. At the 1941 National Nutrition Conference for Defense, a milestone in the history of nutrition, a committee set standards for adequate intake of protein, two minerals (iron and calcium), and six vitamins—thiamine (B_1), riboflavin (B_2), niacin (B_3), and vitamins A, C, and D—as the basis for wartime food supplies.[4]

That committee recommended enriching cereals with these nutrients. The FDA agreed and established standards of identity, rules about what a food can and cannot contain, for enriched grain foods, including cereals; these specified enrichment with thiamine, niacin, riboflavin, and iron at restoration levels.[5] Cereal companies happily complied, and this practice appeared successful. By the 1950s, deficiencies of niacin (pellagra) and thiamine (beriberi) had practically disappeared as public health problems.

Under pressure from manufacturers, the FDA reluctantly allowed them to add higher levels of nutrients—but only if they did not market the products as healthier than natural foods. In 1961, General Mills introduced Total cereal, the first to contain eight added vitamins: "One bowl (1 oz) of Total gives you 100% of every minimum daily adult vitamin requirement now officially established." And although the FDA had not yet established minimum DVs for vitamins B_6 and B_{12}, tiny print at the bottom of the box said, "We estimate [Total] will provide 100% of the minimum daily adult needs."

To counter such statements, the FDA began in 1962 to develop proposals to limit fortification to only those nutrients proven to improve overall health. The 1966 proposed rules allowed fortification in only eight categories of foods, breakfast cereals among them. They also allowed cereals to be fortified with the usual four nutrients (thiamine, niacin, riboflavin, and iron) but in slightly higher amounts—up to 10% of their Recommended Daily Allowances.[6]

In addition, the FDA called for restrictions on levels of vitamins and minerals in supplements; the agency viewed nutrient supplements as unnecessary and as being marketed inappropriately (foods are always more complete sources of nutrients). But this action incited an uproar. Almost everyone, not only the food and supplement industries, but also the public health community, strongly opposed restrictions on nutrients. Nutrition surveys conducted in the 1960s had revealed alarming deficiencies in nutrient intake among low-income groups. A 1968 CBS documentary, *Hunger in America*, shocked the nation with its depictions of hungry and malnourished children and adults.[7] These made it appear that Americans needed more nutrients (when what they really needed was more food).

In 1969, President Nixon convened a White House Conference on Food, Nutrition, and Health to address problems of inadequate nutrition. Its industry panel on food manufacturing and processing, which included representatives of General Foods and Kellogg, urged prompt action to block the FDA's fortification restrictions.[8] Such pressures forced the FDA to delay its rulemaking process and gave cereal companies license to add a greater range of nutrients at higher levels.

And then cereal companies got even luckier. Senate hearings in 1970 encouraged them to add more nutrients and to do so immediately. The explicit purpose of those hearings was to promote an increase in the nutrient contribution of breakfast cereals. Their star witness was Robert B. Choate Jr., a wealthy lifelong Republican and "citizen lobbyist" who had developed a personal interest in alleviating poverty and malnutrition. He argued that most breakfast cereals were so heavily sweetened and so deficient in nutrients that their empty calories were no better than those from alcohol or sugar. His message: cereals were ruining the nutritional health of Americans. He called on the FDA, an agency "affected by politics and by a very peculiar morality," to allow manufacturers to fortify their cereals—and to advertise their improved nutritional quality.[9]

Quaker Oats quickly embraced this opportunity and produced King Vitaman cereal (the FDA balked at calling it Vitamin): "Sweet sugary crowns . . . kids love em!" and "The 100% vitamin and iron cereal." General Mills quickly followed in 1969 with circus-themed, vitamin-fortified Kaboom for kids. The cereal industry argued—correctly—that grains have nutritional value, especially when accompanied by milk. But this was the vitamin era, when nutritional health meant vitamins. A follow-up Senate hearing in 1972 celebrated the "improvement" (meaning expansion) in fortification levels. Whereas in 1969, only 16% of cereals were fortified, 80% were fortified by 1972. It only took another year for the Rice Krispies box shown in Figure 10 to boast of its fortification with eight nutrients. By 1979, virtually all cereals were fortified with multiple nutrients of uncertain value for improving health. Following those Senate hearings, supplement supporters convinced Congress to limit the FDA's authority over the amounts of nutrients that could be added to foods, and they forced the agency to back down on its proposed fortification restrictions.[10]

In 1994, Congress passed the Dietary Supplement Health and Education Act (DSHEA), effectively ending the FDA's authority to regulate supplements except in instances of egregious harm, and forcing it to allow more fortification. By 1997, Kellogg could advertise All-Bran as a good source of 16 vitamins and minerals. Effective January 1, 1998, as a means to prevent

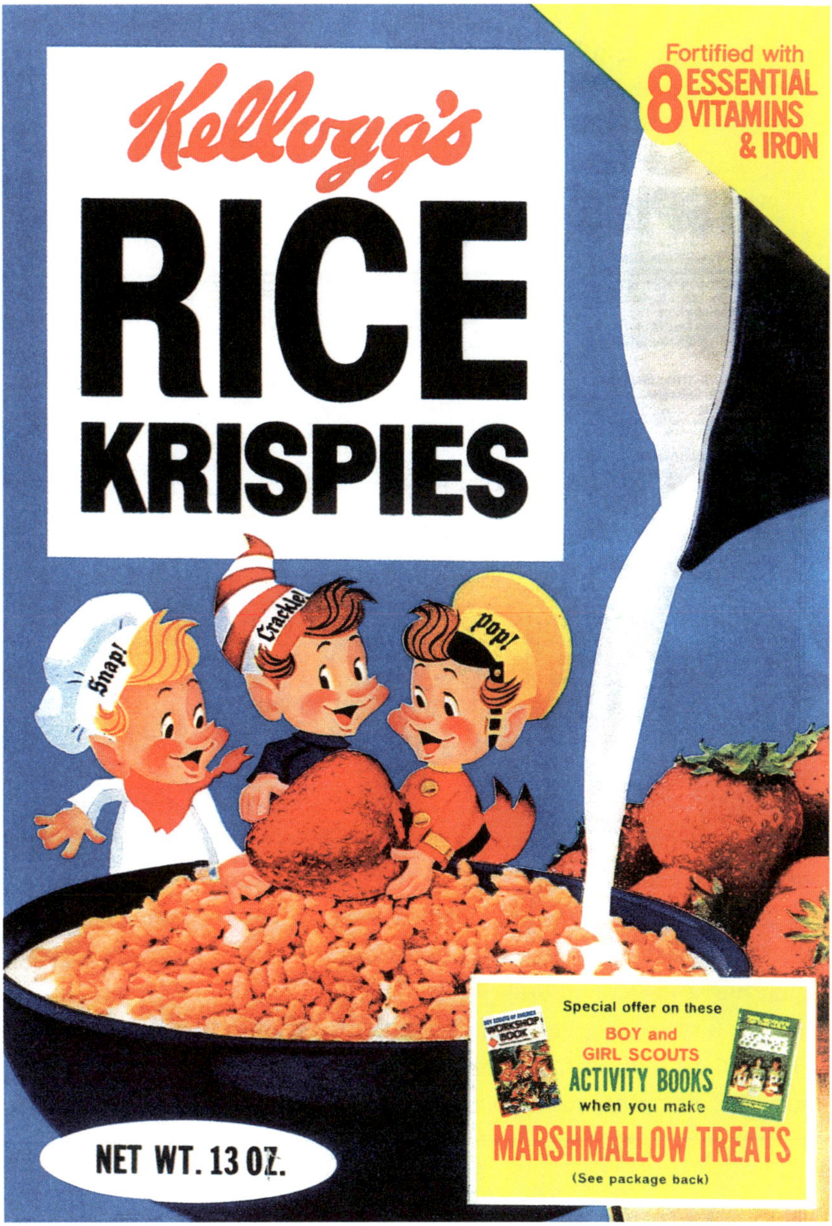

FIGURE 10 This 1973 box of Rice Krispies "Fortified with 8 ESSENTIAL VITAMINS & IRON" celebrates Kellogg's success in overcoming the FDA's long-standing opposition to "indiscriminate" fortification for marketing purposes.

neural tube defects, the FDA required the addition of folic acid to enriched grain products, including cereal.[11]

Today, most breakfast cereals come with long lists of added nutrients at as much as 100% of their DV—the equivalent of a sugar-sweetened one-a-day vitamin pill. Cereal companies claim fortification as an affordable and accessible way to help Americans get more of the nutrients they need or lack. Fortified cereals might make you healthier if you are deficient in nutrients, but *clinical* signs of vitamin deficiencies are remarkably rare among Americans (*deficiencies* are typically considered biochemical indicators below standard).[12]

But the FDA has not given up; it is still trying to regulate fortification. In 2015, the agency advised companies to add nutrients only in order to

- Correct a dietary insufficiency
- Restore nutrient levels to those that existed prior to storage, handling, and processing
- Provide a balance of vitamins, minerals, and protein in proportion to total calories
- Prevent nutrient inferiority in a food that replaces a traditional food in the diet[13]

When the FDA updated the Nutrition Facts label in 2016, it changed serving-size standards to reflect what people might actually eat. The standard breakfast cereal portion increased from 30 to 40 grams for lighter cereals (e.g., Cheerios) and from 55 to 60 grams for the heavier ones (Raisin Nut Bran). This change gave cereal companies the chance to reassess fortification levels, and General Mills doubled its fortification of vitamin D.[14]

As we discuss in later chapters, the FDA continues to discourage companies from adding nutrients for the purpose of making health or nutrient-content claims. But the companies continue to fortify their cereals to the extent they can get away with.

Antioxidants

Eating plant foods is good for health, and scientists would love to be able to pin the health-promoting qualities of plants on their specific components. Plants make hundreds of phytochemicals, many of them antioxidants able to neutralize the effects of oxygen-induced free-radical toxins in the body. Some antioxidants are essential nutrients: vitamins A, C, and E and beta-carotene, a precursor of vitamin A.[15]

Antioxidants are widely touted for their ability to slow the effects of aging, prevent heart disease and cancer, improve vision, promote immunity, and more. Most studies of antioxidants use supplements rather than foods, and early research appeared to confirm such benefits. But when scientists conducted more carefully controlled clinical trials, the results not only showed no benefit, but suggested that antioxidant supplements might actually increase the risk of heart disease or cancer.[16]

Nevertheless, antioxidants retain their health aura. The logic: plant foods are healthy; plant foods have antioxidants; therefore, antioxidants are healthy; therefore, adding antioxidants to cereals makes them healthier. According to FDA regulations, advertising antioxidant nutrients in a food constitutes a *nutrient content* claim, permissible if the nutrients have an established DV, which vitamins do. In the Smart Start cereal shown in Figure 11, Kellogg is not claiming a direct health benefit of antioxidants; it is making a "supports immunity" claim authorized by the 1994 DSHEA. Later, Kellogg had to abandon this claim due to the 2010 legal decisions we discuss in Chapter 9. Never mind. The antioxidant health halo works for marketing. Antioxidants were named a top-10 trend in 2013.[17]

For the record, that 2006 box of Smart Start has 10% of the DV for beta-carotene, 25% for vitamins A and C, and 100% for vitamin E. It also contains 14 grams of sugars per serving. Sugar appears third in the ingredient list (after rice and whole grain wheat), no doubt because sugars of one kind or another appear nine more times on the list.

Because of the sugars, Fooducate, a website that evaluates foods based on their nutritional content, gives Smart Start a D+ grade, ranking it as "one of the worst products in its category." The "Food Babe" Vani Hari, a food industry critic, questioned how Kellogg could get away with advertising the antioxidants in Smart Start. She called the company to confirm that the cereal "only contains a measly 180 micrograms of beta carotene . . . per serving. Way less than what's in one baby carrot!"[18] Late in 2024, this cereal was still available, but with just 10% of the DV for vitamins A, C, and E, along with 18 grams of sugars per serving—probably not the smartest start.

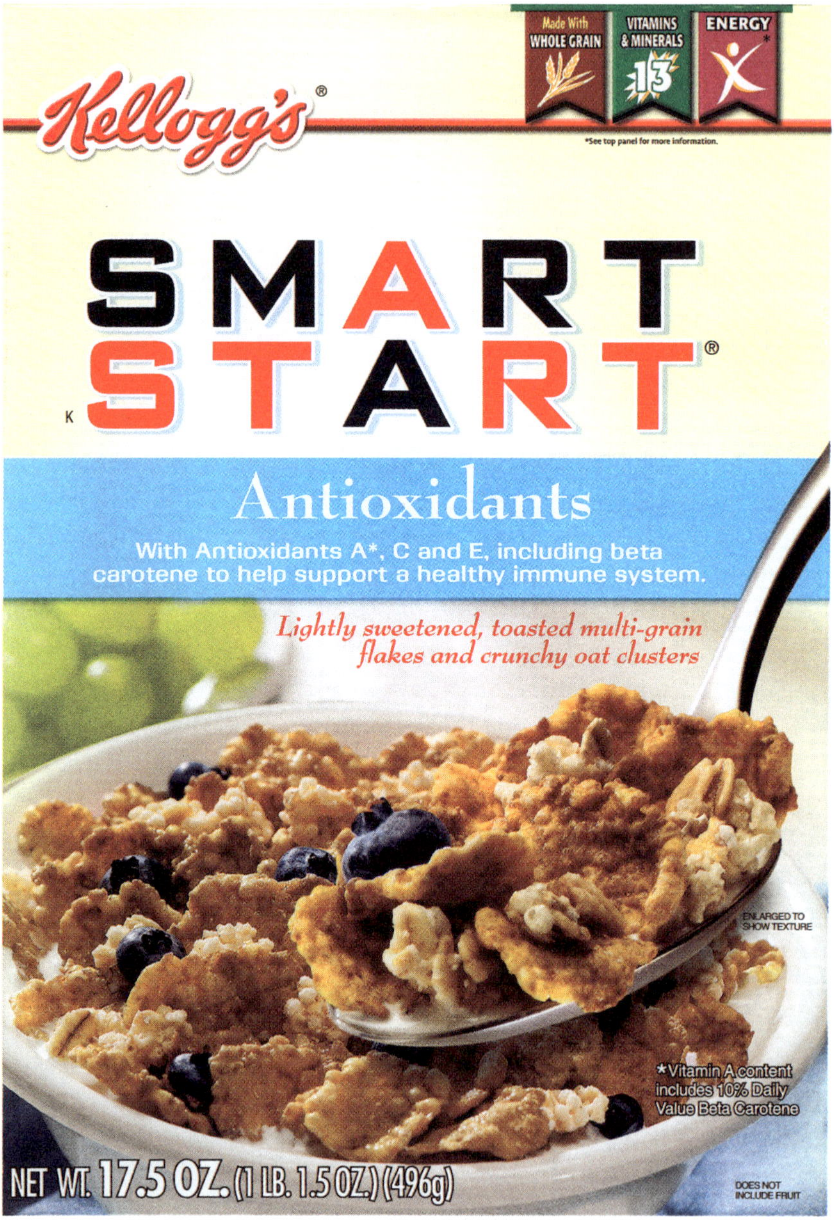

FIGURE 11 This 2006 box of Kellogg's Smart Start "Lightly sweetened, toasted multi-grain flakes and crunchy oat clusters" sports a banner proclaiming its content of "Antioxidants A, C & E, including beta carotene to help support a healthy immune system"—a structure/function claim authorized by an act of Congress.

If you want antioxidants, vegetables are much better sources; one baby carrot offers more than 600 micrograms of beta-carotene.

Something fishy: Omega-3s

Omega-3 fatty acids have been linked to heart health, improved cognitive function, eye health, and infant development. For adults, they first gained popularity in the 1970s when a study revealed low rates of heart disease among the Greenland Inuit.[19] Fish and supplements are the most frequent sources, but you can also find omega-3s in—surprise!—breakfast cereals.

Omega-3 refers to a chemical position in essential polyunsaturated fatty acids. These include ALA (alpha-linolenic acid), which is found in leafy greens and other plants; a longer-chain fatty acid called EPA (eicosapentaenoic acid), found in fatty fish, like salmon, mackerel, and sardines; and long-chain DHA (docosahexaenoic acid), also found in fatty fish. ALA is considered *essential* because we need it, but our bodies can't make it. Once eaten, ALA can be converted to EPA and DHA in the body, but the process is not very efficient. That is why health authorities recommend fish as a source of already synthesized EPA and DHA.[20]

As omega-3s became trendy, cereal companies jumped right in. General Mills launched Total Plus Omega-3s cereal, which "offers all the benefits of Total, plus the benefits of omega-3 fatty acids."[21] But no one wants fishy-tasting cereal, so where did the omega-3 come from? If you followed the asterisks on the "plus+ Omega 3**" banner, you got to microscopic text: "Contains 160 mg ALA from ground flax, which is 10% of the Daily Value for ALA (1.6 mg)." Flaxseed is a rich source of ALA, but not of EPA or DHA.

Kellogg's Raisin Bran Omega-3 followed in 2013: "250 mg ALA from flaxseed." Its small print said "Delicious raisins blended with crisp bran flakes, flaxseeds and a touch of sweetness." That "touch" is 17 grams of sugar, some from the raisins. The back of the box says, in large letters, "Great taste," and in smaller letters it says "Does your heart good." It also provides a puzzle for "Your mental morning stretch"—a plug for the proposed role of omega-3s in cognitive health. Omega-3s must not have sold much cereal. We now only see omega-3 brands occasionally in health food stores.

Protein

Foods have only four sources of calories: fat, carbohydrate, protein, and alcohol (not, to our knowledge, found in cereals). Because many people try to avoid eating too much fat or carbohydrate, only protein remains as a marketing tool. Protein works splendidly for marketing cereals as well as other foods; it has an aura of fitness and health. Surveys report widespread beliefs that high-protein cereals are more nutritious, help prevent age- or diet-related muscle loss, and promote strength, vitality, and longevity.[22]

In 2014, protein was the nutrient of the year, and it has remained a hot trend. Unlike advice to eat less fat, carbohydrate, or calories, the advice for protein is to eat more. When more than 70% of consumers said they wanted more protein in their diets, food companies rose to the challenge. General Mills launched a series of protein-boosted products, including the Cheerios Protein shown in Figure 12. The company's CEO admitted, "Americans don't need more protein in their diet. It is the newest approach to weight management" (but see Figure 15 in Chapter 8).[23]

Really? Cereal grains are already reasonable sources, 7% to 12% protein by weight. Diets based on wheat, rice, or corn supported the protein needs of entire civilizations. Grains do tend to be low in one or another essential amino acid, particularly lysine, but this problem is easily overcome by eating various kinds of grains or beans or some animal-based food.

Americans typically get more than enough protein, about twice as much as needed. The protein requirement for anyone other than an elite athlete is less than 1 gram per kilogram of body weight, meaning a 55-kilogram (120-pound) woman gets more than enough with 55 grams. Most people consume about 40 grams protein per 1,000 calories.[24] If you eat 2,500 calories a day, you are likely to be consuming 100 grams of protein, way more than needed. Hardly anyone needs to be concerned about getting enough protein.

But many people are concerned, and some researchers, and websites, urge you to eat a lot more. Healthline.com, for example, says eating more protein makes you feel full longer, increases muscle mass, helps you lose weight, reduces hunger cravings, and lowers your blood pressure, among other benefits. We are not convinced by the existing evidence. Nevertheless, the 2025–2030 *Dietary Guidelines for Americans* say to "Prioritize Protein Foods at Every Meal," with an emphasis on animal rather than plant sources.

The guidelines recommend reducing refined grains but position whole grains in the "eat less" part of the accompanying food guide, an inverted pyramid.[25]

As for protein excess, that too may not be as harmful as is sometimes claimed, but it is rarely helpful.[26] The Cheerios Protein shown in Figure 12 promotes 11 grams of protein per serving; "with milk" is in small print. The cereal itself got to 7 grams of protein per serving by adding soy protein isolate, almonds, soy flour, and wheat flour to its basic oats and corn. The rest came from the added milk.

But for consumer watchdogs, the advertised total protein count was a red flag. Lawyers for the Center for Science in the Public Interest (CSPI) and some private firms sued General Mills for false advertising and marketing. They argued that because 4 of the 11 grams of protein came from milk, the difference between the 3 grams of protein in regular Cheerios and the 7 grams in Cheerios Protein (minus the milk) was misleading. Oh, and most of the difference could be attributed to the difference in serving sizes. Regular Cheerios used a 28-gram serving size, whereas Cheerios Protein used 55 grams. Two ounces of each cereal had almost the same amount of protein.

The biggest difference between the two cereals, however, was sugar. A serving of Cheerios Protein Cinnamon & Almond had 16 grams of sugars compared with the 2 grams in original Cheerios. Cheerios Protein Oats & Honey had 21 grams of sugars (these appeared in eight places on the ingredient list). A weight-loss strategy? We don't think so. CSPI's director, Michael Jacobson, said, "A serving of Cheerios Protein, with its four teaspoons of sugar, has much more sugar than a typical cereal marketed to kids, such as Trix or Frosted Flakes. . . . They really ought to call the product Cheerios Sugar." The case dragged on for 3 years but finally settled in 2018 when General Mills agreed to stop including the protein from milk in the total protein count and to state the sugars more prominently.[27]

But cereal companies, as we keep pointing out, never give up. A decade later, in 2024, General Mills tried again, this time in partnership with Ghost, a maker of supplements and protein products, to issue Ghost Protein Cereal in marshmallow and peanut butter versions (17 and 18 grams of protein, respectively). A spokesperson for General Mills said, "It's no secret that consumers are looking for more protein choices these days, and the GHOST team has a reputation for the performance nutrition space with

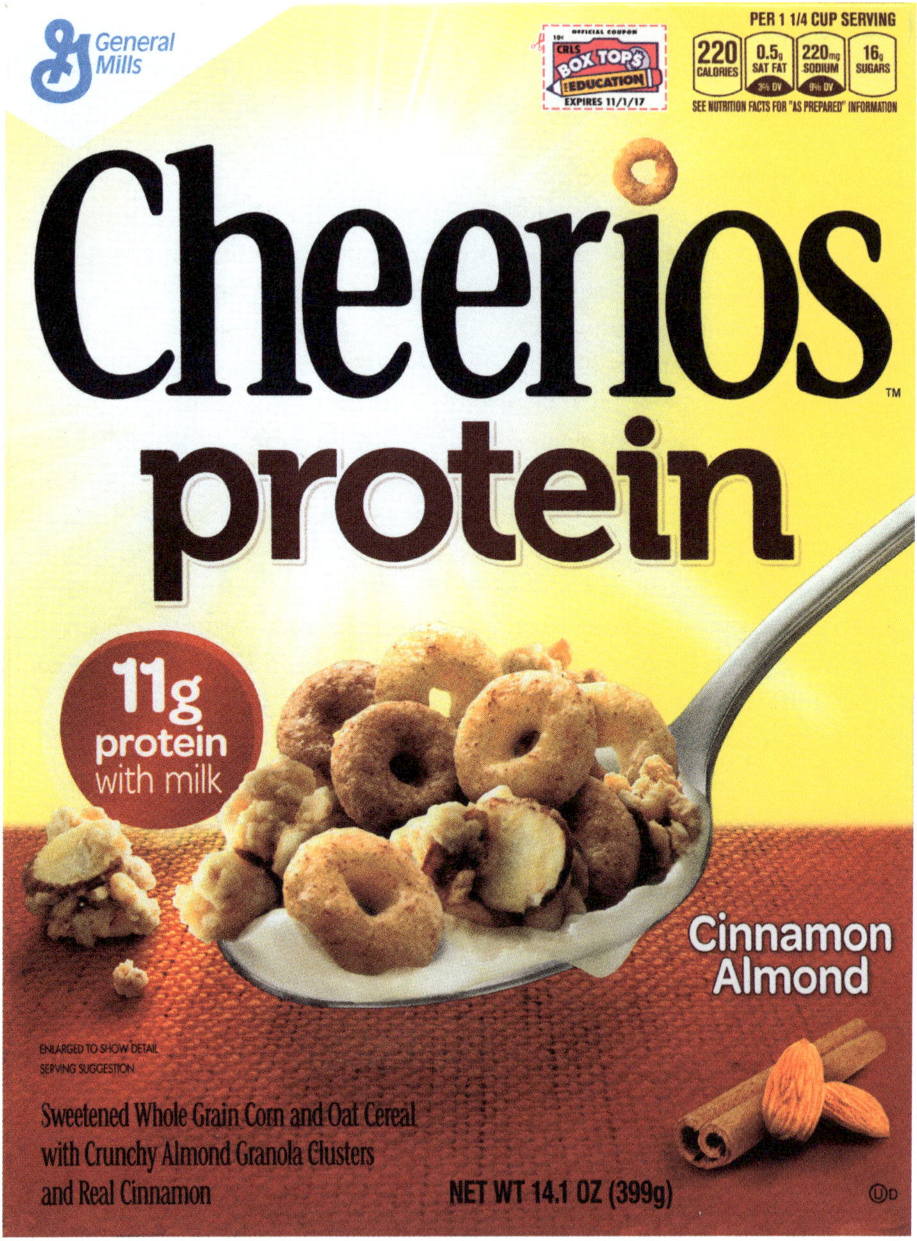

FIGURE 12 General Mills introduced Cheerios Protein Cinnamon Almond in 2014 with "11 g protein with milk" per serving compared with 3 grams in regular Cheerios. Litigation challenged that protein claim, since 4 of those grams came from added milk.

flavors that go beyond the basic chocolate or vanilla." The company hoped that customers would choose protein cereals as snacks.

Also in 2024, General Mills introduced Wheaties Protein, with 21 grams of protein per serving, boosted with vital wheat gluten and soy protein isolate (yum).[28] In 2025, the company launched our favorite example: Cookies & Crème Cheerios Protein (8 grams): a "sweetened oat and pea protein cereal." It adds 11 grams of a combination of sugar (ingredient #2) and corn syrup (#4) to sweeten your pea protein.

Kellogg, not to be outdone, released Eat Your Mouth Off "100% plant based" cereal, aimed at Gen Z (born between 1997 and 2012); it has 22 grams of protein from soy and pea protein isolates and smaller amounts of lentil protein. Kellogg also offers Special K with 13 grams of protein, 6 from milk and 7 from the cereal; the boost is from wheat gluten. This is disclosed in small print, which must be enough to discourage CSPI from suing.

But if you really want protein, go to health food stores. The Happier Grocery on Canal Street in Manhattan did not sell Big Four cereals when we visited in 2025 but instead offered Promix Chocolate Whey Isolate Protein Puffs with 10 grams of whey protein per scoop—at $23.00 for just over 14 ounces (this for isolated whey protein). The store also offered Magic Spoon high-protein (14 grams, also whey-based), no-sugar, artificially sweetened cereal for kids: "as much protein as 10 eggs and fewer net carbs than a typical fruit smoothie, but it's so much more fun to eat." It cost $9 per box (Big Four cereals were about $5 at the time).

What strikes us about trying to use anything other than milk to boost the protein in breakfast cereals is that almost all the ways to do it—isolated soy protein, pea protein, whey protein, or wheat gluten—require sugars or artificial sweeteners to mask the off-tastes. These turn cereals into concoctions of ingredients, as ultra-processed as can be. We prefer food.

Vegetables (sort of)

Early in 2024, we bought a box of General Mills' Cheerios Veggie Blends, intrigued by its claim to contain a quarter cup of "fruit & veggies" and by images of fruit, sweet potato, and carrot on the box, implying loads of nutrients. As previously noted, Cheerios, that old, reliable, and reasonably healthy cereal (4 grams fiber and only 2 grams sugar per serving), now comes in more than 20 options. Veggie Blends (Blueberry Banana or Apple Strawberry) takes advantage of plant-forward diet trends; we doubt this is what proponents of plant-based diets have in mind. Although it is marketed as a way to sneak vegetables into diets, especially for kids, we view this product as particularly misleading.[29]

Consider its fiber. Veggie Blends has only 2 grams of fiber per serving and 8 grams of sugars. Surely, adding a quarter cup of "fruit & veggies" should increase, not decrease, the fiber? This required research. We went first to the Walmart website: "Available exclusively at Walmart, a wholesome bowl of Blueberry Banana flavored Cheerios Blends Cereal contains ¼ cup of fruit and veggies in every serving.*" Uh-oh, an asterisk: "*Cheerios Blends Cereal is made with fruit puree and vegetable powder. . . . It is not intended to replace fruit or vegetables in the diet." OK, but take a look at the ingredient list (our emphasis):

> Whole Grain Oats, Corn Meal, Sugar, **Sweet Potato Powder**, Corn Starch, **Carrot Powder**, Canola and/or Sunflower Oil, **Banana Puree**, **Blueberry Puree Concentrate**, Corn Syrup, Salt, **Spinach Powder**, Vegetable and Fruit Juice Color, Tripotassium Phosphate, Natural Flavor. Vitamin E (mixed tocopherols) Added to Preserve Freshness [vitamins and minerals omitted].

The powders explain the lack of fiber. The concentrates explain the increased sugars. Our advice: if you want the vitamins and minerals in fruits and vegetables, eat fruits and vegetables. If you want Cheerios, we suggest the far less interesting original version.

PART II

CLAIMS

CHAPTER 7

OVERCOMING THE CLAIMS BARRIER

CANCER AND HEART DISEASE

HEALTH CLAIMS are statements or direct implications that a particular food can prevent, mitigate, treat, or cure a condition or disease or can promote a health benefit. Because breakfast cereals were an integral part of early 20th-century health food movements, they were marketed with what the Food and Drug Administration (FDA) defines as a health claim right from the start. When Kellogg introduced Bran Cereal (now All-Bran) in 1919, the box said "Eat it daily—in extreme cases eat it with every meal . . . [as] an easy way to avoid constipation."

But in 1938, Congress passed the Food, Drug, and Cosmetic Act, which, among other things, prohibited health claims on food labels to protect the public from misbranded and adulterated products. The FDA considered any statement of a food's ability to prevent, mitigate, treat, or cure disease to be equivalent to a drug claim. Drugs had to be proven safe and effective through controlled clinical trials, not easily done for foods. While the act might prevent harmful claims, food companies complained it kept them from informing the public about their products' benefits. For decades, food companies pressed the FDA to allow health claims, but the agency consistently refused.[1] In 1984, this would all change, prompted by none other than Kellogg.

Kellogg did an end run around the FDA's restrictions when it partnered with the National Cancer Institute (NCI) to promote the role of fiber in cancer prevention, thereby opening the door to health claims on food packages. Knowing the marketing potential of health claims, Kellogg wanted to use them to promote its high-fiber cereals, which research was increasingly linking to protection against bowel cancer. In the early 1980s, the company approached the NCI to propose a partnership to develop statements about the benefits of fiber. NCI officials enthusiastically welcomed the Kellogg campaign, viewing the offer as "infusing millions of dollars of private sector funds into the promotion of cancer prevention messages."[2]

The result appeared in supermarket cereal aisles in 1984. All-Bran boxes displayed a large yellow banner with "MAXIMUM FIBER" in bright red letters. The side panel said "ALL-BRAN HAS 9 GRAMS FIBER PER SERVING," also in red letters. Kellogg used the entire back panel of the box to describe the partnership: "The National Cancer Institute believes eating the right foods may reduce your risk of cancer. Here are their recommendations: Eat high fiber foods. A growing body of evidence says high fiber foods are important to good health. That's why a healthy diet includes high fiber foods like bran cereals." With such statements, the NCI appeared to be endorsing a fiber-related health claim (and All-Bran), but a Kellogg official denied it: "We are saying the message is not a health claim. The message is from the National Cancer Institute, and we are simply printing it."[3]

The NCI, like the FDA, is an agency within the Department of Health and Human Services. But Kellogg's partnership with the NCI had not involved the FDA, and it caught that agency by surprise: the "FDA was never consulted, nor . . . did Kellogg ever suggest to NCI that there might be any FDA concern about the matter . . . incredible as it may be . . . it never occurred [to NCI] that there were any regulatory implications of putting what they considered to be a perfectly reasonable public health education message on cereal boxes."[4]

FDA staff realized that the All-Bran statement had undermined their ability to regulate health claims; they would no longer be able to stop companies from using claims in marketing. But Kellogg insisted it had done the country a public service: it would be irresponsible *not* to inform customers about the health benefits of its products. When an FDA analysis demonstrated a 47% increase in the market share of All-Bran within the first 6 months of the campaign, the message was clear: claims sell cereal.[5] Kellogg had broken the health claims barrier. All it had left to do was to get Congress to legitimize this victory over regulators.

Making health claims legal

Kellogg's success with NCI and All-Bran was only its first step in forcing the FDA to permit health claims on cereals. In 1985, Kellogg filed a citizen petition asking the FDA to back off on its opposition to health claims. This document, astonishing for its length (more than 500 pages) as well as for its deeply researched review of the science on diet and health, the history of cereals and the company, the past and current nutritional status of Americans, and dietary advice from expert committees, also provided a tightly argued legal analysis of the FDA's regulatory authority. It provided a basis for congressional approval of health claims by its thorough review of evidence linking components of oats—the bran, soluble fiber, and beta-glucan (a type of soluble fiber)—to reduced blood cholesterol levels. Kellogg proposed the precise wording of guidelines it wanted the FDA to use to regulate health claims, and it backed these statements and proposals with more than 50 pages of scientific references.[6]

The Kellogg petition particularly argued against the FDA's 1973 fortification regulations, which deemed a product misbranded if it claimed to prevent, cure, mitigate, or treat a condition. The petition expressed disappointment that although the FDA had held hearings on this restriction in 1978, its position was unchanged. Change, Kellogg argued, was imperative. The FDA should allow statements from scientific experts that were truthful and not misleading; otherwise, the agency was denying consumers information they could use to improve their health.

Most of Kellogg's arguments seemed well reasoned, if self-serving, but the petition also contained an overt threat: do this—or else. The threat invoked the First Amendment: "The First Amendment imposes substantial limitations upon the FDA's authority to regulate health claims on food labels and advertising. . . . The FDA would, therefore, be well advised to (a) issue a general policy statement . . . that alleviate[s] its most blatant speech-restricting characteristics, and (b) do so by an administrative method that has the least possible chilling effect on speech" (pp. 2–48).

This was the first time we had seen this argument, which paved the way for what is now a common food industry strategy. The FDA got the message loud and clear. It had three choices: continue to deny health claims (not feasible given the NCI ploy, Kellogg's petition, and mounting food industry pressures); allow claims but with tight restrictions (also unlikely given the Reagan administration's deregulatory agenda); or set scientific guidelines for claims that companies would have to follow. It adopted the last one.

In 1987, the FDA began writing "cautious and deliberate" proposals for the level of scientific substantiation required for health claims. It attempted to strike a balance, but it failed. Food companies viewed the proposals as too restrictive, but consumer groups thought they would confuse the public, reduce the credibility of food labels, and be unenforceable by this under-resourced agency.[7]

The FDA's rulemaking process is always slow, but this one was prolonged at the highest levels. Under pressure from food companies, the Reagan administration delayed publication of the FDA's revised proposals twice in 3 years. The delays opened up a free-for-all period of nonregulation in which companies could label their packages with impunity. By 1988, 40% of all new food products displayed health messages of one kind or another.[8] Figure 13 shows one outlandish example: Kellogg's Frosted Flakes.

States take action

With the FDA bogged down in rulemaking, several states filed lawsuits against companies using misleading claims. The companies settled most cases by agreeing to remove the claims and pay court costs. Iowa, for example, sued Kellogg in 1988 for marketing the protein in Special K to dieters as a means to avoid muscle loss, and the fiber and iron in 40+ Bran Flakes to help people over age 40 be healthier.

The side panel on Kellogg's 1988 Frosted Flakes box said, "Just one serving contains more of vitamin A and many B vitamins than two eggs or one serving of granola. . . . one serving has less sugar than many of your favorite fruits: a banana, an orange, an apple, or half a cantaloupe. . . . Frosted Flakes really are a Gr-r-reat way to start your day." It emphasized "less sugar" and "no more calories" in bold red text. Litigation followed.

A Texas official participating in the Frosted Flakes lawsuit said of those statements, "I consider that a lie. It's 40 percent sugar." Kellogg retaliated

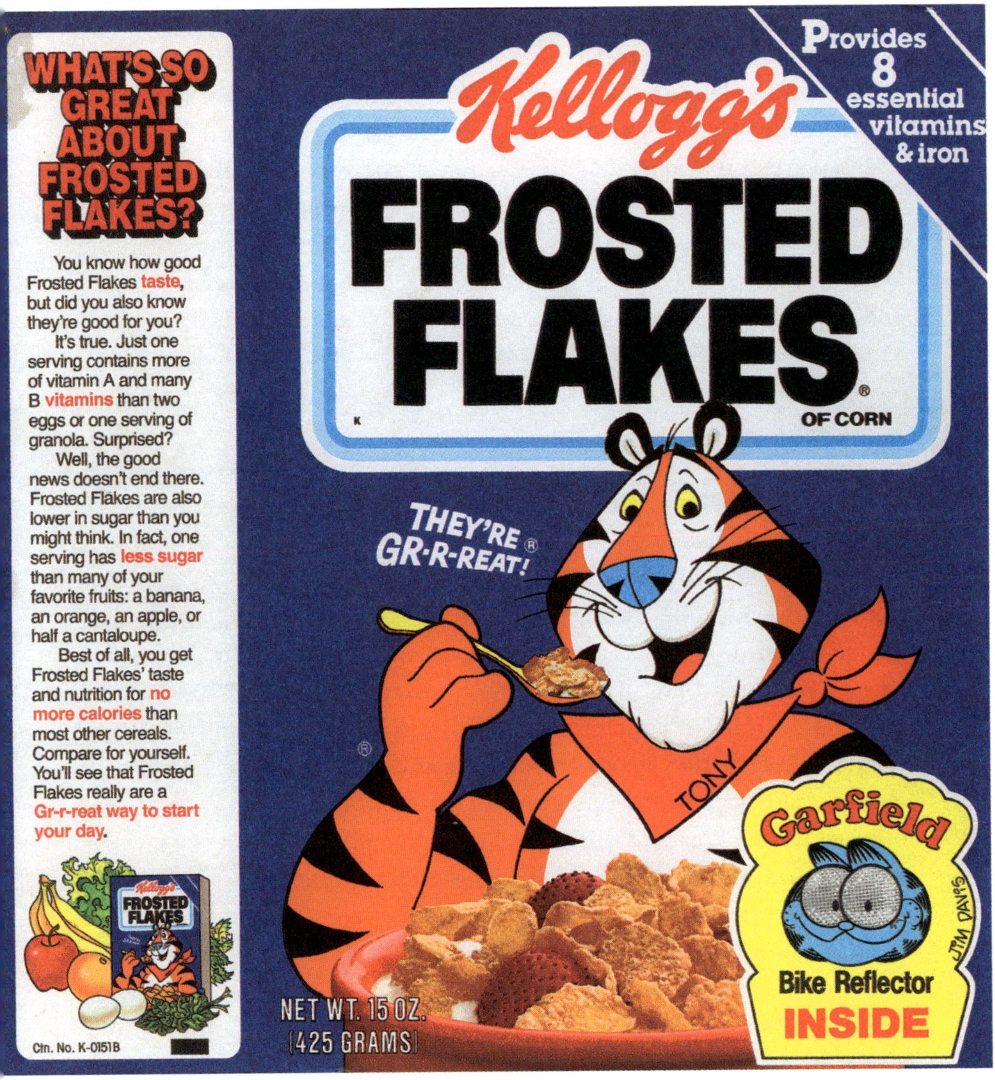
WHAT'S SO GREAT ABOUT FROSTED FLAKES?
You know how good Frosted Flakes taste, but did you also know they're good for you?
It's true. Just one serving contains more of vitamin A and many B vitamins than two eggs or one serving of granola. Surprised?
Well, the good news doesn't end there. Frosted Flakes are also lower in sugar than you might think. In fact, one serving has less sugar than many of your favorite fruits: a banana, an orange, an apple, or half a cantaloupe.
Best of all, you get Frosted Flakes' taste and nutrition for no more calories than most other cereals. Compare for yourself. You'll see that Frosted Flakes really are a Gr-r-reat way to start your day.
Ctn. No. K-0151B
Kellogg's
FROSTED FLAKES
OF CORN
Provides 8 essential vitamins & iron
THEY'RE GR-R-REAT!
TONY
Garfield
JIM DAVIS
Bike Reflector
INSIDE
NET WT. 15 OZ.
(425 GRAMS)

FIGURE 13 While the FDA was working on regulations for health claims, companies took the risk and started using them. The side panel of this 1988 Kellogg's box claimed Frosted Flakes were more nutritious than eggs or fruit. Consumer advocates argued otherwise.

by suing that official for slander. It also asked the court to prohibit the Iowa attorney general's office from interfering with its advertising, saying this was the Federal Trade Commission's jurisdiction. Eventually, Kellogg settled out of court with Iowa and five other states, agreeing to remove or significantly modify claims on its cereals; it paid each state a modest settlement fee of $30,000.[9] Kellogg's revenues were $5.7 billion that year.

Finally, in 1990, the health claims issues got resolved, although in the most politically messy way. The White House lifted its block and allowed the FDA to propose rules for health claims again. But 3 months later, the White House reversed course and once more held up the proposals, ostensibly because its Office of Management and Budget favored the rights of states to make their own food-labeling laws.[10]

The Nutrition Labeling and Education Act of 1990

As if these events were not confusing enough, Congress preempted everything the FDA had been doing by passing the Nutrition Labeling and Education Act (NLEA).[11] Although the act's primary purpose was to put uniform nutrition information on food labels, it also dealt with health claims. In wording remarkably—and surely not coincidentally—similar to that of Kellogg's 1985 petition, the act *required* the FDA to authorize health and nutrient content claims for both foods and supplements. It further directed the agency to consider authorizing ten specific health claims, among them three relevant to cereals: fiber and coronary heart disease (CHD), fiber and cancer, and saturated fat and CHD. The law left it to the FDA to decide how much science was required to support the use of those claims for specific foods.

At that point, the FDA had to scrap what it had been doing about health claim regulation and switch to writing regulations to implement the NLEA. In 1991, it issued preliminary proposals for definitions, portion sizes, and health claims for packaged foods. But later that year, President Bush called for a moratorium on all pending regulations that might adversely affect industry, including rules for labels and health claims. The following year, the FDA agreed to some concessions and revised its proposed rules to make them more acceptable to industry.[12]

Finally, on January 6, 1993, the FDA published the NLEA implementation rules as an 875-page *Federal Register* notice. The rules authorized health claims based on FDA-defined scientific criteria, which the food industry still viewed as too restrictive. In FDA-speak, health claims would have to be supported by "the totality of publicly available scientific evidence (including evidence from well-designed studies conducted in a manner which is consistent with generally recognized scientific procedures and principles), that there is significant agreement among experts qualified by scientific training and experience to evaluate such claims, that the claim is supported by such evidence."[13] The FDA said seven claims met these criteria, including the three relevant to cereals. It invited companies to petition for further claims. Fifty-five years after the 1938 act, food companies had won the right to make health claims.

Subsequent legislation

In 1994, Congress passed the Dietary Supplement Health and Education Act (DSHEA), which essentially deregulated vitamin, mineral, and herbal supplements by ending much of the FDA's authority over them. If the FDA had a problem with a supplement claim, it would have to take the manufacturer to court. DSHEA further introduced a new class of claims called structure/function claims. These could not refer to a disease or condition, but they could say that a supplement—but not a food or ingredient—supported or maintained some structure or function of the body. Manufacturers could say that calcium "maintains strong bones" but not that it "reduces the risk of osteoporosis," hardly a real distinction in our view.

Food manufacturers argued that they also should be permitted to use structure/function claims. When the FDA objected, the companies sued—and usually won. By 2003 the FDA gave up fighting those cases. As one official put it, "We have lost 8 of 10 First Amendment decisions, and doing business the way we were doing it was unsustainable."[14]

Then came the FDA Modernization Act of 1997 (FDAMA). Although its main purpose was to speed up approvals for drugs and devices, one of its provisions required the FDA to authorize nutrient content and health claims even if they did not meet rigorous scientific standards. Claims no longer needed to be based on the totality of evidence or significant scientific agreement, but only had to be supported by a report from a government committee or the National Academy of Sciences. It was FDAMA that gave the FDA 120 days to deal with petitions for health claims; if the agency missed the deadline, the claim would automatically be authorized.[15] That did it. The FDA began authorizing claims.

Today, congressional acts have authorized three distinct categories of claims that breakfast cereals reduce disease risk:[16]

1. Health claims (1990 NLEA): fiber and coronary heart disease (CHD); fiber-containing grains and cancer; lower saturated fat and cholesterol and CHD; calcium and osteoporosis (approved for foods in 1996)
2. Nutrient content claims (1990 NLEA)
3. Structure/function claims (1994 DSHEA)

In addition, the FDA has authorized three cereal claims in response to industry petitions:

- Soluble fiber from whole oats and reduced risk of CHD (Quaker Oats, 1997)
- Soluble fiber from psyllium seed husks and reduced risk of CHD (Kellogg, 1998)
- Whole-grain foods and reduced risk of CHD and cancer (General Mills, 1999)

Did Kellogg's enormous investment in fighting the FDA on health claims pay off? Yes, practically all cereals now promote nutritional or health benefits, allowing marketers to offset concerns about sugar, artificial colors and flavors, or low fiber content. But Kellogg's actions had a social cost. Ending the FDA's ability to hold claims to high scientific standards created a food-marketing environment loaded with claims for benefits that cannot rationally be attributed to any single food, let alone to a sugary breakfast cereal. Health claims, we insist, are about marketing, not health.

We discuss nutrient content claims and other specific health claims in subsequent chapters. But for now, let's take a look at the classic example of a health claim: cereals and heart health.

Heart health claims

Coronary heart disease (CHD) is the most serious form of cardiovascular disease and the leading cause of death among older Americans.[17] It is caused by the buildup of arterial plaque formed from deposits of cholesterol, fats, and other substances that restrict blood flow. Diets rich in grain fiber but low in saturated fat and cholesterol have long been associated with protection against CHD, and companies have long attempted to market their cereals as heart-healthy. When the 1990 NLEA required the FDA to set conditions for the use of heart-health claims for low-fat or high-fiber foods, the FDA's rules said nothing about sugar. As shown in Figure 14, this omission allowed Post to promote Raisin Bran as heart-healthy despite having 19 grams (nearly 4 teaspoons) of sugars in a 1 cup serving.

Heart-healthy: Low in fats

The history of heart-health claims dates back to the 1950s when Dr. Ancel Keys, a University of Minnesota physiologist, first proposed the diet-heart hypothesis linking dietary cholesterol and saturated fat to increased CHD risk.[18] Margarine companies immediately began to advertise their plant-based fats as a way to reduce intake of both. In 1959, the FDA told the margarine companies they were making illegal drug claims.

But Nabisco ignored this threat. In 1964, the back of its Shredded Wheat boxes proclaimed, "Medical studies would indicate a decrease in the occurrence of heart disease when vegetable fats replace animal fats in the diet," implying that a bowl of this cereal could reduce intake of animal fat (presumably by replacing bacon and eggs).[19] The FDA seized all of the offending boxes. Later, from 1985 to 1993, Rice Krispies boxes said "Fat free, cholesterol free food"—a nutrient content claim. Because it said nothing about reducing CHD, the FDA did not object. Such claims can imply a health benefit but cannot state it explicitly.

Once forced to authorize health claims, the FDA allowed one that linked reduced saturated fat and cholesterol to reduced CHD risk.[20] Eligible foods had to contain no more than 3 grams of fat, 1 gram of saturated fat, and 20 milligrams of cholesterol per serving. This was great news for cereals; grains never contain cholesterol and are naturally low in fat. All companies

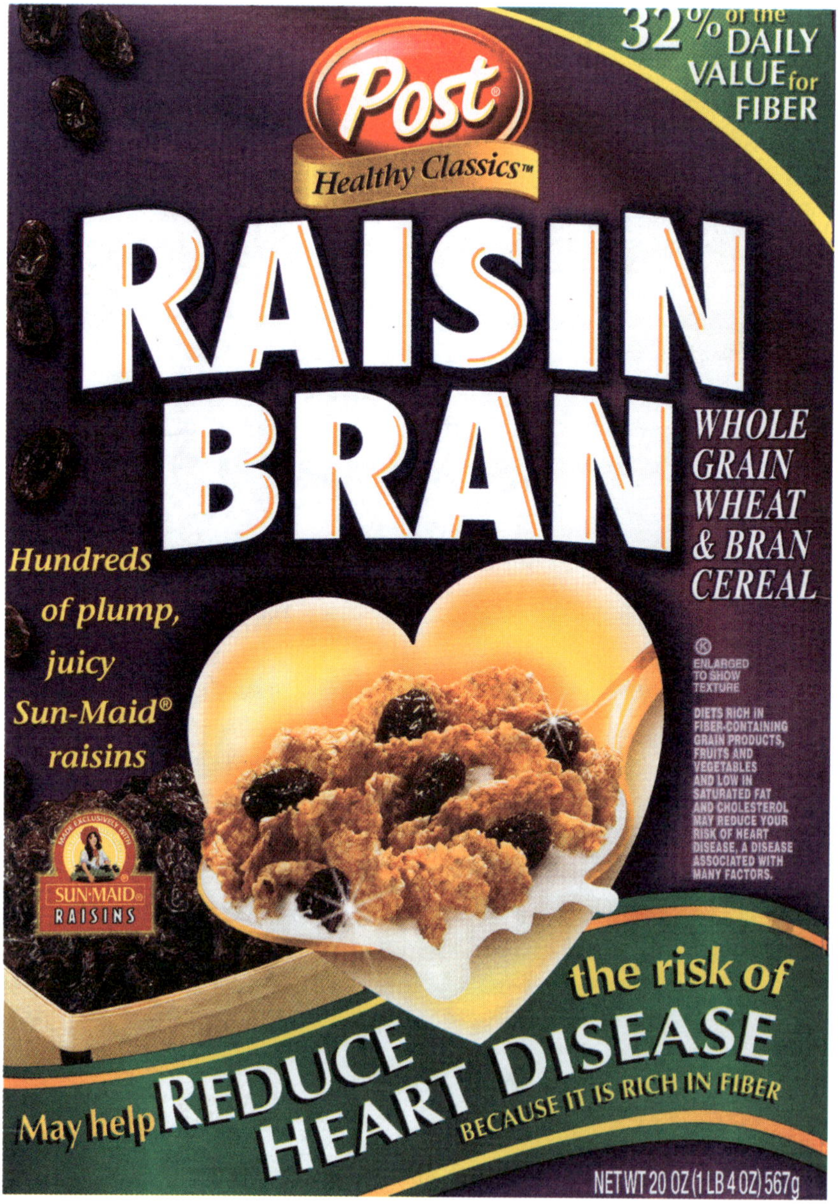

FIGURE 14 Post marketed this 2003 box of Raisin Bran as "May help REDUCE the risk of HEART DISEASE BECAUSE IT IS RICH IN FIBER." The low-fat diet disclaimer above the banner is almost illegible.

had to do was add a disclaimer: "While many factors affect heart disease, a diet low in saturated fat and cholesterol may reduce the risk of this disease."

Heart-healthy: Fiber-rich grains

Cereal grain-fiber claims also date to the 1990 NLEA (other fiber claims came later via petitions). This claim was supported by evidence that people with low blood cholesterol—who also consumed diets high in fruits, vegetables, and grains—had reduced their risk of CHD. The FDA agreed that grain products were protective and "may be a useful adjunct to a low saturated fat and low cholesterol diet."[21] The banner on Post Raisin Bran shown in Figure 14 proclaims: "May help REDUCE the risk of HEART DISEASE" and in smaller capital letters "BECAUSE IT IS RICH IN FIBER," accompanied by the almost illegible disclaimer in minute capital letters: "Diets rich in fiber-containing grain products, fruits and vegetables and low in saturated fat and cholesterol may reduce your risk of heart disease, a disease associated with many factors."

With such claims authorized, cereal companies immediately began using them, emphasizing fiber, whole grains, or low fat. The claims distract from the sugar. Heart-health claims appeared on cereals such as Post Frosted Shredded Wheat, Honey Nut Cheerios, Cocoa Puffs, and Chocolate Cheerios, not exactly foods recommended for CHD prevention. But cereal companies had an even better idea: partnering with the American Heart Association to endorse their cereals' heart-health benefits.

The American Heart Association endorsement

In 1995, shortly after the FDA authorized the heart-health claim, the American Heart Association (AHA) launched its Heart-Check symbol and became the chief heart-healthy endorser of low-fat products—including sugary cereals. This was a surprise. From its beginnings in 1924 until 1988 when it changed the policy, the AHA had not allowed its name to be associated with product endorsements. But here it was, permitting food packages to say, "This product meets American Heart Association dietary guidelines for healthy people over age 2 when used as part of a balanced diet." In 2025, this endorsement appeared on nearly 1,000 products.[22]

In the early 2000s, the AHA's endorsement appeared on the side panels of General Mills' Cookie Crisp, Cocoa Puffs, Count Chocula, and Lucky Charms, none of which are likely to be considered heart-healthy foods. It included the usual qualifying statement about diets low in saturated fat and cholesterol. But the qualification said nothing about sugars; Kellogg's Frosted Mini-Wheats and Quaker Frosted Shredded Wheat also displayed the AHA endorsement.

Almost any cereal can meet the AHA's criteria for cholesterol and fat, but setting a limit on sugars would exclude most of them—as well as the income the AHA derived from the endorsements. Income? Indeed, yes. Food companies pay the AHA for use of its endorsement, raising questions of conflicts of interest.[23] The AHA provided the fee schedule on its website. Companies paid $7,500 per product for the first year of certification and $4,500 for annual renewals, with discounts for more than 10 products. The AHA insisted its pay-to-play program was not an endorsement; instead, it was a "food-certification program or corporate relationship." Perhaps, but this sure looked like a paid endorsement to us.

Subsequently, the AHA reduced its fees. The program's current fees range from $500 to $6,000 per product, depending on overall sales revenues and the number of product brands. More to the point, the AHA has updated its nutrition standards to include a limit on sugars. Cereals qualifying as "good" sources of fiber (at least 3 grams per serving) can contain up to 7 grams of sugars per serving; "excellent" fiber sources (at least 6 grams) can contain up to 9 grams of sugar. The sugars from fruit in the cereal, like the raisins in Raisin Bran, do not count toward the limits.

The AHA also replaced its endorsement statement with a widget seal displaying a red heart with a white check mark and the words "American Heart Association CERTIFIED: Meets Criteria For Heart-Healthy Food" (see Figure 22b). Blame the sugar standard for why our supermarket searches turn up only *one* cereal displaying the AHA seal: General Mills' original Cheerios. Even though all Big Four companies have cereals that should qualify, they have chosen not to participate. Once the AHA updated its criteria to limit sugars, cereal companies no longer needed the paid endorsement. They could continue to make heart-health claims as long as the cereals met the FDA's requirements (which do not address sugars), and they could avoid paying fees to the AHA.

Heart-health litigation

In 2012, Kellogg dropped the AHA symbol and launched its own heart-health widget in time for American Heart Month. This was a red heart inside a green circle with the words "Heart Healthy Selection" along with the usual disclaimer. Kellogg placed this on nine cereal boxes, including Raisin Bran, Smart Start, Fiber Plus, and All-Bran. Kellogg still uses this logo, slightly redesigned. The consumer advocacy group Center for Science in the Public Interest (CSPI) viewed the logo as well-intentioned, but it noted that while some supposedly heart-healthy cereals might technically qualify for the claim, they don't deserve to.[24] CSPI thought qualifying cereals should be higher in fiber and lower in sugar.

Others did too. Soon after the release of the new heart logo, a customer sued Kellogg, complaining that the company falsely advertised its cereals as heart-healthy when Raisin Bran contained 19 grams of sugars per serving and Smart Start had 23 grams. Kellogg asked for dismissal of the case, arguing it had followed federal regulations and made what was "plainly a health claim because it characterizes a relationship between the ingestion of a Breakfast Product and heart health."[25]

The judge disagreed, saying the company's response was "vague" and had not followed proper legal procedure. The case took 3 years to settle. Kellogg agreed to pay $20 million into a class action settlement fund (later revised to $13 million), remove the heart-health claim, and limit the use of the claim on Raisin Bran for at least 2 years. Similar lawsuits were filed against General Mills (dismissed) and against Post (settled for $15 million).[26] Cereal companies should have learned their lesson but have not. Using health claims must be worth the legal risks.

Contemporary heart-health claims

Today, we see heart-health claims on cereals from the Big Four companies: Kellogg's All-Bran and Raisin Bran; General Mills' Basic 4 and Honey Nut Cheerios; Quaker Life and Oatmeal; Post's Raisin Bran and Weetabix; and more. They are meant to reassure you that these cereals are good for health, despite their sugar. Most heart-health claims are displayed as small heart-shaped logos on cereals marketed to older consumers. General Mills has a "hearts matter" web page to promote the benefits of its cereals to aging boomers for whom "the health implications are a bit more real" (compared with millennials). But it also puts low-cholesterol banners on most Cheerios versions and in 2024 released heart-shaped Honey Nut Cheerios labeled for Mom, Dad, Family, and My Bestie: "This year, the special-edition Cheerios name boxes and Happy Heart Shapes are a simple reminder for people to take care of their heart so they can be there for all of life's special moments" (we show one example in Figure 37).[27]

Three decades after the first heart-health claims were authorized, they still help sell cereal. We wish the FDA would set a limit on the added sugar in cereals permitted to make such claims. This, however, would require an amendment to the current regulations and formal rulemaking, which could take years—a task not for the faint of heart.

The diabetes endorsement

Although diabetes is a leading cause of death and disability among Americans, it has never been the subject of a health claim. For cereal companies, this is a lost opportunity. The solution? An "endorsement" from the American Diabetes Association (ADA). In the early 2000s, Post's Raisin Bran, Honey Nut Shredded Wheat, and Frosted Shredded Wheat displayed heart-healthy banners along with a statement on the side panel: "A proud sponsor of American Diabetes Association." Post could not use the AHA's endorsement because the association did not allow partnerships with tobacco companies. At the time, Post was owned by Kraft, which in turn was owned by Altria, the maker of Philip Morris cigarettes.

The ADA had no such compunctions. Post was a member of its "Banting Circle"; companies at that sponsorship level contributed at least $500,000 in 2004. As *The New York Times* science writer Jane Brody observed, the diabetes association seemed like "a surprising bedfellow for a sweetened cereal, even one made from whole grain." The ADA, she said, told her it was changing its policy and would "no longer automatically permit such statements from companies that contribute to it."[28] Perhaps, but we were still seeing the acknowledgment of Post's ADA sponsorship on its cereals through 2006. At some point the ADA partnership stopped; we no longer see it on cereal boxes.

CHAPTER 8

MORE HEART-HEALTH CLAIMS

INGREDIENT PETITIONS

ALONG WITH DIRECTING the Food and Drug Administration (FDA) to authorize several specific health claims, the 1990 Nutrition Labeling and Education Act (NLEA) encouraged food companies to petition for additional claims. Cereal companies quickly submitted one petition after another to use the heart-health benefits of cereal ingredients to help market their brands. In this chapter, we set the stage for this discussion with the pre-NLEA excitement over oat bran.

The oat bran craze

We lived through the astonishing oat bran craze of the late 1980s—countless products, skyrocketing sales, the banner on Cheerios, and oat bran seemingly added to everything. This began in response to Robert Kowalski's best-selling diet book, *The 8-Week Cholesterol Cure.* Kowalski maintained he had dropped his blood cholesterol by 115 points in only 2 months by adhering to a diet containing less meat, supplemented with daily doses of niacin (vitamin B_3), and, you guessed it, oat bran.[1]

Oat bran is the outer, inedible husk of the oat seed; it contains soluble fiber, the cholesterol-lowering ingredient (insoluble fiber helps bulk up the digestive system). Studies were linking oat bran to measurable reductions in blood cholesterol levels. Kowalski's personal account launched a frenzy of new products, including more than two dozen oat bran cereals.[2]

Figure 15 shows one example. Its "Excellent Source of OAT BRAN" banner appeared in the wake of Kellogg's 1984 deal with the National Cancer Institute, and the FDA could do nothing to block the implied cholesterol claim—or the serving size issue. One Cheerios serving contained 8 grams of oat bran, but studies showed it took at least 25 grams to produce a measurable cholesterol-lowering effect.[3]

During this period, oat bran product sales reached eye-popping levels, increasing by 900% annually. Customers stripped shelves bare, and oat farmers could not keep up with the demand. Per capita consumption of oats went from 4.4 pounds per year in 1987 to 6.6 pounds in 1991. As a tribute to oats' popularity, *Saturday Night Live* spoofed oat bran in a not-to-be-missed sketch about a new cereal, "Colon Blow," with "more fiber than anyone could possibly guess."[4]

Oat bran became an *expected* ingredient. A 1989 Cheerios television ad featured breakfast eaters utterly dismayed by the lack of oat bran in Corn Flakes, Rice Krispies, and Raisin Bran. Kellogg's versions, Cracklin' Oat Bran and Common Sense Oat Bran, could not compete. Common Sense held a mere 2% of the market, while Cheerios rose to 10% of all US cereal sales, and General Mills' overall market share increased by 3%. Collectively, oat bran cereals were said to account for $1.5 billion of the $7 billion cereal market in 1989. Market share is serious business, and with Kellogg's decline, its president, Horst Schroeder, resigned amid this market turmoil.[5]

All good crazes must come to an end, and this one ended abruptly. In 1990, Harvard researchers found oat bran to be no better than any other high-fiber cereal in reducing blood cholesterol. They concluded any effect of oat bran was most likely the result of its substitution for dietary fat. Quaker Oats' officials objected that the study was uncontrolled, atypical, and too small to be taken seriously, as did others with less of a vested interest.[6]

Vested interests matter; industry-funded studies almost invariably produce results profitable to the funder. Quaker quickly announced it would fund its own studies of the health benefits of oat bran. Unsurprisingly, the Quaker-funded studies, among them an analysis of the combined results

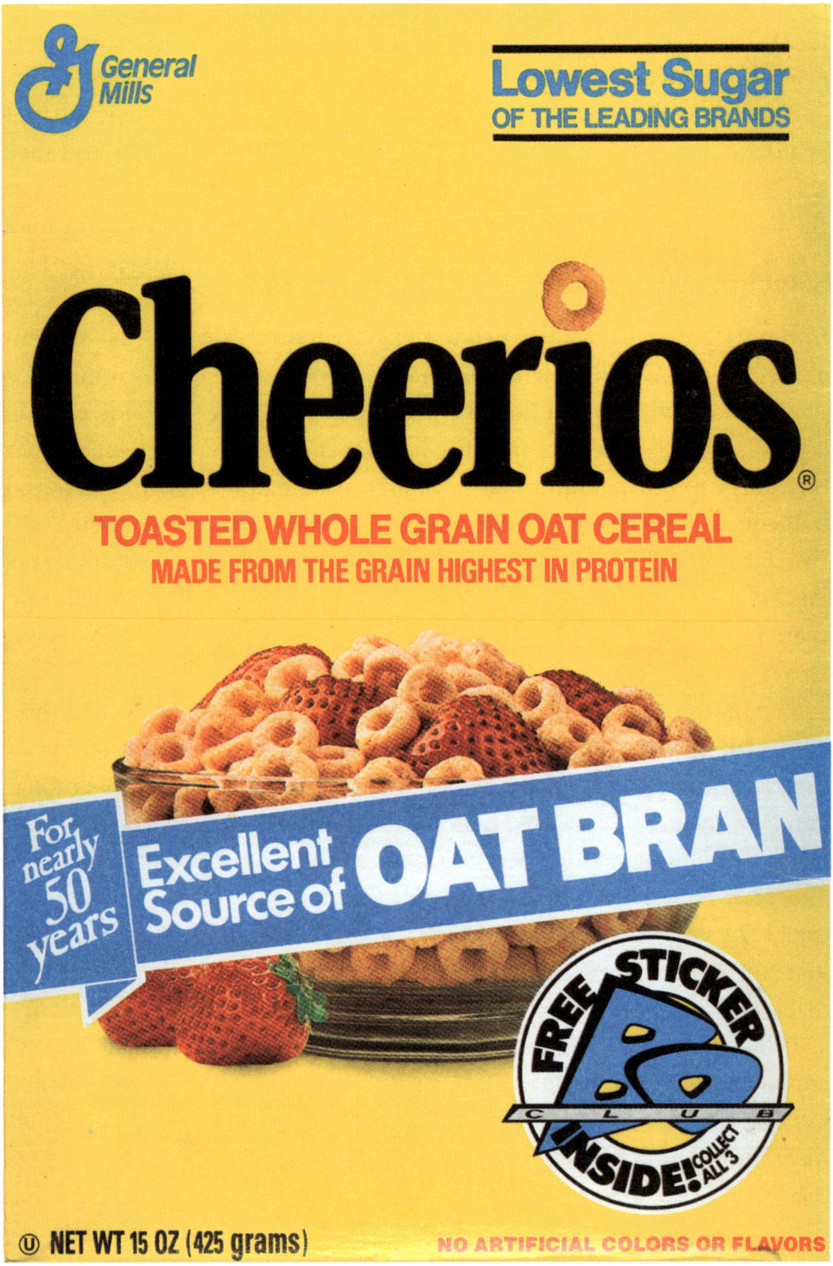

FIGURE 15 This 1988 Cheerios box exemplifies General Mills' contribution to that era's enthusiasm for oat bran as a means to reduce blood cholesterol. It contained 8 grams of oat bran per serving, requiring three daily servings to produce a "modest" cholesterol-lowering effect.

of 20 clinical trials, did indeed find benefits, although the researchers characterized them as "modest."[7]

If nothing else, the oat bran craze provided convincing evidence that health claims sell products. Once the NLEA claims petition option took effect in 1993, Quaker Oats was quick to take advantage.

Soluble fiber from oatmeal (Quaker)

In 1995, Quaker Oats petitioned the FDA to approve a claim that oat cereals reduced the risk of coronary heart disease (CHD). It submitted a review of 37 studies conducted since 1980. The FDA responded a year later with a 43-page analysis discounting most of the studies for poor methods or equivocal findings, although it agreed that 9 studies found that eating oatmeal or oat bran along with typical diets reduced the CHD risk factors—total cholesterol and LDL (low-density lipoprotein—the "bad" cholesterol). On that basis, "the agency tentatively concluded that there is significant scientific agreement that diets high in oat bran or oatmeal may help to reduce blood total and LDL cholesterol levels."[8]

The FDA allowed companies to say that oat bran or oatmeal could reduce CHD risk, as long as they also stated that they worked best in diets low in saturated fat and cholesterol. The FDA put all this out for public comment. Ten days later, on January 14, 1996, Quaker Oats celebrated the FDA's proposed but not yet final decision, with a full-page advertisement in *The New York Times*: "Why is this man [the Quaker pictured on the box] smiling? FDA proposes first food-specific health claim: diets high in oatmeal and low in saturated fat and cholesterol may reduce the risk of heart disease."

During the next year, the FDA collected and evaluated more than 1,450 comments filed in response to the proposed claim. Its final rule included significant revisions. Companies would not be able to claim that oats, oatmeal, or oat bran reduced CHD. Instead, the FDA would permit claims related to beta-glucan, a specific component of oat soluble fiber.

The FDA had concluded that most of the cholesterol-lowering effect was due to beta-glucan, with a dose effect: the more beta-glucan consumed, the greater the cholesterol reduction. Studies suggested the minimum amount of beta-glucan needed: 3 grams of beta-glucan per day, an amount provided by 40 grams of oat bran or 60 grams of oatmeal (1.5 servings). The FDA conceded significant scientific agreement among qualified experts and allowed this precisely worded claim: "Beta-glucan soluble fiber from whole oats, as part of a diet low in saturated fat and cholesterol, may reduce the risk of coronary heart disease." But because people are unfamiliar with beta-glucan, the FDA allowed companies to substitute the phrase "soluble fiber from oats."[9]

On January 23, 1997, Quaker Oats again celebrated with another full-page ad in *The New York Times*: "Now he has another reason to smile . . . Quaker oatmeal. Oh what those Oats can do." General Mills placed its own ad the same day: "FDA announces heart healthy news. So go ahead. Eat to your heart's content . . . the one and only Cheerios."

A year later, Quaker Oats launched an advertising campaign, "Warms Your Heart and Soul" based on its beta-glucan research. One ad showed 100 people happily holding boxes of oatmeal. After eating Quaker Oats for a month, it said 98 of them reduced their cholesterol, thus "redefining oatmeal as a soul food." Subsequent ads in professional journals referred to Quaker Oats' review of the literature (without mentioning the FDA's dim view of most studies): "More than 37 independent clinical studies have documented the cholesterol-lowering effect of soluble fiber (beta-glucan) from oats."[10]

As intended, the claim paid off. Before 1996, oatmeal sales had been declining by up to 4% per year. Publicity about the claim led to an immediate 5% increase in sales as well as an increase in the share prices of Quaker, General Mills, and Kellogg. Once the claim actually started appearing on cereal boxes in 1997, sales continued to increase at around 5% per year. But even this boost was not enough.[11] Once PepsiCo bought Quaker Oats in 2001, it pushed even harder for health claims, as we soon discuss.

Cheerios for reducing cholesterol (General Mills)

Once Quaker convinced the FDA to allow oatmeal to claim that soluble fiber could reduce blood cholesterol and CHD risk, other companies could do the same. In 2003, General Mills put "Can Help Lower Cholesterol" inside a red heart on boxes of Honey Nut Cheerios, followed by "& Reduce the Risk of Heart Disease" and, in the usual barely legible print, "As part of a low fat diet with the soluble fiber in Honey Nut Cheerios." Figure 16 illustrates this point.

But in 2007, General Mills went further. It put a banner over a heart-shaped bowl of Cheerios: "you can Lower Your Cholesterol 4% in 6 weeks (see back for details)." The details: "Cheerios is the only leading cold cereal clinically proven to lower cholesterol. A clinical study showed that eating two 1½ cup servings daily of Cheerios cereal reduced cholesterol when eaten as part of a diet low in saturated fat and cholesterol.*"

We love asterisks. This one referred to a study in which researchers gave people with high cholesterol levels either 3 ounces a day of whole-oat Cheerios or 3 ounces of a control cereal, cornflakes. Cheerios eaters reduced their total cholesterol by 3.8% and their LDL ("bad") cholesterol by 4.2% compared with those eating cornflakes. The investigators concluded: "These findings translate to a simple and practical approach to help reduce blood cholesterol levels," obviously implying "Eat more Cheerios." Guess who paid for the study: "This project was supported in part by a grant from General Mills, Inc."[12]

The Center for Science in the Public Interest (CSPI) examined the science behind the claim: "The truth: Cheerios doesn't lower cholesterol very much."[13] CSPI pointed out that participants had to eat 450 calories of the cereal a day (excluding the milk) to reduce LDL cholesterol from an average of 160 points to 153, still well above the optimal level of 100. But the industry-friendly Better Business Bureau's National Advertising Division supported General Mills as having substantiated the claim.[14]

The FDA disagreed. In 2009, the FDA warned General Mills to stop using the claim, because it was positioning the cereal as equivalent to cholesterol-lowering drugs. Cheerios, the FDA pointed out, "is not generally recognized as safe and effective for use in preventing or treating hypercholesterolemia or coronary heart disease. Therefore . . . it may not be legally marketed with the above claims in the United States without an approved new drug application."[15]

Nevertheless, General Mills soon launched a new box design claiming that Cheerios "helps lower cholesterol 10% in one month." This claim was based on yet another study funded by the company, published only as an abstract (the full study did not appear until the following year).[16] General Mills also put a banner on Honey Nut Cheerios proclaiming cholesterol

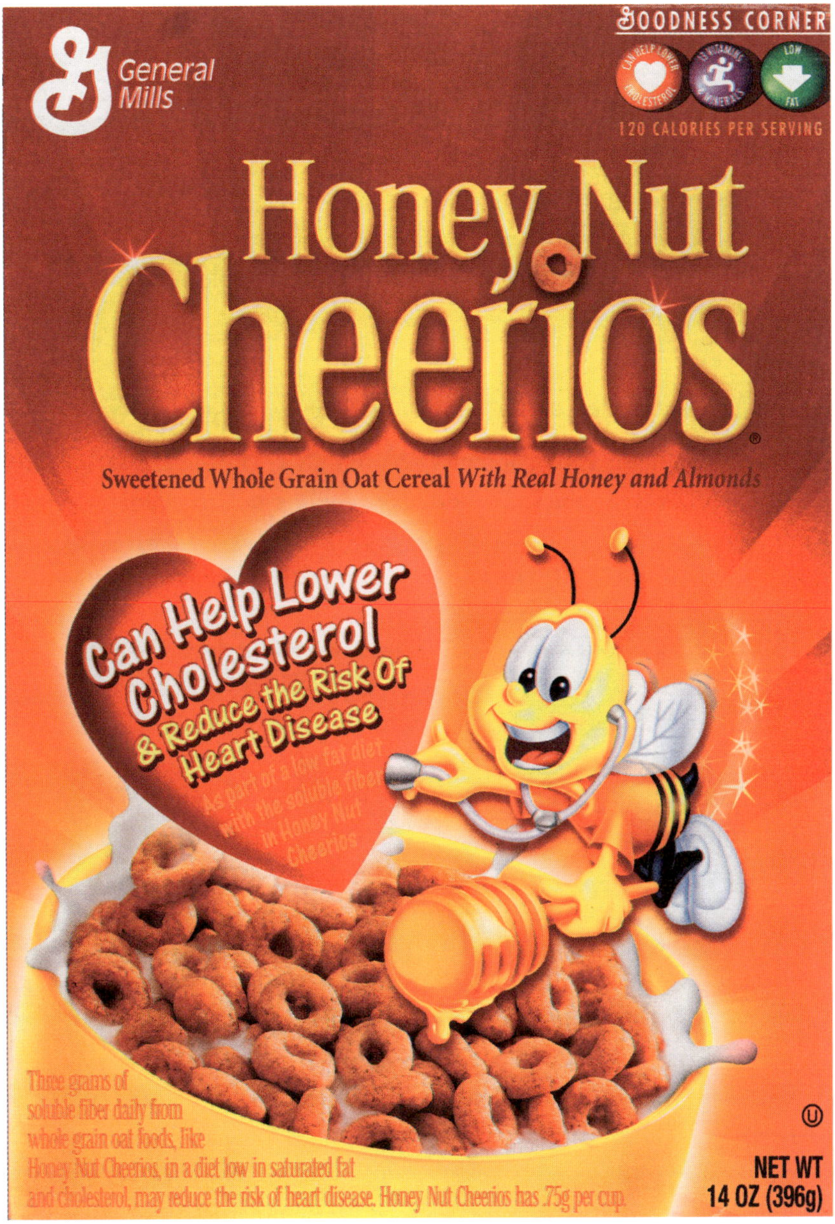

FIGURE 16 Once Quaker Oats won the soluble fiber claim, General Mills used it in 2003 to promote Honey Nut Cheerios for reducing cholesterol and heart disease risk. But when the boxes made more specific claims, the FDA objected that General Mills was positioning Cheerios as an unapproved drug.

reduction as an ostensible "non-challenge." However, the FDA's warning applied to all such claims, and General Mills had to drop them.

The National Consumers League, concerned about misleading advertising, took full credit for this result. In September 2008, it had complained to the FDA about Cheerios' drug-like claims. It applauded the FDA's warning letter in May 2009, and in September, it filed a suit against General Mills (which became moot once the boxes disappeared).[17] Today's Cheerios cereals still have banners saying "Can Help Lower Cholesterol" but no longer specify by how much or how fast, nor do they claim "clinically proven."

More cholesterol lowering: Psyllium fiber (Kellogg)

Oat bran is not the only source of soluble fiber. During the late 1980s, when the FDA was unable to stop rule-bending health claims, General Mills and Kellogg developed new cereals using psyllium seed husk to boost the fiber and claim heart-health benefits, such as the Heartwise cereal shown in Figure 17.

Psyllium is derived from *Plantago* species grown worldwide but mainly produced in India. Its husk fiber is 80% soluble. Psyllium is the active ingredient in over-the-counter laxatives such as Metamucil. General Mills named its psyllium-supplemented cereal Benefit: "What makes Benefit so remarkable is the psyllium grain. Ounce for ounce, this natural grain contains 8 times more soluble fiber than oat bran. . . . Reduce cholesterol. Get the Benefit."[18]

Claims like these rarely go unchallenged. Procter & Gamble (P&G), the maker of Metamucil, raised the first objection. The FDA had denied P&G's petition to use a cholesterol-lowering claim for Metamucil. P&G demanded the FDA "eliminate the inconsistency in allowing these new cereals to make cholesterol-reduction claims while Metamucil cannot." General Mills, it complained, was marketing Benefit as a cholesterol-lowering drug.[19]

The FDA asked General Mills to respond. But the dispute was soon irrelevant. After 8 months of unsuccessful market testing, General Mills withdrew Benefit cereal in 1990. You will be pleased to know that the 50 tons of unsold cereal did not go to waste. They were sent to South Dakota farmers to feed to less picky pigs and cows.[20]

Kellogg introduced Heartwise, "The natural, multi-grain psyllium cereal," in 1989. It contained 3 grams of soluble fiber and 6 grams of total fiber

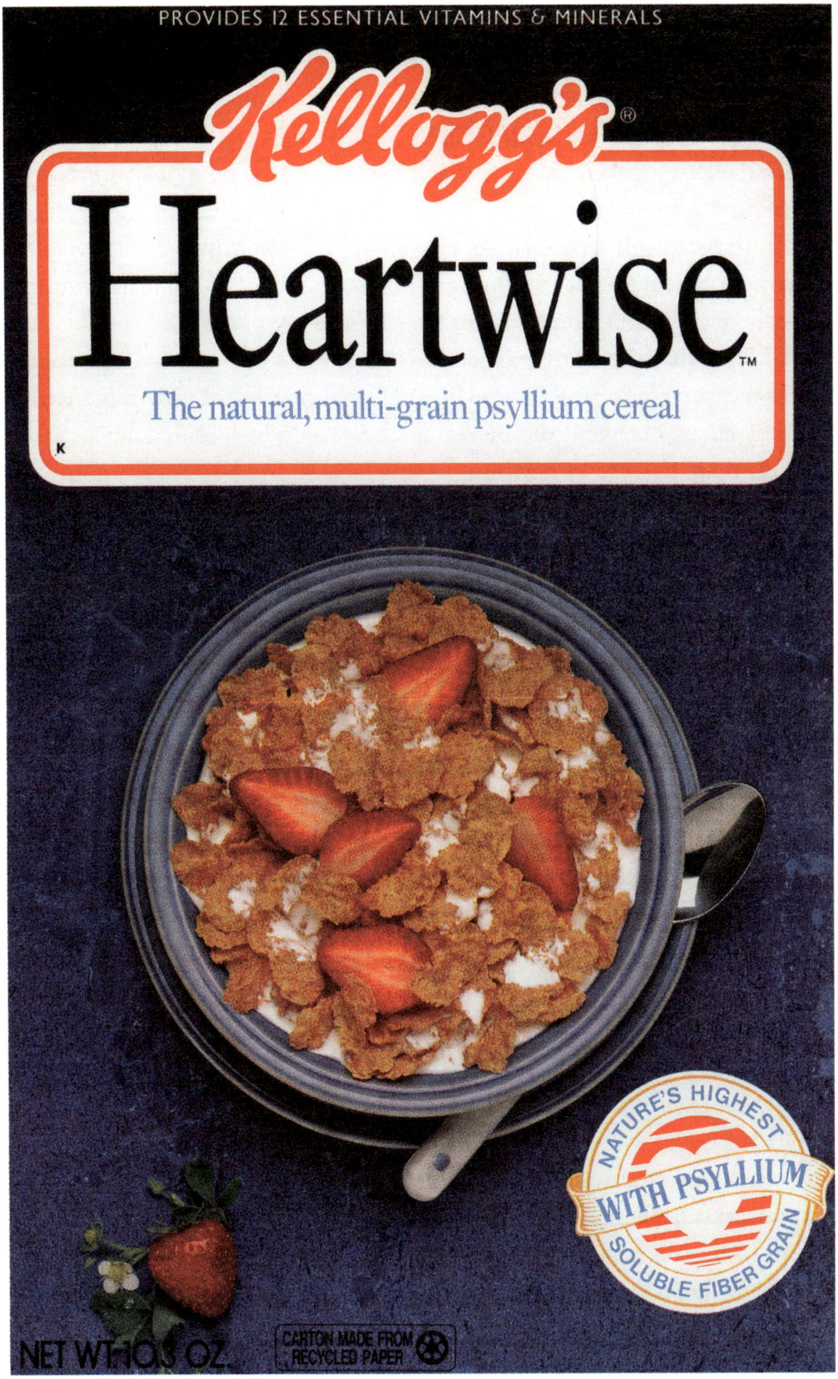

FIGURE 17 When studies in the late 1980s linked soluble fiber to reduced blood cholesterol and heart disease risk, companies created cereals with added psyllium, such as this 1989 Heartwise from Kellogg. The FDA questioned the safety of such cereals and the science behind the claims.

(whereas most cereals offer 2 grams), and it was promoted as "NATURE'S HIGHEST SOLUBLE FIBER GRAIN." But Kellogg said it would not make a health claim for it; it would instead use what it called a health *message*: "According to medical research, a diet low in fat and high in soluble fiber can help lower cholesterol. At the Kellogg company, we believe that Heartwise can be part of that diet."[21] This was right out of Kellogg's National Cancer Institute fiber-and-cancer health message playbook.

Late in 1989, the FDA warned both General Mills and Kellogg that it had "serious concerns" about psyllium. Psyllium was not GRAS (generally recognized as safe), and the FDA was unaware "of any scientific data that would justify the use of psyllium at this level in food."[22] Additionally, six states filed lawsuits against Kellogg to block the use of its "health message."

In 1990, Texas banned Heartwise, stating it did not warn buyers that psyllium husk could sometimes cause laxative and allergic reactions in susceptible people. Kellogg added a warning statement, but a Texas official characterized it as "backhanded . . . in mice type" and said "Kellogg constantly lies about its products. . . . Companies under investigation by states these days feel they have First Amendment rights to lie to their customers."[23] Kellogg strongly objected to these statements and sued the Texas official for slander, saying: "It has taken 85 years to build one of the best corporations in the world, and we will not allow an arrogant, irresponsible public official to attack our reputation."[24] The Texas official countered, calling the lawsuit out for what it was, "a bully-boy tactic."

The FDA also objected to the word *heart* in the cereal's name. Kellogg backed down and said it would change the brand to Fiberwise. We have a Fiberwise box from 1991; it did not last much longer. But Kellogg did not give up on psyllium. Once the NLEA went into effect, Kellogg petitioned the FDA to authorize a claim. The FDA did so in 1998, stating, "The agency has concluded that soluble fiber from psyllium seed husk, similar to beta (β)-glucan soluble fiber from whole oats, when included as part of a diet low in saturated fat and cholesterol, may reduce the risk of CHD by lowering blood cholesterol levels."[25]

With that decision in hand, Kellogg promptly created a $65 million functional foods division to introduce an entire line of psyllium-supplemented products. The company named the new line of products Ensemble: "Great food that does great things." Because lowering cholesterol requires three daily servings of psyllium, and few people were likely to eat that much cereal, Kellogg created 21 additional psyllium-containing food items such as potato chips, minicakes, and pastas. One of us (MN) sampled those products at a Kellogg-sponsored breakfast for heads of nutrition departments and thought they tasted chalky, reminiscent of Metamucil. Regardless, Ensemble failed, and Kellogg soon abandoned the project.[26]

Psyllium, to our amusement, is still with us. A niche company called Fiber Champion Brands has produced a line of psyllium-supplemented cereals amusingly called Poop Like a Champion ("Eat cereal. Poop. Repeat.") with the mission to "get you pooping again." With 19 grams of fiber (4 soluble, 15 insoluble), this ought to work. Psyllium is the fourth ingredient after corn bran, sugar, and sorghum flour. In 2024, we could buy the cereal online for around $14 for a 10.2-ounce box, but we could not find it in any of our local supermarkets.

Oatmeal again (Quaker Oats)

The oatmeal story is a good example of the unrelenting persistence of companies to be allowed to claim health benefits for their products. You might think claims for soluble fiber and oat bran would be enough for marketing purposes, but no. Quaker Oats wanted health claims on many more of its products, particularly oatmeal.

This saga began shortly after PepsiCo acquired Quaker Oats in December 2000. The company immediately petitioned the FDA to expand the "soluble fiber from certain foods and heart disease claim" to include a fourth beta-glucan source, Oatrim, a food additive marketed as a fat replacement in flour. Quaker Oats and Rhodia Inc., a French chemical firm, jointly filed the petition and pushed to make the claim apply exclusively to Oatrim under the trademark BETATRIM, the brand name for its food ingredients containing beta-glucan. After an exhaustive review, the FDA approved the claim in 2003—but not the brand exclusivity. Instead, it determined that *any* fat replacement made from Oatrim was eligible for the health claim as long as it was "the soluble fraction of alpha-amylase hydrolyzed oat bran or whole oat flour with a beta-glucan soluble fiber content."[27]

But in 2005, Quaker Oats again petitioned the FDA, this time to allow *all* of its oatmeal products to claim heart-health benefits when the fat came from the oats themselves. It did this because while its flavored (sugar-added) instant oatmeal qualified for the heart-health claim, the reduced-sugar version did not.[28]

This is a perfect example of why we so enjoy labeling issues. Recall that under FDA rules, heart-health claims can only be made for foods low in fat and cholesterol. Oats are naturally low in both; their fat is about 3 grams per serving. One more rule: for foods that need to be reconstituted before eating (like by adding water or milk to oatmeal), all nutrients must be calculated by rounding up the serving size to 50 grams (don't ask). When Quaker Oats reduced the sugar to create the lower-sugar variety, the serving size also decreased, but rounding it up increased the proportion of oats in the oatmeal, thereby boosting the fat per serving to exceed the FDA's 3-gram limit for low fat.[29] Whatever.

Quaker argued that having different rules for regular and reduced-sugar oatmeal confuses customers. The FDA agreed and in 2007 proposed to exempt oats from the low-fat requirement; its final rule appeared in 2008. Quaker Oats went to work. It described oatmeal as uniquely "able to actively find cholesterol and remove it from the body," as illustrated by a graph demonstrating oatmeal's cholesterol-lowering ability. CSPI, ever on the job, viewed these statements as highly exaggerated and threatened to sue. The company agreed to delete words and phrases like *unique*, *actively find*, and *remove from the body* and to add the qualification "3 grams of soluble fiber daily may help reduce heart disease risk as part of a heart healthy diet."[30]

Michael Jacobson, CSPI's director, issued a statement: "Of course, the Food and Drug Administration should be the one policing food labels, but the agency is so short-staffed and dysfunctional that officials won't take action even when a neatly wrapped complaint is handed to them with a ribbon around it and a bow on top."[31] That was in 2007, by no means the last time consumer advocates urged the FDA to block misleading health claims on cereal boxes.

CHAPTER 9

NUTRIENT CONTENT AND STRUCTURE/FUNCTION CLAIMS

HEART-HEALTH CLAIMS authorized by the Food and Drug Administration (FDA) typically appear on cereals promoted to adults, but kids' cereals mostly feature nutrient content or structure/function claims. Nutrient content claims promote the beneficial levels of a cereal's "positive" nutrients (vitamins, minerals, fiber, protein), qualifying the cereal as a "good" or "excellent" source of those nutrients. Or they describe the cereal as "low in" the "negatives" (fat, sugars, sodium). Claims like "excellent source of fiber" or "good source of calcium" make cereal seem like an ideal nutrient source—even when the nutrients come from fortification, and the cereal contains added sugars.

Structure/function claims, in contrast, tout the nutrient benefits for a bodily structure or function, using words like *supports*, *maintains*, or *promotes*, as in "fiber promotes digestive health." As a result of the Dietary Supplement Health and Education Act of 1994 (see Chapter 7), cereal companies do not have to notify the FDA about these claims, and they do not have to include disclaimers, as they must for other kinds of health claims.[1] As long as the claims are "truthful and not misleading," they are fair game, until they are not. As we explain here, Kellogg learned this the hard way—not once but twice.

But before getting to examples of nutrient content and structure/function claims, let's look at Kellogg's ill-fated use of an unauthorized health claim: Frosted Mini-Wheats help improve kids' cognition.

Unauthorized health claim: Kids' attentiveness

Early in 2008, you could buy Frosted Mini-Wheats that Kellogg boasted had been "Clinically Shown to improve kids' Attentiveness by nearly 20%." This sounded impressive, but in clinical trials the important question is always, Compared to what? The fine print gave the answer: "Based upon independent clinical research, kids who ate Kellogg's Frosted Mini-Wheats cereal for breakfast had up to 18 percent better attentiveness three hours after breakfast than kids who ate no breakfast." Well, yes. Not eating breakfast of course makes kids hungry and distracted.[2]

While Kellogg's research report is no longer available online, accounts at the time described it. To establish a baseline measurement, the researchers used unspecified tests on an unspecified number of children to assess their attentiveness before eating breakfast. They gave the children either Kellogg's Frosted Mini-Wheats or water. They tested the kids again over the next 3 hours, long enough for them to feel hungry again.[3] But this was an unauthorized health claim, and it soon got the attention of the Federal Trade Commission (FTC), the agency responsible for ensuring that statements are "truthful and not misleading," including those on cereal boxes.

Someone must have filed an objection with the FTC, which soon issued a complaint. To our surprise, the FTC did not argue that the claim was inherently absurd, even though the kids in the control group had not eaten breakfast. Instead, it took the study at face value and charged Kellogg with exaggerating the results, creating false advertising, and violating federal law:

> In the clinical study referred to in respondent's advertisements, for example, only about half the kids who ate Frosted Mini-Wheats cereal showed any improvement after three hours as compared to their prebreakfast baseline. In addition, overall, only one in seven [14%] kids who ate the cereal improved their attentiveness by 18% or more, and only about one in nine [11%] improved by 20% or more. Therefore, the representation . . . was, and is, false or misleading.[4]

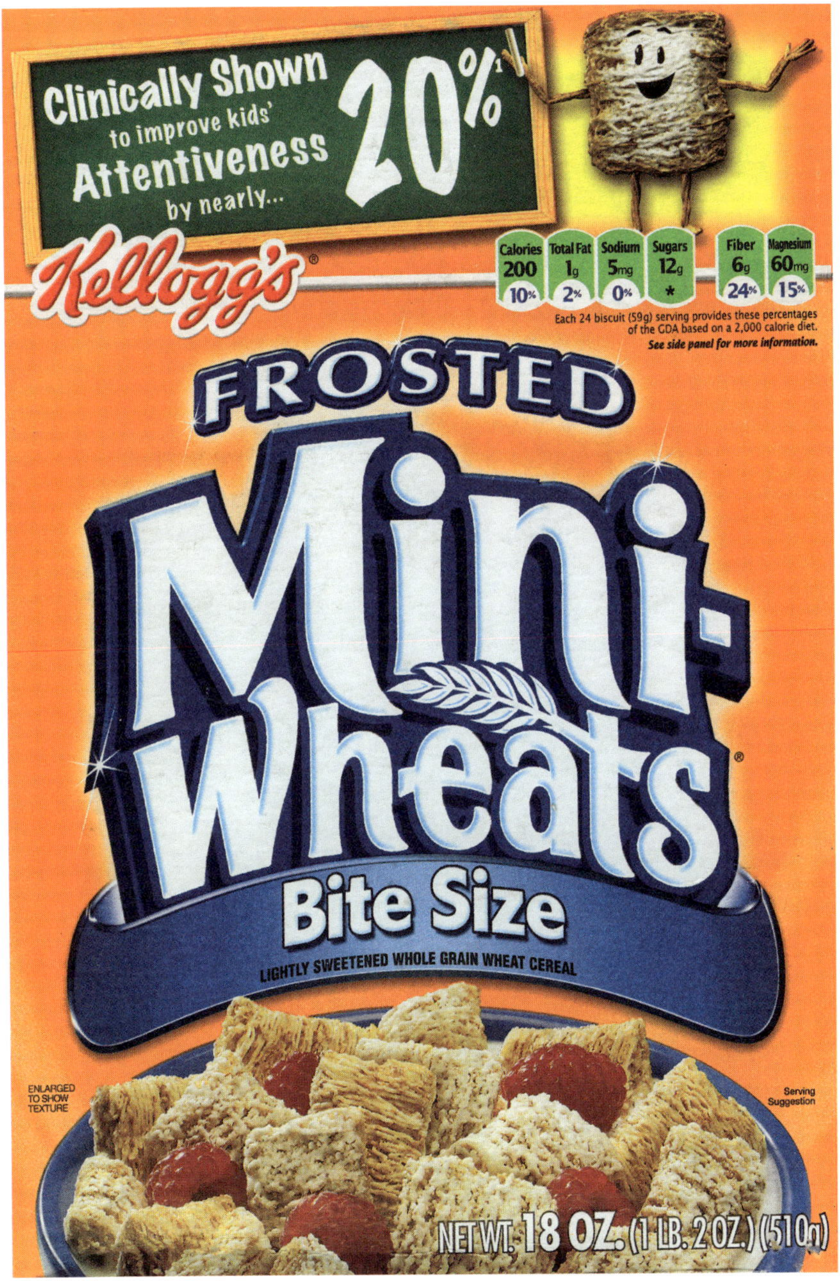

FIGURE 18 The banner on this 2008 box referred to a clinical trial purporting to show that kids who ate Frosted Mini-Wheats improved their attentiveness. When the Federal Trade Commission objected and advocates filed lawsuits, Kellogg settled the suit and withdrew the claim.

Kellogg agreed to settle the federal charge that it falsely advertised the attentiveness claim, but it maintained it had not violated any laws. The FTC issued a consent agreement that barred Kellogg from making misleading cognitive health claims for any of its cereals and misrepresenting tests or studies in advertising and product packaging. But it did permit Kellogg to make further claims for cognitive health, process, or function provided the claims were "substantiated and true."[5]

This, however, did not end the matter. In 2010, Kellogg agreed to settle a consumer class action lawsuit over the claim, initially agreeing to pay $2.75 million to claimants, $5.5 million to charities, and $2 million in costs and to cease making improved attentiveness claims for 3 years. After more than 2 years, a federal appeals court rejected the deal, ruling that the money intended for charities would not benefit the class action. Eventually, Kellogg settled the suit for $4 million. In 2016, class action members were mailed checks for a grand total of $3.81 for one box, $7.63 for two, and $11.44 for three boxes of the cereal.[6] We could only hope this taught cereal companies a lesson, but no such luck, as we soon explain.

Nutrient content claim: Calcium and vitamin D

While Kellogg was focusing on kids' cognition, General Mills was busy helping kids grow up strong. Calcium and vitamin D are nutrients essential for kids' growth and development. The back of the box shown in Figure 19 says "75% of kids don't get the recommended levels of calcium and vitamin D." General Mills has a solution to this problem: "Grow up strong with Big G kid cereals."

The widespread fortification of cereals with these particular nutrients dates to the mid-1980s, when the food industry began adding calcium to every product it could. Food companies, knowing that nutrients increase sales, found calcium especially useful for this purpose; its role in bone health is widely understood. Dairy products may be the major source of calcium, but when Coca-Cola added calcium to its diet soft drink Tab, sales nearly doubled. *Fortune* advised, "If your product contains calcium, flaunt it. If it doesn't, add it and flaunt that."[7] The FDA authorized a health claim associating calcium with a reduced risk of osteoporosis specifically for dietary supplements following passage of the 1990 nutrition labeling act; it allowed the same claim for foods in 1996.[8]

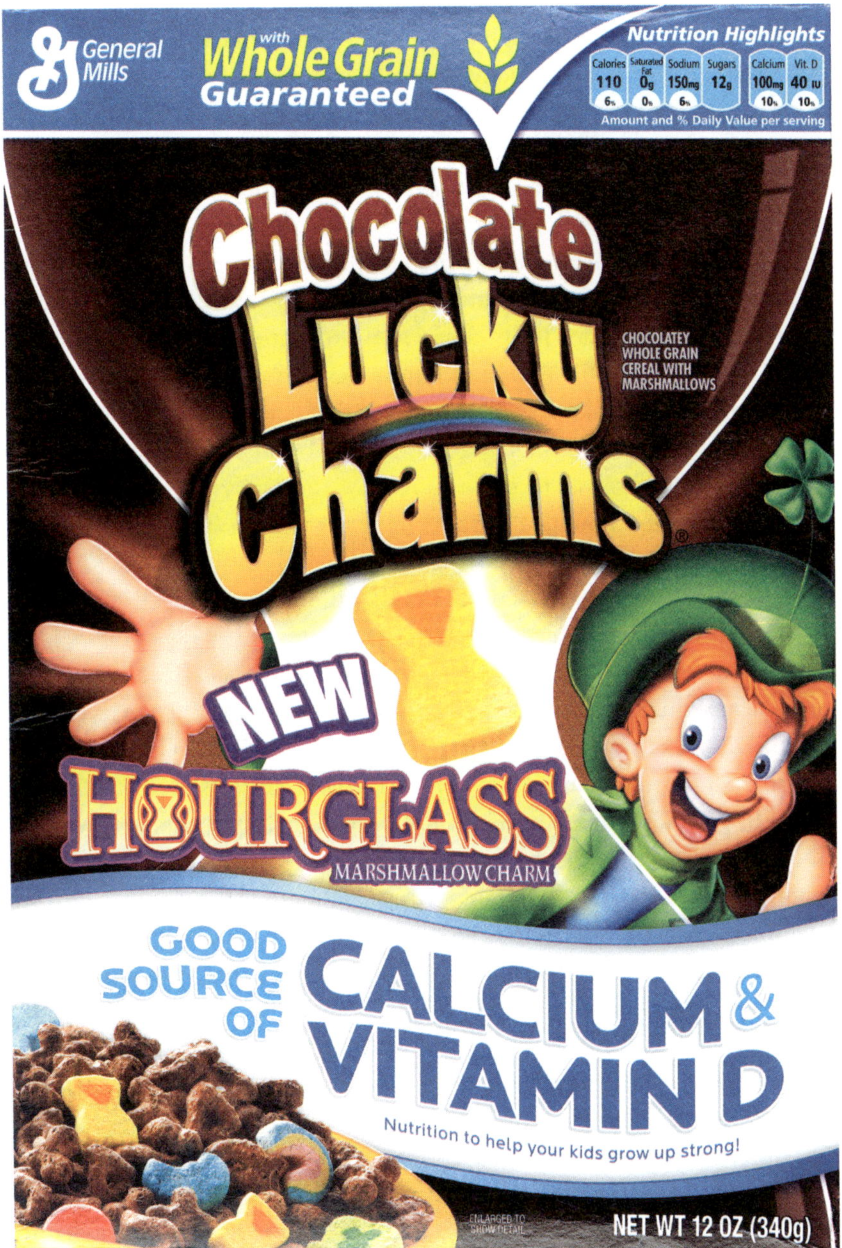

FIGURE 19 In 2008, cereal companies began touting their candy-laden products as good sources of calcium and vitamin D. This FDA-authorized nutrient content claim from General Mills implies but does not explicitly state benefits for bone health.

Vitamin D is also critical to bone health; it is required for calcium absorption. But cereals are an unlikely source of vitamin D. Indeed, "vitamin" D is not a vitamin as usually defined; it is actually a hormone synthesized in the body in a process initiated by the action of sunlight on the skin—the best source. Unless foods are fortified with vitamin D, few are sources, let alone good ones.

In 2008, the FDA amended the calcium and bone-health claim to include vitamin D.[9] The new rule did not take effect until January 1, 2010, but General Mills went right ahead and promoted the dynamic duo as shown in the banner displayed in Figure 19: "Nutrition to help your kids grow up strong!" General Mills was advertising Chocolate Lucky Charms—with marshmallows yet—as a "good" source because it had added both calcium and vitamin D to provide 10% of the Daily Value per serving, despite the cereal having 12 grams of sugar per serving, or 44% of its calories.

In 2019, Kellogg petitioned the FDA to allow greater levels of vitamin D fortification in breakfast cereals.[10] When the FDA finally approved the petition in 2023, General Mills quickly took advantage of its competitor's success, announcing it would double the amount of vitamin D in its cereals. It launched a renewed campaign, "Goodness We Grow Up On." Lucky Charms could now claim "2X VITAMIN D HELPS BUILD STRONG BONES." As one company official put it, "the more things change, the more things stay the same."[11] Apparently so. Two years later, Quaker introduced Mighty Life cereal as an "excellent source of vitamin D & calcium," sporting a banner across the box front: "SUPPORTS HEALTHY BONES."[12]

Structure/function claim: Immunity

You are not alone if your mind boggles at the thought that Kellogg's Cocoa Krispies and other such cereals might protect your child against the flu and other infectious diseases, as we show in Figure 20. Almost as soon as this box appeared in supermarkets, the San Francisco attorney general (AG) sent a warning letter to Kellogg:

> Specifically, the Immunity Claims may falsely suggest to parents that cereals like Cocoa Krispies are more healthy for their children than

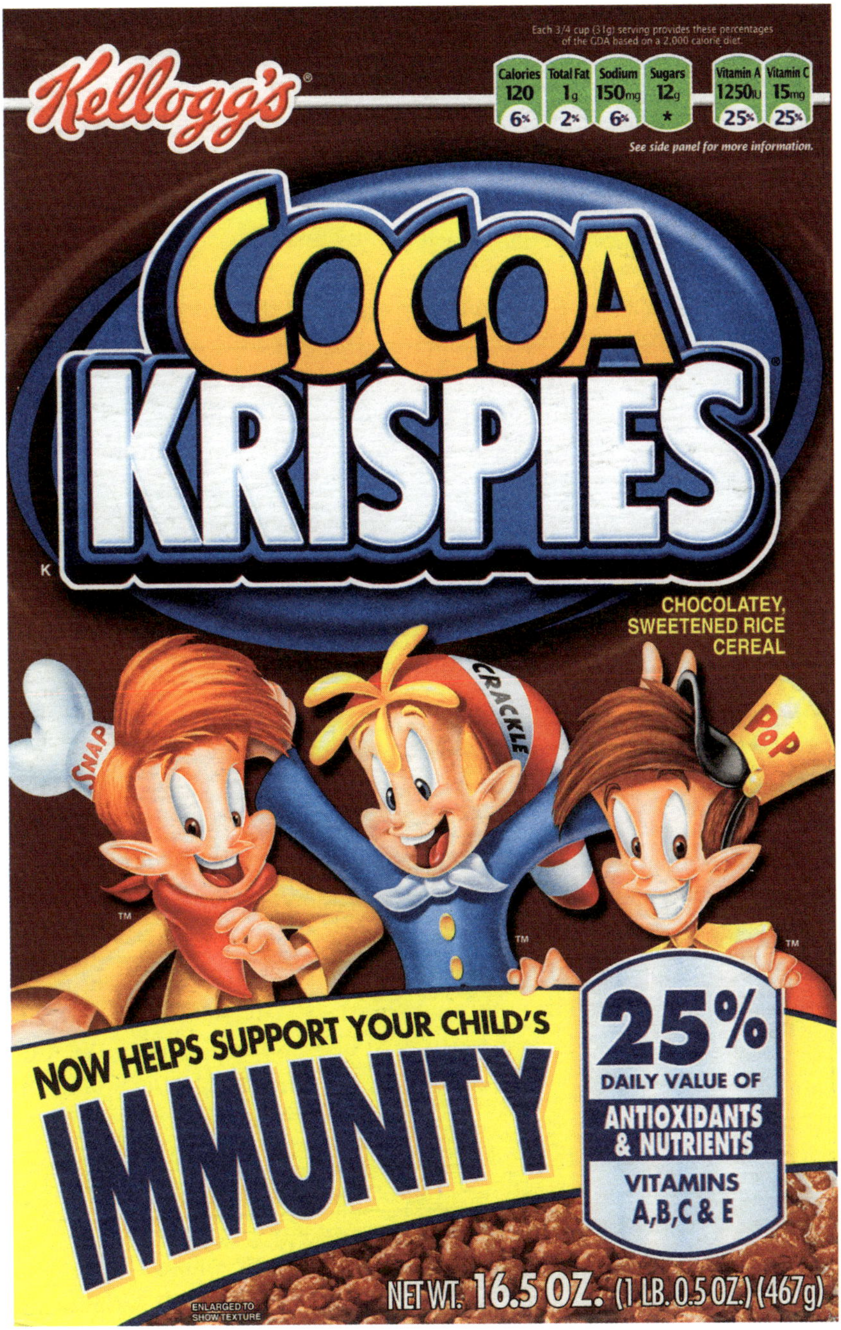

FIGURE 20 In 2009, Kellogg's Cocoa Krispies boxes displayed an immunity banner. This elicited public outrage at the idea that sugary cereals could protect children against the then-concurrent outbreak of H1N1 swine flu.

> other breakfast foods that are not high in sugar and not highly processed. The Immunity Claims may also mislead parents into believing that serving this sugary cereal will actually boost their child's immunity, leaving parents less likely to take more productive steps to protect their children's health. At a time when parents are increasingly worried about the spread of the H1N1 virus ("swine flu"), it is vitally important that parents receive accurate information about what they can do to protect their children's health.[13]

The letter demanded that Kellogg provide copies of all research used to establish the claim. If the evidence was not immediately forthcoming, the AG threatened to "seek an immediate termination or modification of the advertising claim." A few days later, a reporter learned of the letter and turned it into national news: "Critics blast Kellogg's claim that cereals can boost immunity."[14] Kellogg got the message. Within days, the company announced it would phase out all boxes displaying the immunity claim. It did this even though the FDA had not taken action, which it could not. The wording of the immunity claim, "NOW HELPS SUPPORT YOUR CHILD'S IMMUNITY," makes it a structure/function claim, which does not need FDA approval.

But the FTC objected. From its stance, the size of the word "IMMUNITY" on the box was sufficiently misleading to constitute false advertising and a violation of the settlement reached in the Mini-Wheats kids' attentiveness case discussed earlier. Under that settlement, Kellogg was not supposed to be making claims about its cereals' benefits to cognitive health, process, or function. The FTC, sufficiently annoyed, revised the settlement order in 2010 to make it even more restrictive. Kellogg was to stop making any health claims on any of its products unless substantiated by the totality of competent and reliable scientific evidence, of sufficient quality and quantity, and meeting the standards of qualified experts. The FTC order would apply to Kellogg products until 2030.[15] As one commentator said, maybe Kellogg "should have just stuck with Snap, Crackle, and Pop."[16]

But this was not the first time a cereal company promoted an immunity claim, nor would it be the last. In 2003, General Mills' Total Raisin Bran cereal displayed a banner, "Help maintain a healthy immune system with 100% of Vitamin E and Zinc." The explanation on the back of the box: "One important function of nutrients like vitamin E and zinc, is to help maintain a strong immune system. Where can you find this combination of nutrients? One place is your cereal bowl." The word *maintain*, like *support*, signals that this is a structure/function claim. Perhaps because the brand name, Total, was in a much bigger font than the claim, neither the FDA nor the FTC raised objections.

And then in 2025, Quaker launched Mighty Life IMMUNITY SUPPORT: "Helps maintain healthy immune function with vitamins C, D, & Zinc."[17] We'll see if anyone objects this time.

Structure/function claim: Sleep

When a cereal called Sweet Dreams hit supermarket shelves in 2023, as shown in Figure 21, we were amazed. It had the first new claim we'd seen since cereals proclaimed their antioxidant ingredient content 8 years earlier. And this was quite a claim: "Supports Natural Melatonin Production with Zinc, Folic Acid, and B Vitamins." In case you are unfamiliar with melatonin, the box says "part of a healthy sleep routine."

What is this really about? The obvious explanation: expanding cereal eating occasions (and cereal sales) and taking advantage of the growing $5 billion sleep aid market. One in three adults says they don't get enough sleep, and 50 to 70 million Americans report having chronic sleep disorders. Sweet Dreams to the rescue! An industry newsletter made that point: "Post Consumer Brands is turning the day on its head, encouraging sleep-poor Americans to eat cereal for dinner."[18] For this cereal to work, you are supposed to eat it at dinner or bedtime, preferably both.

Right away, we bought the box shown in Figure 21. Its back was worth reading:

- "Sleep . . . We want to help you enjoy it. With delicious wholesome ingredients, curated vitamins and minerals, and a specially formulated night-time herbal blend, our dreamy cereal is part of a healthy sleep routine."
- "Made with a night-time herbal blend containing a touch of lavender and chamomile."

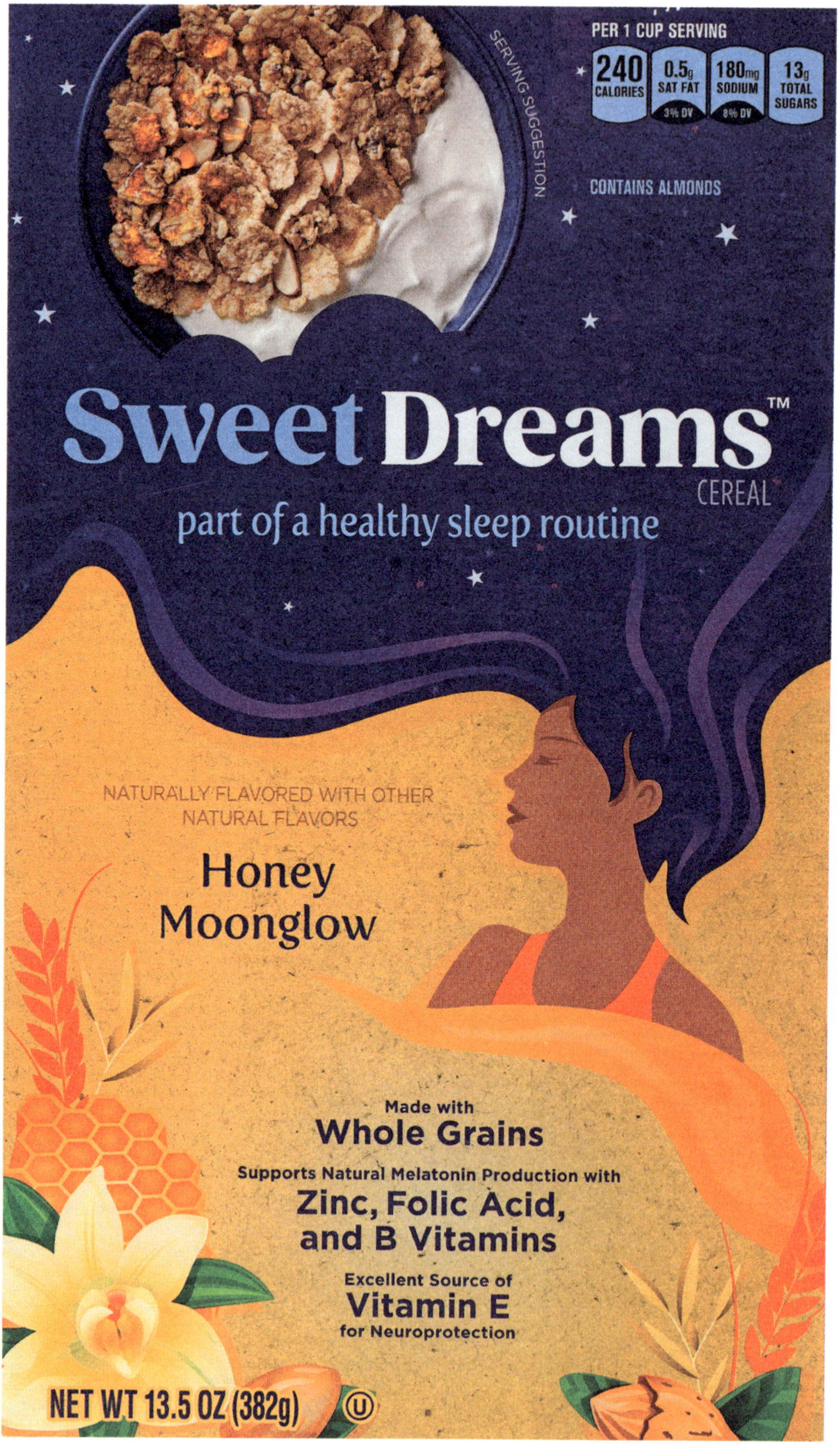

FIGURE 21 Post launched this vitamin-fortified cereal in 2023, advertising its ability to help you sleep better. Cereals are not just for breakfast anymore.

"Curated" vitamins and minerals? We guess that means carefully selected for their melatonin-boosting effects. As for "Supports Natural Melatonin Production," this is yet another structure/function claim protected against FDA complaints and any need for serious scientific substantiation. Curious to know what Post said about the science, we checked the website: "Melatonin is a hormone released by the brain when it starts to get dark. It helps set circadian rhythms, the timing of the internal biological clock. After a few hours, it makes you sleepy."

The site did not review the science, understandably; there isn't much. A 2004 Agency for Healthcare Research and Quality review deemed melatonin ineffective for treating most sleep disorders, jet lag, or shift work disorders. Another review published in 2013 put a more positive spin on the results. It found melatonin to decrease sleep onset latency, increase total sleep time, and improve overall sleep quality, but "modestly." The authors advised trying it. Melatonin, they concluded, "*may* [our emphasis] have a role in the treatment of insomnia given its relatively benign side-effect profile compared to these [pharmacological] agents."[19] The NIH National Center for Complementary and Integrative Health currently says there is "not enough strong evidence on the effectiveness or safety of melatonin supplementation for chronic insomnia to recommend its use."[20] *Consumer Reports* says it *may* (that again) help some people get some relief—not exactly a ringing endorsement.[21]

We tried Sweet Dreams. The crunch was good but the cereal was way too sweet, not surprising given that five different sugars appear seven times in the ingredient list. And where is the promised "touch of lavender and chamomile"? *Touch* must be meant literally; neither herb appears on the ingredient list, but perhaps they are part of the listed natural flavor.

This cereal contributes to two larger marketing trends: the growth in products designed to help people sleep and the attempt to get people to eat cereals more often.[22] We ate the cereal in the morning; it did not make us feel sleepy. Its sales, however, were indeed sleepy, putting it to bed. Late in 2024, it was no longer available at our local supermarkets and had disappeared from the Post Consumer Brands website.

CHAPTER 10

WIDGETS

NUTRITION AT A GLANCE

IF YOU CLOSELY INSPECT cereal boxes, you will surely find what we call widgets, for lack of a better collective term. These are the symbols, icons, logos, seals, stamps, or endorsements attesting to the cereal's production method, its ingredient or nutritional content, or its contribution to specific conditions or overall health. Figure 22 displays several examples. We discussed some of these in connection with whole-grain ingredients (Chapter 4, Figure 22a) and heart-health claims (Chapter 7, Figure 22b). And we will discuss others later: the low FODMAP diet claim (Chapter 11, Figure 22g), production methods such as organic and non-GMO (Chapter 12, Figures 22h and i), and philanthropic partnerships (Chapter 16, Figure 22j). In this chapter, we talk about the four in between, Figures 22c to f.

Unless you are looking for widgets, you might not notice them, but they are important marketing tools. They appeared on cereal boxes as early as 1912, when Uncle Sam cereals (now owned by Post) proclaimed that the American Medical Association endorsed their laxative-inducing wheat flakes. Later, a 1963 box of General Mills Sugar Jets displayed the "Recommended by Betty Crocker" seal of approval, directly targeting moms. Such symbols appeared hit or miss until the 1990s, when cereal companies began to display self-designated nutrition-at-a-glance symbols to help

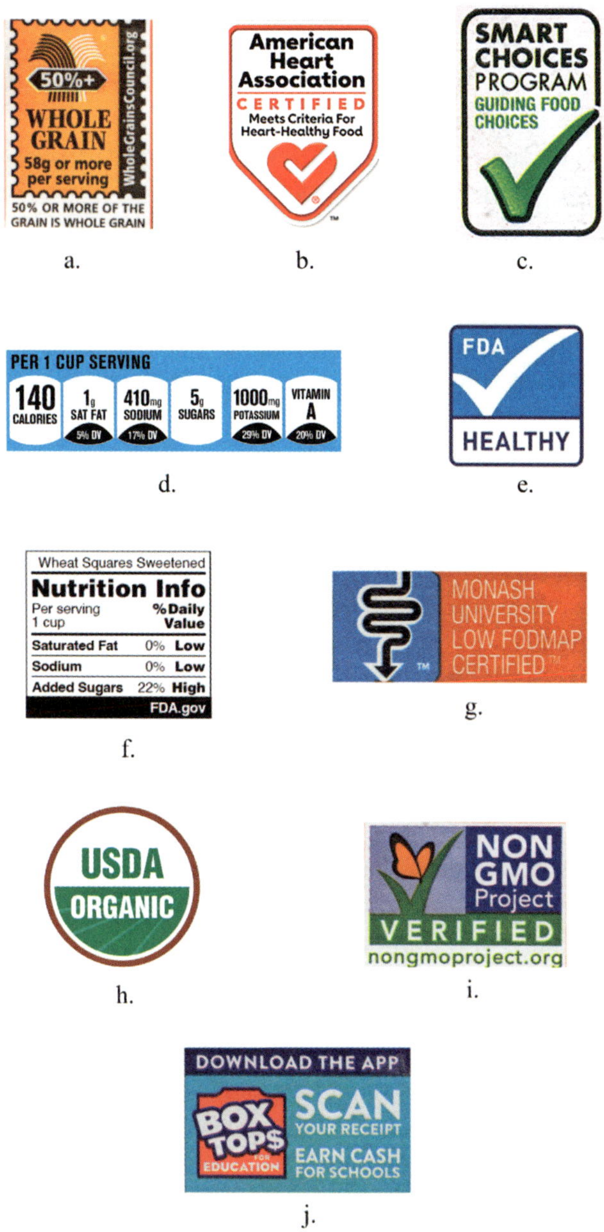

FIGURE 22 These nutrition icons and symbols—"widgets"—have appeared (c), currently appear (a, b, d, g, h, i, j), or have been proposed to appear (e, f) on cereals to promote benefits for nutrition and health. These are listed in the order of their discussion in the chapters. Four (c, d, e, and f) are discussed in this chapter. Sources: (a) Oldways Whole Grains Council; (b) American Heart Association; (c) Smart Choices Program; (d) Consumer Brands Association; (e) and (f) FDA; (g) Monash University; (h) USDA; (i) Non-GMO Project; (j) General Mills.

consumers quickly identify the supposedly healthiest products without having to decode Nutrition Facts labels.

Of the four widgets discussed here, the food industry designed two: the now-defunct SMART CHOICES (Figure 22c) and the current Facts Up Front (Figure 22d). The Food and Drug Administration (FDA) designed the other two: the voluntary HEALTHY icon (Figure 22e), which evaluates only good-for-you (positive) nutrients, and the proposed mandatory front-of-package icon, based only on the negatives (Figure 22f). We start with SMART CHOICES, which turned out to be not so smart.

The ill-fated Smart Choices program

This widget is history, but it created a cautionary tale worth retelling. Following the passage of the Nutrition Labeling and Education Act of 1990, cereal boxes displayed Nutrition Facts labels on their side panels, but these were difficult for many people to understand. Soon after the American Heart Association established its Heart-Check certification program in 1995 (Chapter 7), food companies began inventing their own systems for self-designating "better-for-you" products. For example, PepsiCo put a "Smart Choices Made Easy" logo on hundreds of its snack and drink products, Kraft Foods developed a "Sensible Solution" icon, and Unilever had a "Choices" logo. Front-of-package widgets like these seemed ubiquitous and competed for marketplace attention.[1]

Adding to the competition, supermarkets began using their own systems and symbols. Hannaford introduced (and still uses) the Guiding Stars ranking system (0, 1, 2, or 3 stars); Tops Markets used the now defunct NuVal system (score 1—100); Supervalu Inc. (which includes Albertsons) implemented the color-coded NutritionIQ system; and Giant Foods launched a Healthy Ideas stamp. In 2006, the United Kingdom Food Standards Agency introduced the voluntary red, yellow, and green traffic light label system to indicate high, medium, and low levels of calories, fat, saturated fat, sugar, and salt in food products. Kellogg cereals in the UK displayed such labels. When they led to reduced sales of red-lighted products, food companies knew they had a problem with front-of-package warning labels.[2]

In 2007, in an attempt to resolve this chaos, 14 food companies joined together to develop an industry-wide system for identifying healthier products. They recruited the Keystone Center, a nonprofit consensus-building organization, to facilitate the process. Keystone, in turn, convened a roundtable with participants mainly from the food industry (including nutrition experts from General Mills and Kellogg) but also from retail, academic, health, and consumer groups. To make the process appear even more credible, it hired two groups to manage the process: the American Society for Nutrition (ASN), a professional organization for nutrition researchers and scientists, and NSF International, a nonprofit health-consulting organization that, among other things, performed third-party certifications. Even so, we could not imagine how this group could possibly reach consensus on nutrition standards, and we eagerly awaited its outcome.

For 2 years, the roundtable worked to develop nutrition standards for a symbol to replace those of the member companies: "a single, trusted symbol that could help consumers make smarter food and beverage choices within product categories." Its working group, composed mainly of food company representatives, organized food and beverage products into 19 categories, including breakfast cereals. They set minimum requirements for the "positives" to encourage: nutrients (vitamins, minerals, fiber) and food groups (fruits, vegetables, whole grains, low-fat dairy foods). They also set upper boundaries for the "negatives" to limit (total fat, saturated fat, trans fat, cholesterol, sodium, and added sugars). Qualifying breakfast cereals could not exceed standards for the negatives but also had to contain at least one positive nutrient or food group. Most pertinent, the roundtable set the upper limit for added sugars at 25% of total calories.[3]

The Smart Choices Program and its symbol launched in August 2009. *New York Times* food business reporter William Neuman headed right to a supermarket, immediately spotting the SMART CHOICES green checkmark symbol (Figure 22c) on, of all things, Froot Loops, shown on the box in Figure 23. His early September headline: "For Your Health: Froot Loops."[4]

How was this possible? The added sugars in Froot Loops provide 44% of its calories. But the industry-controlled roundtable, which included nutrition experts from General Mills and Kellogg, had exempted breakfast cereals from the 25% limit. Instead, they set the standard at 12 grams of added sugars per serving under an allowance for "food specific variations."

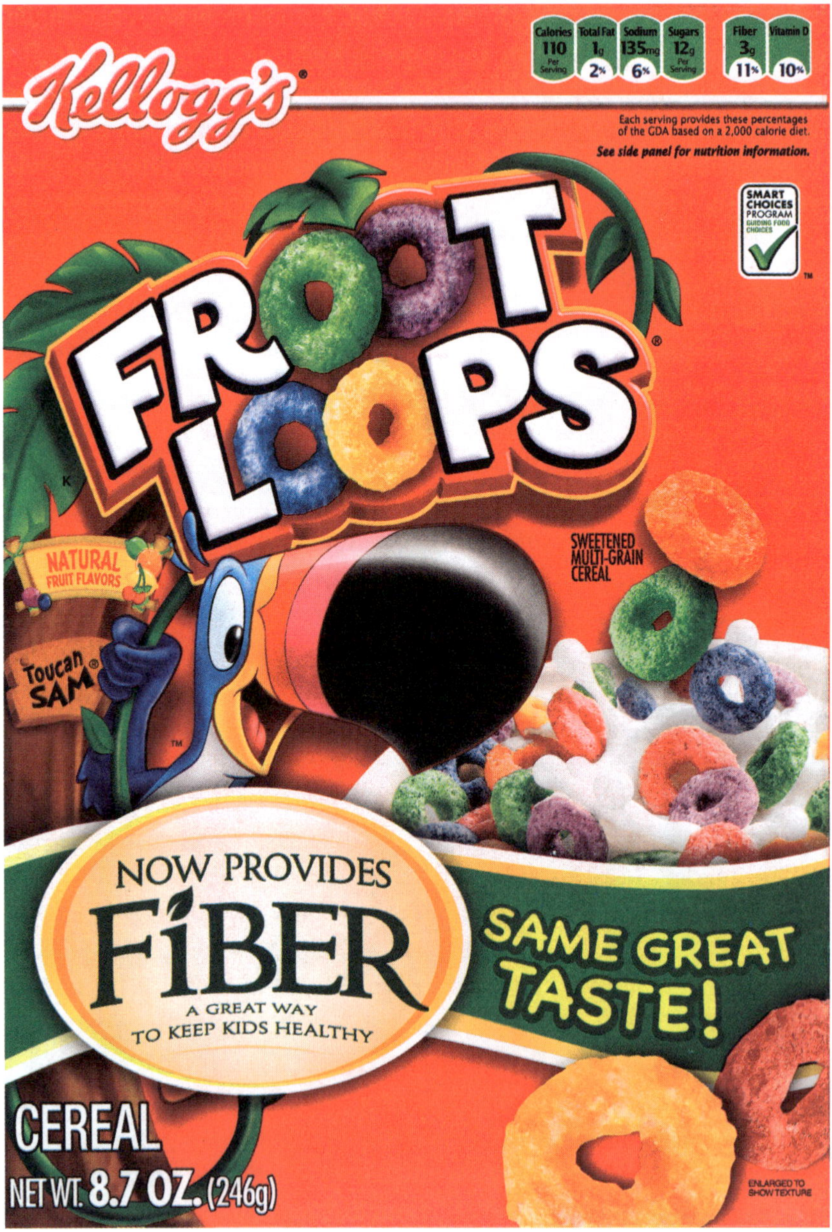

FIGURE 23 The SMART CHOICES check mark in the upper right corner of this 2009 box identified Kellogg's Froot Loops as an especially healthful choice—despite its sugar. Public ridicule ended the program within a few months of its launch.

Neuman's article quoted Eileen Kennedy, then dean of nutrition at Tufts University and chair of the roundtable's board: "Froot Loops was better than other things parents could choose for their children . . . you have a choice between a doughnut and a cereal . . . so Froot Loops is a better choice." This was soon rephrased as "better than a doughnut" or, as *The Economist* explained, "it's practically spinach."[5] Neuman also quoted the response from Celeste Clark, Kellogg's senior vice president for global nutrition: "Froot Loops is an excellent source of many essential vitamins and minerals, and it is also a good source of fiber with only 12 grams of sugar. . . . You cannot judge the nutritional merit of a food product based on one ingredient."

Michael Jacobson, the founding director of the Center for Science in the Public Interest (CSPI), was an original member of the roundtable but had resigned from it a year earlier. He explained to Neuman: "It was paid for by industry and when industry put down its foot and said this is what we're doing, that was it, end of story."

Other reporters revealed that the industry roundtable members paid fees ranging from $5,000 to $100,000 each, for a total of $1.47 million. Of this, $680,000 went to the groups managing the program, and the rest went for consumer testing. The funding explains why the ASN and others permitted generous nutrition standards. The more products that qualified for the Smart Choices symbol, the more money the program received—a blatant conflict of interest. Kellogg paid $50,000 or more but denied any conflicts: "Kellogg joined many others in the industry in investing in the development of the Smart Choices program to help consumers make informed food choices."[6]

Froot Loops is hardly a paragon of nutrition; at the time, sugar was its first ingredient; it had no whole grains and only 1 gram of fiber. Kellogg quickly addressed these last deficiencies; it raised the fiber to 3 grams (via whole-grain corn and oats, oat fiber, and soluble corn fiber) and produced a new box with a fiber banner shown in Figure 23.[7] Whether adding fiber converts Froot Loops into a health food is debatable; it's still a sugary cereal aimed at kids.

The fallout from the bad press happened right away. The FDA warned the Smart Choices board that the agency would be concerned if Smart Choices "used criteria that were not stringent enough to protect consumers against misleading claims; were inconsistent with the Dietary Guidelines for Americans; or had the effect of encouraging consumers to choose highly processed foods and refined grains instead of fruits, vegetables, and whole grains." Change.org, "the world's platform for change," organized a letter-writing campaign to express outrage that nutrition experts were supporting Smart Choices and to demand that they "stop shilling for Kellogg's" and its "better-than-a-doughnut" program.[8]

Change.org was especially troubled by the endorsements of Smart Choices by major nutrition organizations. It sent letters to the presidents of the American Diabetes Association, the American Dietetic Association (now the Academy of Nutrition and Dietetics), and Tufts University's School of Nutrition Science and Policy calling for them to withdraw. All three groups did so—to the program's further embarrassment.[9]

Board chair and Tufts University Dean Kennedy wrote a letter to alumni saying *The New York Times* had "grossly misquoted" her and that Smart Choices should be valued for its rigorous scientific underpinnings, focus-group testing, replacement of multiple symbols, and ability to reach millions of consumers. She regretted the negative response and asked nutritionists to "have a respectful and open dialogue about these issues."[10] This did not help.

In October, Richard Blumenthal, then the Connecticut attorney general, threatened an investigation. The FDA announced it would start working on proposed standards for front-of-package labels. Faced with this level of opposition, the Smart Choices board said it was putting the program on hold. The ASN, which had managed to escape criticism despite its conflicted involvement, commended the decisions made by the FDA and Smart Choices: "ASN will continue to provide nutrition science expertise within the dialogue on front-of-pack labeling in order to best serve the interests of the health of Americans."[11]

By late October, it was all over. Smart Choices issued a public statement saying it would "voluntarily postpone active operations" but welcomed the opportunity to collaborate with the FDA on front-of-package labeling. Blumenthal announced that all the food companies involved in the Smart Choices Program had agreed to abandon it. The companies issued a final statement: "Our initiative should send a message to other food manufacturers that labeling must be completely truthful and accurate without hype or spin, especially when appealing to children." Tufts distanced itself: "Dr. Kennedy participated in the process as a nutrition scientist, independent of her role at Tufts. Tufts University is not involved in the Smart Choices Program."[12]

We leave the final word on this debacle to Tom Laskawy, then a reporter for *Grist*: "It's hard to see the 'Smart Choices' process as anything other than classic groupthink. . . . How else could a bunch of well-educated, presumably perfectly 'reasonable' people start a process that ends with Froot Loops, Frosted Flakes and Cocoa Puffs as 'Smart Choices'? . . . What's becoming clear is that the 'Smart Choices' program looks like it's turning out to be a very dumb move."[13]

The industry's response: Facts Up Front

In the wake of the Smart Choices fiasco, the food industry tried again. The Grocery Manufacturers Association (GMA, now the Consumer Brands Association, representing the consumer-packaged goods industry) and the Food Marketing Institute (FMI, now the Food Industry Association, representing food companies and retailers) created yet another voluntary front-of package (FOP) labeling initiative, Facts Up Front, in 2011 (Figure 22d); cereal boxes in 2026 still display it. They said its purpose was to improve the accessibility of critical nutrition facts, promote nutrition literacy, and help consumers achieve their unique dietary goals.

They created Facts Up Front by drawing on systems already in use by cereal companies. General Mills began using Nutrition Highlights icons on its boxes as early as 2007, and Kellogg used similar icons (shown in the upper right of the box in Figure 23) for Nutrition at a Glance, later called Nutrition Keys. These pulled information from the Nutrition Facts panel for calories and the negatives (saturated fat, sodium, and sugars) and allowed companies to include icons for up to two optional positive nutrients (fiber, protein, calcium, potassium and iron, and vitamins A, C, and D).

You might wonder why all this was needed, given that Facts Up Front provides no new information and is difficult to read and interpret. The explanation requires some history, but to get right to the point: the purpose of Facts Up Front was to preempt the FDA from developing its own FOP scheme that might reduce sales of the least nutritious products. The GMA and FMI had reason to be worried. Following the demise of Smart Choices, the FDA had started work on a new FOP scheme to supersede the symbols of individual companies.[14] It asked the Institute of Medicine (IOM) to evaluate the universe of FOP labeling systems and to develop one, unified system to replace all others.

The IOM committee appointed to take on this charge proceeded in two phases. First, it reviewed research on public understanding of about 20 FOP systems then in use, and it reported these findings in 2010 (phase I). Its unsurprising conclusion: the systems were inconsistent. One oat cereal, for example, earned three different scores in three systems: two stars in one system, an 84 out of 100 in another, and a score of 37 in a third. The IOM strongly recommended that labels display *only* calories and the negative nutrients. It cited two reasons for not using the positives: Using them would confuse consumers, and it would encourage unnecessary addition of nutrients for marketing purposes. *The New York Times* translated these decisions as "tell us how your products are bad for us."[15] While the IOM committee was working on phase II recommendations for a new FOP system, the FDA held off taking further action until release of that report.

With the FDA stalled, the GMA and FMI moved right in and introduced Facts Up Front in January 2011, first calling it Nutrition Keys, as did Kellogg. Later that year, GMA and FMI rebranded it to Facts Up Front to align with their concurrent "consumer education" (public relations) campaign.[16]

The reason for the industry's preemptive strike was obvious; food companies did not want the FDA to impose anything like the UK's recently developed traffic light system. That, in fact, was much like what the IOM committee had in mind; its phase II report also appeared in January 2011. It again recommended that any FOP system use only calories and nutrients to discourage. It suggested a point system based on levels of saturated fat, sugar, and sodium, as well as a symbol including zero to four check marks or stars, with calories highlighted in a circle. Under this system, unsweetened cereals like oatmeal would qualify for up to four checks or stars, but sugary cereals would not qualify for any.[17]

The GMA reacted to the threat of FDA action by defending its just-released Facts Up Front and accusing the agency of nanny state overreach: "Food and beverage companies have developed a real-world program that delivers real value to real consumers in real time . . . consumers have said repeatedly that they want to make their own judgments, rather than have government tell them what they should and should not eat."[18] In the face of intense industry opposition, the FDA ignored the two IOM reports—never referring to them again—and told GMA and FMI that it would use "enforcement discretion" (meaning do nothing) about Facts Up Front. Soon after, the FDA added a new objective to its strategic plan for 2012 to 2016: "Explore front-of-pack nutrition labeling opportunities."[19] Explore? Didn't the IOM just do that?

And in 2014, to one-up the Obama administration's forthcoming revision of the Nutrition Facts panel, GMA and FMI put $50 million into promoting Facts Up Front.[20] Although cereal boxes continue to display these icons, the rest of the food industry mostly ignores them; they must not boost sales. The successor to GMA, the Consumer Brands Association, argues otherwise. In 2025, it did its own study, which conveniently revealed "overwhelming awareness, usage and trust of the Facts Up Front (FUF) label."[21] We have our doubts.

As for what is wrong with Facts Up Front, we think there's plenty. The IOM wanted FOP labels to be simple (easy to understand), interpretive (putting judgments in context), and scaled (indicating good, better, and best). Facts Up Front does none of these. It is a tool for selling, not buying.[22] Its purpose is to make cereal companies appear to be providing consumers with information to make better choices, but its real purpose was to head off FDA initiatives that might emphasize negative nutrients and discourage sales. In that, it succeeded—until late in 2024.

The FDA's "healthy" logo

Early in 2023, representatives of General Mills, Kellogg, and Post wrote to the FDA to object to its proposals for a revised definition of the term *healthy* and a symbol to go with it. They argued that setting minimums for whole grains and maximums for sugars would "exclude more than 95% of the major RTE [ready-to-eat] cereals on the market from making the healthy claim." The excluded cereals, they pointed out, included those currently eligible for the WIC program, and their exclusion "would potentially discourage the consumption of a top breakfast food choice in the US that provides many nutritional benefits."[23]

Even more, this letter contained an implied threat: The rule "would be open to legal challenge because it violates the First Amendment by prohibiting truthful, non-misleading labeling claims in an unjustified manner and also exceeds FDA's statutory authority in several ways." The companies called on the FDA to amend *healthy* to refer only to the content of *positive* nutrients and to raise the limit on added sugars.

The FDA had first defined *healthy* in 1994, permitting manufacturers to voluntarily use the term as an implied nutrient content claim—as long as their products did not exceed cut points for negative nutrients (total fat, saturated fat, cholesterol, and sodium) and did contain at least 10% of the Daily Value for one or more of the positives (vitamin A, vitamin C, calcium, iron, protein, or fiber). It said nothing about sugars. The FDA explained that it lacked a method for distinguishing between added and naturally occurring sugars and had no way to enforce a limit.

A further problem emerged in 2015 when the KIND company labeled some of its fruit-and-nut bars as healthy. The FDA objected; nuts were too high in fat to qualify. In response, KIND filed a citizens petition arguing that nuts are real foods and, therefore, healthy, which they are (in moderation). The absurdity of the existing definition of *healthy* induced *The Wall Street Journal* to produce a video demonstrating how the FDA considered Frosted Flakes to be healthy because the cereal is low in fat, but avocados to be unhealthy because their total fat exceeds the cut point.[24]

The FDA got the message, reexamined its definition, and told KIND it could use the term. But it planned to reevaluate its rules for nutrient content claims and solicit public comment on a revised definition of healthy. It spent the next several years conducting further research and working on a revised definition of *healthy* and design of its new symbol.[25]

In 2022, the FDA announced the proposed rule. To qualify as healthy, products must contain a meaningful amount of food from one of the food groups recommended by the Dietary Guidelines and adhere to limits for saturated fat, sodium, and added sugars.[26] Total fat and positive nutrients would no longer count, but food groups and added sugars would.

The FDA's 2022 proposal required cereals to contain at least ¾ ounce of whole grains and no more than 1 gram of saturated fat (5% of the DV), 230 milligrams of sodium (10% of DV), or 2.5 grams of added sugars (5% of DV). No wonder the cereal companies wrote that letter in 2023. Cereals like Honey Nut Cheerios (12 grams of added sugars) and Raisin Bran (9 grams) would not make the cut, nor would any WIC-eligible cereals with 6 grams.[27] The cereal companies proposed a far more favorable framework that would allow positive nutrients (read "fortification") as an alternative to the whole-grains requirement and would allow added sugars at 20% of the DV—four times the FDA's recommendation.

At the end of 2024, just before the newly elected Trump administration was about to take office, the FDA issued its final rule updating the healthy nutrient content claim, to take effect by February 2028. Despite vehement objections from cereal companies, the FDA kept the whole-grain requirement intact (pun intended). It granted a slight concession on added sugars, doubling the limit to 10% of the DV, allowing cereals to have up to 5 grams per serving—still below the WIC cut point. Under this rule, regular Cheerios could be labeled as healthy, but Honey-Nut Cheerios could not. For the first time in 30 years, the *healthy* definition would largely align with nutrition science and dietary guidelines. Overall, the healthy symbol emphasizes the positives and appears likely to summarize the positive criteria in a simple check mark.[28]

But to complicate the matter, as discussed next, the FDA was also working on another FOP label initiative based only on negative nutrients. How the Trump administration would reconcile the differences between the FDA's healthy/all-positive and FOP/all-negative proposals remained uncertain at the time of this writing. But the relevance of the updated *healthy* term and symbol is clear; few cereal brands can qualify for it.

The FDA's proposed Nutrition Info icon

In 2022, a White House Conference on Hunger, Nutrition, and Health released its *National Strategy* to end hunger and reduce diet-related disease. This urged the FDA to propose an FOP labeling scheme that would empower consumers, particularly those with little nutrition knowledge, to quickly and easily identify healthier foods—10 years after the FDA had commissioned those now forgotten IOM reports.[29]

With this mandate, the FDA once again set to work. It reviewed the recent literature on FOP labels, particularly on international labels warning about excessive saturated fat, sugar, salt, calories, and, sometimes, caffeine and artificial sweeteners (see Figure 44 in Chapter 17). In 2022 and 2023, the FDA developed designs and tested them in focus groups. The Reagan-Udall Foundation, which supports the FDA, held a public meeting to present the designs and gather opinions about them.[30]

This meeting was part of the foundation's Nutrition Partnership Project, which Kellogg and Nestlé underwrite. The proposed designs for an icon ranged widely; some resembled Facts Up Front, some were black and white, while others used traffic light colors.[31] The meeting revealed surprising levels of agreement among participants from industry and academia. The icon should be mandatory, be easy to understand, and focus only on nutrients to avoid—the negatives (sodium, saturated fats, and added sugars).

While the FDA was testing designs, the CSPI petitioned for a mandatory FOP label, and the FDA published initial proposals for just that in July 2024. Immediately after the November 2024 election, which gave Donald Trump a second term as president, the FDA sent its completed proposal to the lame-duck Biden White House, hoping to get it released for public comment before the new administration took over. Just days before Trump's inauguration, the FDA got the go-ahead to release its proposal.[32] The FDA's new Nutrition Info icon ranks the negatives as low, medium, or high and gives DV percentages. Figure 22f shows one possible option for the icon.

We view this proposal as a baby step forward. An icon like this is better than Facts Up Front, but it looks too much like it to be much of an improvement. We consider it inferior to traffic lights and also to the warning labels now in use in Latin American and other countries, by now well established to discourage sales of products high in undesirable nutrients. Other researchers consider it inferior to comparative labels such as *good*, *better*, or *best*.[33]

One month after the Trump administration took office, it implemented a "regulatory freeze pending review." But on February 28, 2026, Secretary of Health and Human Services Robert F. Kennedy Jr. appeared on the influential *Joe Rogan Experience* podcast to announce that the administration would define ultra-processed foods by April, "and as soon as we do that, we're going to do front-of-package labeling. So every food in your grocery store will have will have a label, maybe a green light, red light, or a yellow light telling you whether or not it's going to be good for you." We can't wait to see it.

CHAPTER 11

DIET CLAIMS

FADS AND FANTASY

BREAKFAST CEREALS MIGHT well be the first diet foods. Since Dr. Kellogg served bran flakes at The San, diet fads have come and gone. Cereal companies rarely miss chances to capitalize on the latest diet fad by creating new cereals or finding clever new ways to market old ones. Analysts project that the weight-loss and diet-management market will be worth $628 billion by 2032, driven by obesity, cardiovascular disease, and the quest for health.[1] In 2023, the food industry made up two-thirds of this market, with Kellogg among the top diet-market leaders. This chapter presents some of our favorite examples.

Weight loss: The Special K way

Kellogg's Special K started out as a basic cereal in 1955. Today, it is a billion-dollar brand primarily marketed to women, who comprise 65% of its eaters. In the early 1960s, Kellogg promoted the cereal to everyone, men and women, as a "low-fat, protein breakfast that fits so many modern diets." But by 1970, the brand was in full weight-loss mode with ads saying, "If you're watching your weight, we've got breakfast figured out for you." A 1991 Special K box had a "fat-free" claim on the front, and you could write for a free personalized diet offer. A 1997 box offered customers a coupon for a free pack of Equal, the zero-calorie, artificial sweetener.

Weight loss became the sole brand focus in 2003 when Kellogg launched its "Special K Challenge," promising women they could lose 6 pounds in 2 weeks, as the box from 2006 shows in Figure 24. All dieters needed to do was to replace breakfast and lunch with a bowl of Special K. Indeed, yes. Replacing two full meals with a small bowl of cereal without eating much else should help anyone lose weight.

A company official said, "Our mission is to be a weight-loss partner, to go along with women for their whole day and whole week and give them solutions." As proof that replacing regular meals with calorie- and portion-controlled cereal could result in weight loss, the company promoted the results of a 2002 study (guess who paid for it).[2] With this, Kellogg kicked off a cereal weight-loss competition.

Weight loss: Calcium

We could hardly believe the claim on the Total Corn Flakes box from 2003 shown in Figure 25:

- "Lose More Weight" [in big print]
- "with 100% Daily Value of Calcium" [in smaller print]
- "As part of a reduced calorie diet" [in tiny print]

The back of the box explained: "For years, you have heard that calcium is important for strong bones. Now a recent study from a major university suggests that increasing calcium intake while cutting calories may help you lose more weight than dieting alone. Scientists believe that a calcium-rich diet may enhance weight loss while dieting by helping control how much fat we store and burn." Special K may have promoted cereal as a meal replacement, but Total Corn Flakes drew on dairy industry research to promote calcium as a weight-loss nutrient (if only).

The National Dairy Council was funding research to demonstrate the benefits of eating dairy foods, which are naturally high in calcium. Some studies measured how much weight people lost when consuming low-calorie diets supplemented with various levels of dairy foods and calcium.

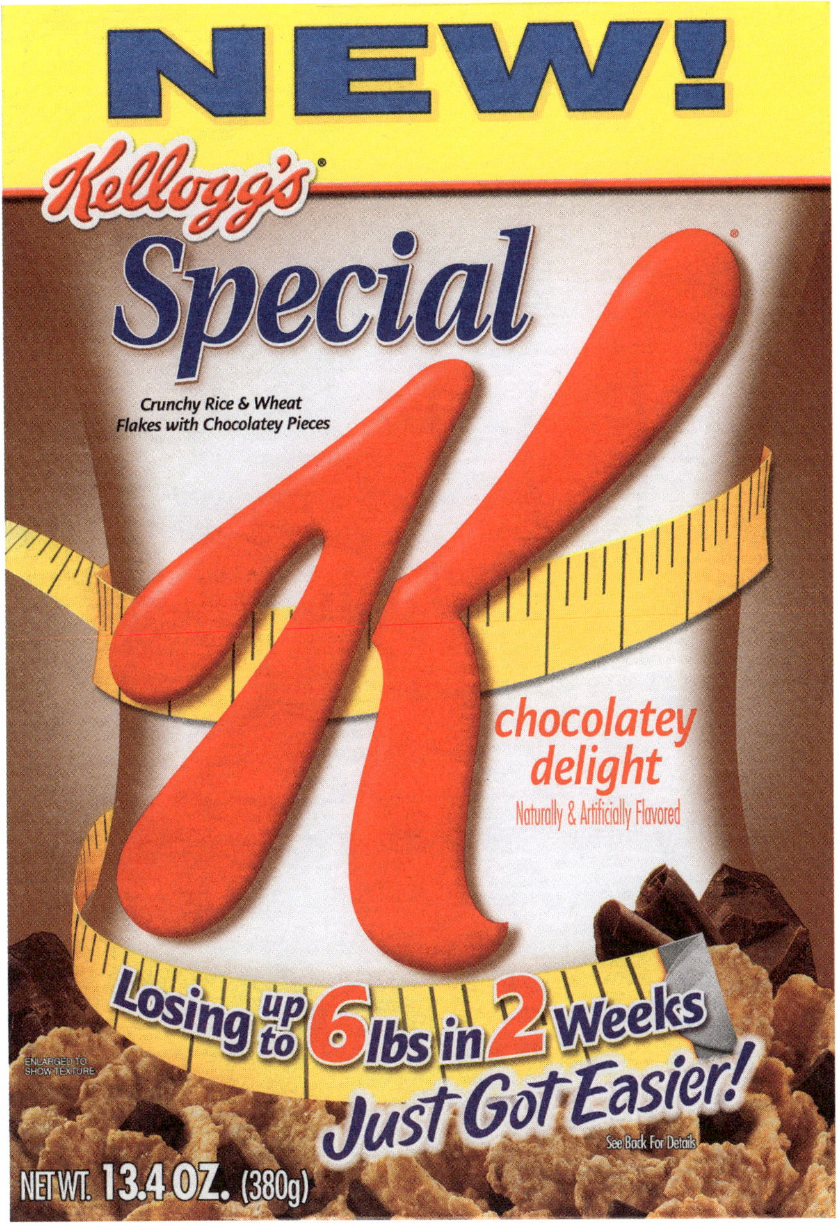

FIGURE 24 In 2006, Kellogg's Special K promised a 6-pound weight loss in 2 weeks—if this chocolatey delight cereal replaced two meals a day.

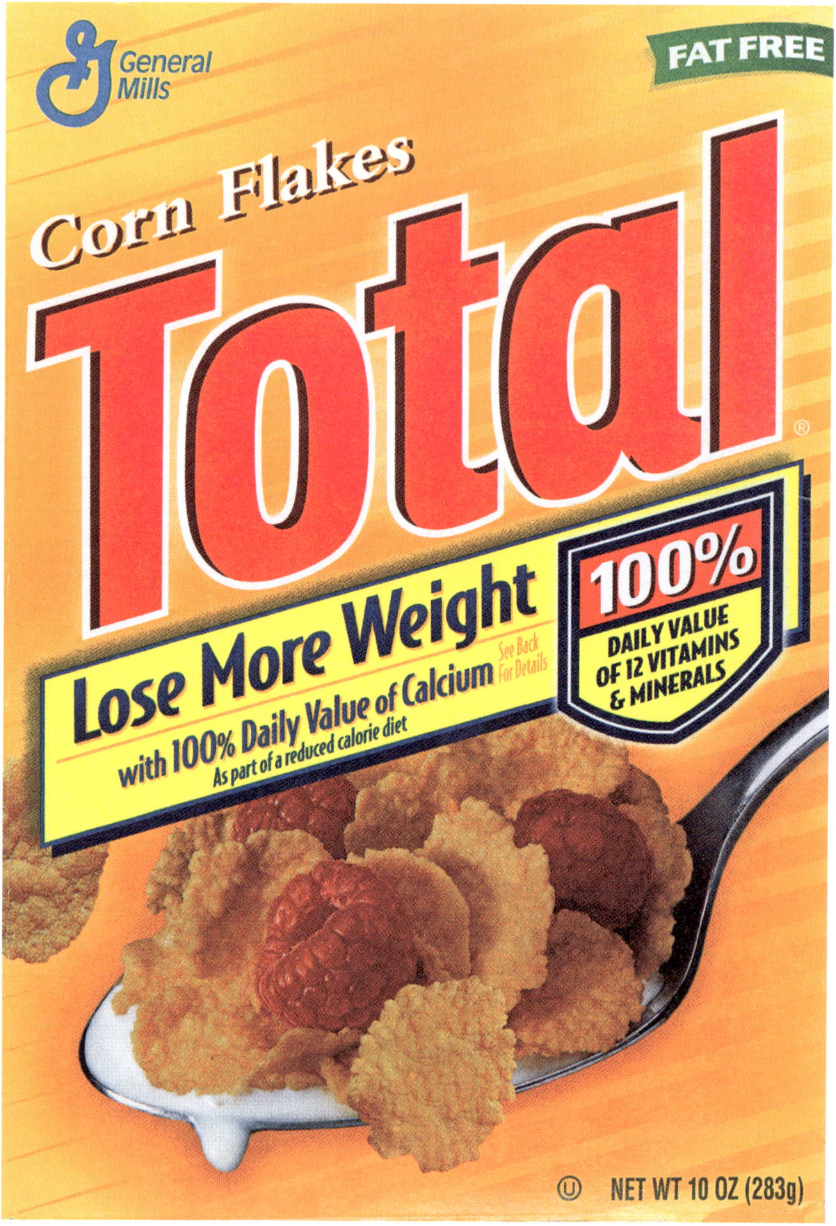

FIGURE 25 This 2003 Total Corn Flakes box from General Mills says calcium can help you lose more weight, but the small print advises, "As part of a reduced calorie diet."

The result: people who ate dairy foods experienced more weight loss, as did those who consumed more calcium.[3]

In July 2004, the National Dairy Council advertised these results in journals for dietitians: "Milk, cheese, and yogurt may help your patients lose weight." An ad in *The New York Times* (January 23) said, "Drink milk. Lose weight. Looking to drop a few pounds? Emerging research suggests that drinking 3 glasses of milk daily when dieting may promote body fat loss." The ads failed to mention calcium, the National Dairy Council's role in the research, or the lead investigator's patent on calcium as a weight-loss strategy, a conflict of interest characterized as a blurring of "the lines between science and marketing . . . for growth-desperate food marketers."[4]

Taking advantage of this research, General Mills launched calcium-fortified Total Corn Flakes, in competition with Kellogg's Special K. Television ads showed a woman stepping on a scale. She eats Special K until she is shown that Total has 100% of calcium's Daily Value whereas Special K has only 45%; this convinces her to switch to Total.

Post, not to be outdone, launched Bran Flakes with a banner: "Lose 10 lbs. the heart healthy way." How? The back of the box explains: "That's right! Research by a leading cardiologist shows that people who ate 2 bowls of Post Health Classics cereal each day, as part of a reduced calorie diet, LOST 10 LBS and reduced their risk factors for heart disease by decreasing blood pressure, lowering triglyceride levels (fat found in the blood), trimming waistlines." The explanation did not cite the research study, but by then, weight loss when cereals replaced meals had been demonstrated by several studies, most of them paid for by cereal companies, as had a more recent review of the topic.[5]

We must confess to particularly enjoying the idea of sugary cereals as weight-loss aids. A box of Post Frosted Shredded Wheat from 2007 (12 grams of sugar per serving but an "excellent source of whole grain & fiber") says, "Why diet hungry? Help satisfy your hunger while you lose weight." This statement is followed by, in typically illegible print, "as part of a reduced calorie diet and exercise plan." That should work.

The weight-loss claims, absurd as they were, did not last long. Post eventually abandoned them, General Mills discontinued Total Corn Flakes, and by 2014, sales of Special K were declining after a decade of gaining market share. In 2015, Kellogg's CEO said Special K would end its 2-week challenge because it was "basically asking people to deprive themselves where they have less calories."[6] We thought that was the point. Today, Special K focuses on "weight wellness," which still sounds like dieting to us. Sales for the brand continued to decline in 2024.

Weight loss: The South Beach way

Would you believe a South Beach Diet cereal? The South Beach Diet was one of the most popular diet trends of the early to mid-2000s. Created in the 1990s by cardiologist Dr. Arthur Agatston, it was originally intended to help reduce cardiovascular risk. His 2003 book was a *New York Times* bestseller and sparked the development of a line of South Beach foods. This included cereal, surprising because the diet required limiting almost all carbohydrates for 2 weeks. After that, the complex kinds could be added back, making room for whole-grain cereals.[7]

But by the end of 2004, low-carb weight-loss diets were less popular. Nevertheless, Kraft Foods tried to capitalize on the trend by launching a line of foods that included South Beach Diet Toasted Wheats cereal. It attempted to position the brand beyond low-carb as a "whole health" solution, marketing it as an "excellent source of whole grains."[8] The "lightly sweetened whole grain" cereal contained 210 calories per serving—hardly low in calories—but did provide 6 grams of protein and 8 grams of fiber.

But by 2009, this cereal had disappeared. In 2015, Nutrisystem, a weight-loss company, bought the South Beach Diet brand for $15 million, planning a relaunch. *U.S. News & World Report* recognized both weight-loss brands as among the "10 best commercial diets" (meaning best-selling).[9] But South Beach Diet cereals are no longer in the supermarket aisles. This particular fad faded away—for now.

Special diets: Gluten-free

Since 2015, original Cheerios have been labeled gluten-free, a designation that ought to be redundant, since oats do not contain gluten proteins. But the claim takes advantage of the growing popularity of gluten-free products, and it alerts people with celiac disease (who must avoid gluten) and those who would like to avoid gluten that Cheerios are safe to eat. But are they? Not everyone thinks so.

Gluten is one of the proteins responsible for the elasticity of yeast breads. Wheat is its major source, although it also appears in rye, barley, and triticale.[10] But oats can be grown, stored, processed, or transported in places where wheat or other gluten-containing grains or derivatives (wheat starch, barley malt) have also been stored, processed, or transported. Companies making gluten-free cereals must use meticulous operating procedures to keep gluten and non-gluten ingredients firmly separated. Gluten is seriously toxic to people with celiac disease.

Individuals without celiac disease digest gluten proteins into small chains of amino acids (peptides) and then into single amino acids with no ill effects. But celiac disease, generally understood to be a genetically determined gluten-induced autoimmune condition, causes the peptide fragments to induce a toxic reaction that destroys the lining of the intestinal tract, making it difficult or impossible to digest and absorb nutrients. People with celiac disease must scrupulously avoid eating even the tiniest trace of gluten. Under no circumstances should they be "glutened," unwittingly exposed to gluten in a food they had been assured was gluten-free.[11]

Celiac disease affects about 1% of the population, or roughly 3.3 million Americans. But many other people are allergic or sensitive to wheat—one of the nine food allergens required by law to be disclosed on food labels. And some people believe they are sensitive to gluten and avoid it. The market for gluten-free products is large and growing; by 2032, it is expected to be worth $14 billion, a doubling since 2022. Around 14% of millennials report eating gluten-free diets, the largest of any generational cohort.[12] To all these groups, "no gluten" is an important—and sometimes lifesaving—selling point. General Mills' introduction of gluten-free Cheerios, shown in Figure 26, appeared as a gift, and it came with an implied endorsement: "Proud sponsor of Celiac Disease Foundation, celiac.org."

But some members of the gluten-free community questioned the effectiveness of the method used by General Mills to remove contaminating grains from oats. This mechanical/optical sorting method involves sifting out optically identified contaminants and repeatedly testing for gluten during processing, to ensure that oats meet the gluten-free standard of the Food and Drug Administration (FDA): a gluten level of no more than 20 parts per million (ppm).[13] This standard converts to 20 milligrams of gluten per kilogram (2.2 pounds) of food, a minuscule amount. A serving of

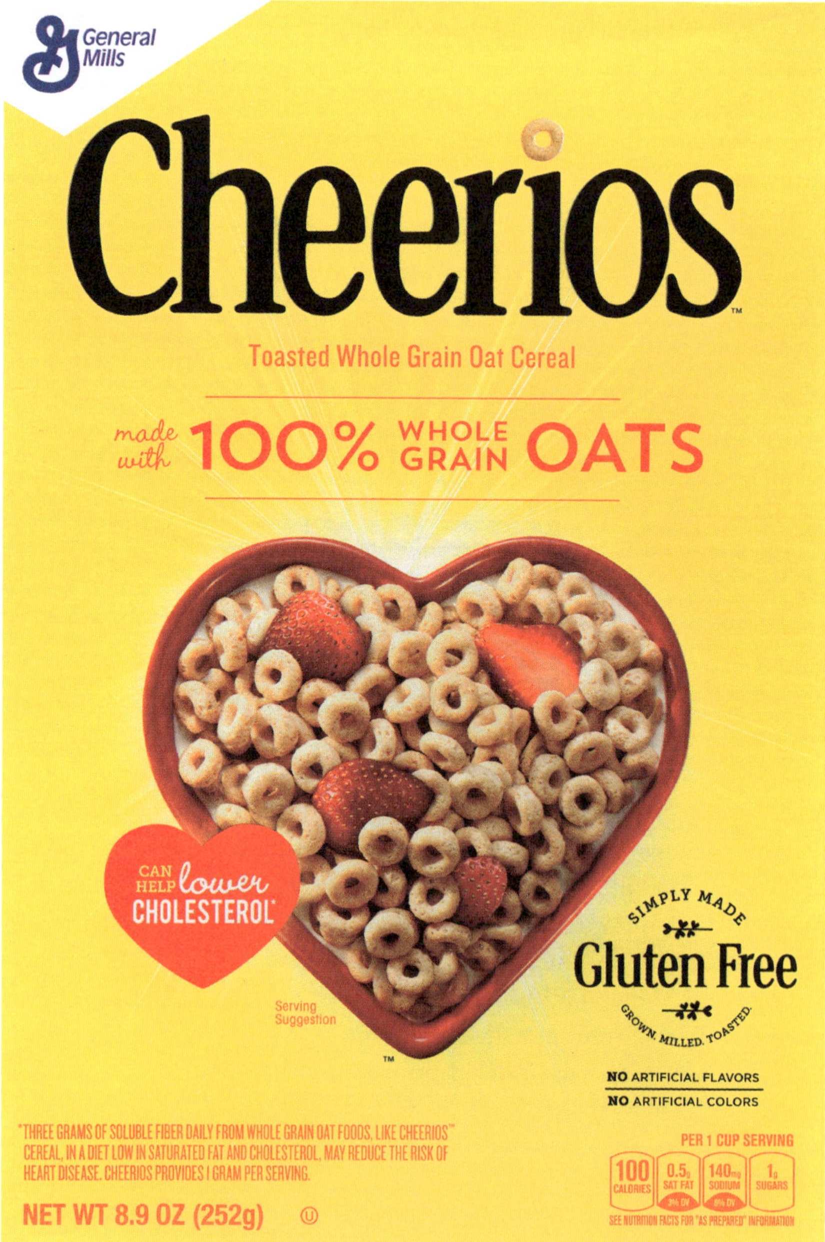

FIGURE 26 General Mills introduced gluten-free Cheerios in 2015. Oats do not naturally contain gluten but can become contaminated by gluten-containing grains during transportation and processing. It is possible to remove gluten contaminants, but some groups challenge the reliability of the methods used to do this.

Cheerios at that level would contain about half a milligram of gluten, which the National Celiac Association says should not cause problems for anyone. Its recommendation for people with celiac disease is to restrict daily total gluten intake to an amount 20 times higher—no more than 10 milligrams per day.

But the advocacy group Gluten Free Watchdog argues that the 20 ppm standard is too high; it prefers 5 ppm. In 2015, out of concern about the sorting method, it said it could not recommend gluten-free Cheerios to the celiac community. This was prescient. Within just a few months, General Mills had to recall 1.8 million boxes of Cheerios due to cross contamination with wheat during manufacturing. The FDA had received 136 complaints about adverse reactions to the cereal, 46 from people with celiac disease or gluten sensitivity. Although the company said it was embarrassed and "truly sorry" for the human error, lawsuits ensued.[14]

How likely are oats to be contaminated with gluten? The FDA says 20 ppm is the lowest level of gluten detectable by current methods and is tolerable for most people with celiac disease. In 2017, when the FDA tested more than 700 samples of products labeled gluten-free, only 1 exceeded the standard. Scientists at PepsiCo, which owns Quaker Oats, did a study to determine the potential for inadvertent gluten exposure. It found 10 of 132,000 lots of oats to have more than 20 ppm gluten. Whether this minute level of contamination is acceptable depends on point of view. Under pressure from the Canadian Celiac Association, General Mills removed the gluten-free label from Cheerios sold in Canada in 2017, but it retains the label in the US.[15]

Gluten Free Watchdog monitors this situation closely. In 2021, its own testing found occasional boxes of Cheerios to exceed 5 ppm gluten, but none exceeded 20 ppm. On this basis, it said, "Whether or not you choose to eat Cheerios is your personal decision." In 2023, difficulties with the oats supply chain caused the group to update its advice: "First and foremost, everyone with celiac disease or a gluten-related disorder must make their own decision whether to eat gluten-free oats and what brands to eat. . . . As of now, Gluten Free Watchdog cannot recommend any brand of gluten-free oats."[16]

Its highly cautious position is understandable. In 2024, another private group, Consumer Lab, tested several brands of rolled oats (not Cheerios) for gluten. Most brands had gluten levels below 2.5 ppm, as gluten-free as possible. But it found Quaker 100% Whole Grain Oats to have a gluten level approaching 700 ppm, a potentially unsafe level.[17]

What to advise? Most people with celiac disease should do fine with gluten-free Cheerios or any of the dozen-plus other General Mills cereals labeled gluten-free. We wish that gluten were listed along with other allergens on Nutrition Facts labels and that manufacturers of products labeled gluten-free would test them for gluten and make the test results readily available.

Special diets: Keto

Like many diets, the keto fad goes in and out of style every few years. This one attracts endorsements from celebrities, which bring it more attention than it deserves. But cereal companies never pass up a good diet trend that might boost sales. Kellogg introduced Special K Zero in 2022 to help satisfy the "food mood" of its consumers.[18] This cinnamon-flavored puff cereal is marketed as "keto-friendly" and claims 2 grams of net carbs, 0 grams of added sugars, and 20 grams of protein.

The ketogenic (keto) diet emerged in the 1920s as a treatment for epilepsy. Typically, this diet provides 70%–80% fat, 10%–20% protein, and only 5%–10% carbohydrate (in contrast, recommended diets allow up to 35% fat and range from 45% to 65% carbohydrate). If followed diligently, the keto diet is so low in carbohydrates that it forces metabolism to replace sugars with ketones (acid by-products from fats) as brain fuel, helping to resolve seizures in people with epilepsy. This fat-burning metabolic shift allows the diet to be promoted for weight loss, blood sugar control, and mental clarity, but its value for these purposes has limited—and much contested—research support.[19] As with any diet, people on keto diets will lose weight any time they reduce calorie intake below expenditure.

The keto diet soared to popularity in the 1970s in the form of the Atkins diet—a low-carbohydrate, high-fat, ketone-producing, and ostensibly weight-loss-inducing diet. The Atkins diet became popular again in the 1990s, faded out, and experienced a resurgence in 2019. A *U.S. News & World Report* survey found 84% of people on keto diets were doing so to lose weight. Although keto diet research rarely shows long-term benefits for weight loss, *keto* had over 24.5 million searches on Google in 2020, making it the leading food-related topic of interest. And in January 2026, Walmart lists "Keto-friendly" as one of its six featured food and diet trends. A quick search returned over 100 keto-tagged cereals. The keto diet market is expected to reach $15.6 billion by 2027.[20] No wonder cereal companies want in.

General Mills introduced three varieties of Wonderworks keto-friendly cereals in 2020, each containing 3 grams "net carbs"—referring to digestible and usable carbohydrates.[21] The back of the boxes said, "Remember how happy you were when you got to dig into your favorite bowl of cereal as a kid. Wonderworks Keto Friendly Cereal is like that except with 3 grams of net carbs." The cereals contained milk protein, whey protein, inulin (indigestible fiber), palm oil, corn fiber, and rice starch, and they were sweetened with allulose, erythritol, and stevia, none of this sounding delicious. Perhaps for that reason, the cereals disappeared by 2024. That year, General Mills launched a new brand—:ratio Trio—with the tagline "We do the math so you don't have to," referring to the net carb calculation. The :ratio Trio Maple Almond Crunch has 9 grams of net carbs and 7 grams of fat.

We wish there were a magic diet for weight loss, but the math is straightforward: eat fewer calories than you expend in basal metabolism and physical activity. If keto diets help you reduce calories, they will do the trick. Like all diet fads, this one is unlikely to last long, leaving cereal companies to move on to the next.

Special diets: Low-FODMAP

Early in 2025, we spotted a new widget—a stylized intestine with a blue background—on boxes of Kellogg's Frosted Flakes and Cocoa Krispies: Monash University's certified low-FODMAP seal (Figure 22g in Chapter 10). This required some investigation. The seal refers customers to a statement on a side panel: "One serving of this product is low in FODMAPs. A low FODMAP diet does not treat disease. Monash University receives a license fee for the use of the Monash University Low FODMAP Certified trademarks." Kellogg, we discovered, had arranged to have seven cereals certified as low-FODMAP in 2019 but didn't put the seal on the boxes until 6 years later.

Low-FODMAP is yet the latest diet said to promote gut health. The global low-FODMAP food category—yes, this exists—is projected to exceed $10 billion by 2027, due to worldwide complaints about digestive and gastrointestinal disorders, some of them brought on by the new anti-obesity drugs.[22]

FODMAP is the acronym for "fermentable oligosaccharides, disaccharides, monosaccharides, and polyols [sugar alcohols]"—short-chain carbohydrates or sugars that resist human enzymes but are readily digested and fermented by microorganisms in the large intestine. Microbial fermentation produces gas and water that can lead to gastrointestinal discomfort: bloating, cramping, and altered bowel habits. These symptoms can be especially debilitating for people with irritable bowel syndrome (IBS), which affects up to 15% of the US population.[23] While the cause of IBS is unknown, certain foods can trigger the symptoms through mechanisms believed to be mediated through the microbiome. Hence FODMAP diets.

Nutritionists at Monash University near Melbourne, Australia, developed a low-FODMAP diet aimed at minimizing symptom-triggering foods. The main sources of FODMAPs are wheat, rye, onions, garlic, legumes, dairy foods, foods high in fructose (honey, apples, and other fruits), and the artificial sweeteners sorbitol and mannitol. Diets low in these foods reduce symptoms in most people with IBS.[24] Symptomatic people are to switch to low-FODMAP foods (e.g., almond milk, Cocoa Krispies, or Corn Flakes) for a few weeks, then slowly reintroduce high-FODMAP foods to discover which foods they can safely eat.

Cereals derived from corn, rice, and oats—but not wheat—are naturally low in FODMAPs. To qualify products for the low-FODMAP seal, Monash tests them using sophisticated laboratory methods. Companies pay fees for a pre-assessment application, the testing, and annual licensing. The application fee is minimal ($16 per product), but the size of the other fees is not publicly available; companies must contact Monash for that information. Kellogg must think the cost of this certification is worth the price in reassuring customers that its low-FODMAP cereals, like "chocolatey sweetened" Cocoa Krispies (15 grams of digestible sugars per serving), will not add to their discomfort.

As obesity, heart disease, type 2 diabetes, and other health issues continue to increase, especially in parts of the world that have been transitioning to a Western diet, this creates new markets for diet-promoting cereals. We cannot predict the next trend, but have no doubt that cereal companies will find ways to profit from the global weight-loss and diet market.

CHAPTER 12

"GREEN" CLAIMS

NATURAL, ORGANIC, AND NON-GMO

CEREAL COMPANIES use the terms *natural*, *organic*, and *non-GMO* (non-genetically modified organisms) to convince you to buy their products. These "green" claims imply that cereals have been produced in ways that are healthier for the environment and for you. Many people care about how food is produced and are willing to pay higher prices for products grown in line with their own values. Companies can, and do, charge more for cereals using such terms.

Green claims were first used in the 1950s when concerns about the effects of industrial agriculture gained public attention. The increase in agricultural consolidation and consequent loss of small farms in the 1970s led to recognition of the hazards of "foodopoly"—corporate control of the food system, which resulted in deteriorating food quality and displacement of real foods by food products. "Crunchy granola" stores proliferated and attracted countercultural customers who wanted to eat food produced organically, without chemical pesticides, herbicides, and fertilizers.[1] Later, participants in this food movement protested against genetically modified foods and called for organic certification. They founded small cereal companies responding to such calls. Larger companies eventually snapped up many of them.

The meaning of *natural*

Kashi brand cereals, owned by Kellogg, came under fire in 2011 for its claims of "all natural"—but use of this term dates to the origins of Kellogg's Corn Flakes and All-Bran. To say the least, the meaning of *natural* is subject to interpretation. The Food and Drug Administration (FDA) does not help. It has not exactly ignored *natural*, but also has not defined what it means on food labels. Even for the notoriously sluggish FDA, defining *natural* sets a record. It began working on a definition in 1991, recognizing that the term was used "on a variety of products to mean a variety of things." Two years later, it published its first guidance: *natural* would simply mean "nothing artificial or synthetic (including all color additives regardless of source) has been included in, or has been added to, a food that would not normally be expected to be in the food."[2]

This left considerable leeway for food companies to use the term as they wished. But some wanted clarification. The Sugar Association, for example, petitioned for a definition that would permit it to advertise sugar as a "natural" sweetener. But in 2008, the FDA declined to provide further guidance. Doing so, it said, was not a priority.[3]

As for advertising, the Federal Trade Commission (FTC) also is no help. In 2010, it proposed Revised Green Guides, guidelines first published in 1992 to help marketers make truthful environmental statements about their products. Typically, the FTC goes along with FDA labeling decisions, so its green guidance followed the hands-off approach. The Natural Products Association was happy about that; it much prefers to let its member companies define *natural* however it best serves them.[4]

Natural serves them well. It has become the Wild West of food claims. In 2010, "natural" was among the most used claims on food packages and constituted a $22 billion industry.[5] Consumers conflated the term with *organic*. Enter Kashi, a California company founded in 1984 by two health food enthusiasts, acquired by Kellogg in 2000. Kashi set out to do what the FDA and FTC had not done—define *natural*—and use it to build brand loyalty, generate sales, and protect its slipping market share in the natural cereal space.

Kashi positions itself as a health-food brand. It started out in food co-ops and independent grocers but under Kellogg's ownership is now a Big Food brand. Kashi spent months creating a working definition of *natural* to use in marketing: "food that's minimally processed, made with no artificial colors, flavors, preservatives or sweeteners."[6] Kashi then conducted consumer research, drafted guiding principles, examined how other companies used *natural*, reviewed government and nongovernment position statements, and drafted technical standards for reviewing ingredients. It shared its definition and technical standards with professional and consumer advocacy groups like the Center for Science in the Public Interest. This was all part of Kashi's "Real Food" marketing campaign to win back customers who thought the brand had sold out to Kellogg and become too mainstream.

In 2011, Kashi labeled its cereals with "all natural" and "no artificial" claims, but these immediately came under fire. An independent health-food grocer in Rhode Island announced that his store would no longer sell Kashi cereals because, despite the "natural" claim, they contained GMOs. The response: "Kashi has done nothing wrong. . . . The FDA has chosen not to regulate the term 'natural.'"[7]

Then came the lawsuits. The first, filed in California courts, asserted that Kashi cereal was not "all-natural" because it contained not only GMOs, but also synthetic vitamins and soy ingredients processed with hexane (used in gasoline but considered safe for food by the FDA). The lawsuit named 10 Kashi cereal and granola products, among them Kashi GoLean Crunch, Kashi Honey Sunshine, and three granolas. All contained GMO ingredients from soy, corn, or canola. A similar lawsuit was filed in Florida.[8]

Kashi and its parent company, Kellogg, insisted they were merely following FDA guidance. But to avoid litigation, they agreed in 2014 to settle the first lawsuit and remove the claims from their cereals and other products. They also agreed to establish a $5 million settlement fund to allow consumers to recoup $0.50 per package for Kashi products with proof of purchase. The Florida case settled in 2015 with a similar $3.99 million fund. Kellogg continued to defend its position: "We stand behind our advertising and labeling practices. We will comply with the terms of the settlement agreement by the end of the year and will continue to ensure our foods meet our high quality and nutrition standards, while delivering the great taste people expect."[9]

If the lawsuits did nothing else, they induced further calls for a definition. In 2014, the Grocery Manufacturers of America (GMA), the trade group representing most Big Food companies and, since 2020, renamed the Consumer Brands Association, filed a citizens' petition asking the FDA to issue binding regulations that would define the meaning of *natural.* The group particularly wanted the FDA to allow products containing GMO ingredients to be labeled "natural." In contrast, Consumers Union (later called Consumers Union Action Fund) petitioned the FDA to ban "natural" claims altogether on grounds that they are misleading. Several federal district courts asked the FDA for an administrative decision on the term. In 2015, the FDA requested public comments on the matter. Three years later, again in response to citizens petitions, the FDA again called for comments on three pressing questions: whether it should define *natural*; if so, how; and how it "should determine appropriate use of the term on food labels."[10]

But by 2018, "natural" claims on food products had dropped by more than 50%, and the pressures seemed less intense.[11] In 2026, the FDA continues to be silent on the topic, no doubt hoping the matter will go away. More than 30 years after the FDA first began working on the claim, *natural* remains legally undefined. We suspect this no longer matters: "natural" claims can be risky—and costly—for food companies, and cereal companies have moved on to less contentious trends and claims. Kashi, for example, now uses the other "green" production claims we discuss here, USDA organic and non-GMO.

USDA certified organic

In 2006, Kellogg launched the Organic Raisin Bran box shown in Figure 27 with "Organic" covering its top third and a staff of wheat—the grain in this cereal—underlining the word. The USDA ORGANIC seal in the lower left corner of the box indicates that nearly all, at least 95%, of its ingredients are organic. Kellogg introduced organic versions of three popular cereals that year—the others were Rice Krispies and Frosted Mini-Wheats—but soon discontinued them.[12] We can only assume that the higher costs of organic production increased their prices, resulting in disappointing sales compared with conventionally produced cereals. The cost differential largely explains why so few organic cereals are in mainstream supermarkets. We mainly find them in health-food stores, where customers expect to pay higher prices.

What does *organic* even mean? To be labeled and marketed as organic, foods must be produced according to principles established by the Organic Foods Production Act of 1990 and regulations set by the USDA's National Organic Program in 2002.[13] Yes, it took the reluctant USDA 12 years to figure out how to define organic foods and set rules for their production. Why reluctant? Organic production methods are an explicit critique of conventional industrial agriculture. The organic standards require three main practices. Producers must

- not use any synthetic pesticides, herbicides, or fertilizers except those permitted by the National List of Allowed and Prohibited Substances,
- not plant genetically modified seeds, use fertilizer derived from sewage sludge, or treat the seeds or foods with irradiation, and
- keep records of everything they do and use and show the paperwork—and their farms—to inspectors from a USDA-accredited state or private certification agency, any time they are asked to, whether or not announced in advance.

Under the organic rules, farms are inspected at least once a year, and producers must keep records for 10 years. These requirements raise costs for farmers, and also for food manufacturers, retailers, and consumers.

Consider the Raisin Bran cereal shown in Figure 27: 95% of its ingredients must be organic. Wheat is the first ingredient, and sugar is second. In the United States, most wheat is grown according to standard practices, and most sugar beets are GMO; neither meets organic standards. For this cereal, Kellogg had to source organic versions of wheat, sugar, and raisins, but supplies of these are limited. Hence its higher cost compared with nonorganic Raisin Bran.

The USDA ORGANIC seal and labeling

The USDA also dictates how the term *organic* can be used for labeling and marketing, and it developed the seal along with the organic production standards. The National Organic Program website describes four categories for organic labeling and use of the seal:

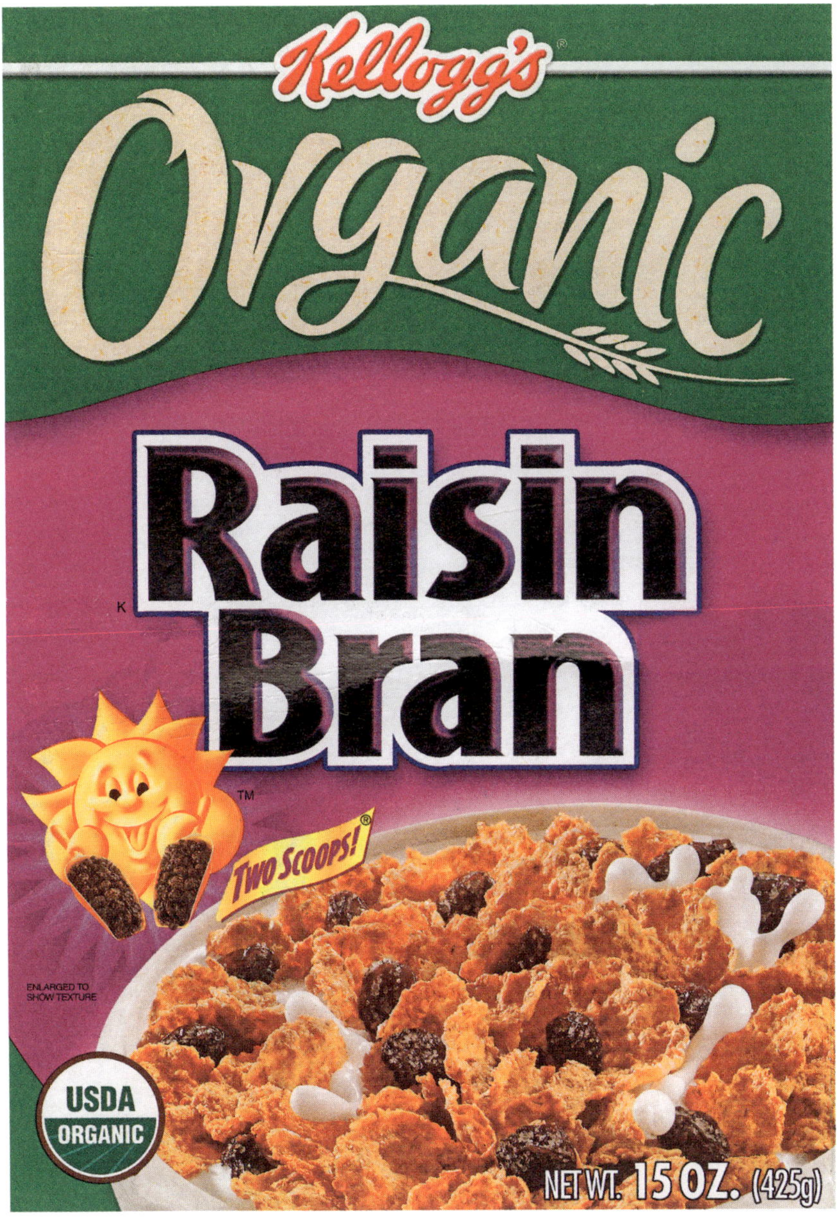

FIGURE 27 The name of this Kellogg cereal, released in 2006, tells consumers its ingredients are mostly organic, as does the USDA ORGANIC seal in the lower left corner.

100% organic: Foods with 100% organic ingredients (excluding salt and water) can use the USDA ORGANIC seal (shown in Figures 22h and 27) and "100% organic" claim.

Organic: Foods with at least 95% organic ingredients can use the USDA ORGANIC seal and "organic" claim (as in Figure 27).

Made with organic: Foods with at least 70% organic ingredients can use this claim and list up to three organic ingredients on the front of the pack; they cannot use the seal or be labeled as organic.

Specific organic ingredients: Foods containing less than 70% organic ingredients can only mention them in the ingredient list (e.g., Ingredients: organic wheat, organic brown sugar). They cannot display the seal or use "organic" elsewhere on the box.

To repeat: for a cereal to qualify for the seal, at least 95% of its ingredients must be organic, and all of its nonorganic ingredients, such as salt or vitamins, must be permitted by the USDA's National List of Allowed and Prohibited Substances. By regulation, organic cereals are never GMO (although some brands redundantly display the NON GMO seal). Most organic cereals are never 100% organic, because they contain synthetic vitamins or other approved additives. We think these are a minor concern and that 95% to 99% organic is worth buying if you can afford it.

In our supermarket explorations, we do not see the USDA ORGANIC seal on any of the best-selling Big Four mainstream cereals, although it does appear on the natural and health-food brands owned by those companies: General Mills' Cascadian Farm and Annie's, Kellogg's Kashi, Quaker/PepsiCo's Organic Oatmeal, and Post's Better Oats Organic. The organic seal can also be found on retailers' store brands, such as Good & Gather at Target, Simple Truth Organic at Kroger, and Full Circle at Tops, as well as on cereals from smaller companies sold in the organic sections of some large retailers or in food co-ops and natural food stores where the organic movement started.

Consumer Reports ranks certification seals according to what they require, how they operate, and how well they verify standards; it gives the USDA ORGANIC seal its highest rating, "excellent."[14] The seal is an easy and reliable way to identify organic cereals, and we wish manufacturers would produce more of them.

Are organics healthier?

Everyone asks us whether organics are healthier, but this question remains widely debated and is still unsettled. It might seem obvious that foods produced on healthier soils and without synthetic pesticides are healthier to eat, but the research is difficult to conduct and produces mixed results. For example, a Stanford evaluation of 233 studies examined nutrient intakes and health outcomes in people consuming organic versus conventional foods, but it found no significant differences. Another review of 35 studies found organic eaters to have reduced risks of infertility, birth defects, allergies, ear infections, metabolic syndrome, obesity, and non-Hodgkin's lymphoma, but the differences were small; the researchers said they could not make a definitive statement about organics' health benefits. More recently, a review of 25 years of research concluded that organic foods contained higher levels of iron, magnesium, and vitamin C, but again it concluded that the differences were too small to affect health.[15]

Our view is that growing food organically is not just about nutrition; it is about producing food in ways that are demonstrably better for the environment, exposing farmworkers—and eaters—to fewer harmful chemicals, and reducing ultra-processed ingredients and synthetic additives in foods. These are all good reasons to choose organic. We hope that one day organic foods will be democratized so all Americans can afford to eat them.

Big Four promotion (exploitation?) of organics

Big Four cereal companies have committed some of their "healthier" or "natural" brands to increased use of organic ingredients. They began doing this in the 2010s in response to class action lawsuits over the "natural" claims, as well as to meet consumer demands for more organic products.

In 2012, Kellogg-owned Kashi committed to purchasing 35 million pounds of organic ingredients and, in 2016, further promised to use "certified transitional ingredients" in their nonorganic cereals. *Transitional* refers to the 3 years required for conventional producers to grow foods organically before they can qualify for USDA certification. Kellogg pledged to work directly with farmers to provide financial and technical support during the transition years, to purchase transitional crops at a fair price, and to provide farmers with market access. This was good news for the organic movement.

Kashi also partnered with Quality Assurance International, a USDA-approved organic certifying group, to develop a Certified Transitional program, the first such standard. Kashi launched the first-ever cereal made with wheat grown on transitional farmland in 2016—Dark Cocoa Karma Shredded Wheat Biscuits—marketed as "Made with Transitional Wheat" with the Transitional Certified icon. The back of the box has a picture of a farmer accompanied by the statement "This cereal is not organic" and a description of Kashi's commitment to organic production methods. In 2018, Kashi launched its first line of organic kids' cereals, Kashi by Kids, but soon discontinued them.[16]

General Mills has done much the same. In 2016, it announced support for the transition of 53 square miles of farmland in South Dakota to help expand its organic Cascadian Farm brand. Despite these efforts, only around 1% of all US farmland is certified organic—hardly enough to make a dent in supermarket food aisles.[17]

The good news is that organic sales are increasing. Globally, organic cereals brought in $38.8 billion in 2023, and revenues are projected to grow to more than $50 billion by 2032. In 2023, the top three organic cereal brands were Kellogg's Kashi, General Mills' Cascadian Farm, and Kroger's private label. Organic Trade Association surveys find millennials and Gen Z (born 1997 to 2012) to be more interested in buying organic foods than older generations.[18] Such "conscious consumers" increasingly care about health, sustainability, and knowing where their food comes from and what goes into it.

We predict the Big Four will eventually consider sourcing organic ingredients for mainstream brands. In mid-2025, Kroger was selling a 12-ounce box of Cascadian Farm Organic Raisin Bran for $4.69 (39 cents per ounce) but selling a 16-ounce box of Kellogg's conventional Raisin Bran for $4.99 (31 cents per ounce). In early 2026, Kroger's Simple Truth Organic cereals cost less per ounce than Honey Nut Cheerios and many other of its mainstream equivalents. The narrowing of the Kroger price gap is good news for the organic movement. As organic crops become more widely available, and consumer demand continues to increase, we expect the price differential to continue to narrow. This will make organic foods accessible and affordable for everyone.

Non-GMO Project Verified

In 2014, in response to petitions and pressures from "green" consumer groups and anti-GMO advocates, General Mills said it would no longer use genetically modified ingredients in its original Cheerios. The side panel said (and still did in 2026), "Not made with genetically modified ingredients." While some critics applauded the announcement, and others created a satirical cartoon version of the box with a big blue "NEW! No GMOs!" banner across the front, still others questioned General Mills' motives, suggesting that the company was only doing this to improve its bottom line.[19] GMOs are on the foods-to-avoid lists for many people. One distinction worth noting: a food can be non-GMO but also not organic; in contrast, all organic foods are non-GMO.

The term *GMO* is commonly (and pejoratively) used to describe plants, animals, or microbes containing DNA from the same or other organisms deliberately inserted to confer desired traits or benefits. In the US, the most common GMO foods are crops—corn, soybeans, sugar beets—modified to resist glyphosate (Roundup weed killer) or other herbicides, or to resist insect pests, or to do both.[20]

The GMO ingredients in cereals are most likely to be corn, corn syrup, or sugar. Indeed, unless corn and sugar are stated as organic, you have to assume they are GMO. Sugar beets, for example, account for more than half of US sugar; 95% of US sugar beets are GMO. Oats are not genetically modified, but because sugar beets and corn are, General Mills has to use cane sugar (not a GMO crop) and non-GMO cornstarch in its non-GMO Cheerios.[21] The company has not committed to sourcing non-GMO ingredients for its other cereals (including its 20-plus other Cheerios varieties), perhaps because of the cost and limited availability of non-GMO crops.

GMOs do not seem to be unsafe on their own, but genuine concerns exist about the potential carcinogenicity of the herbicides and pesticides used with them, the effects of the chemicals on nontarget insects and the environment, and the disproportionate economic and political power of the agricultural corporations that own this technology. In addition, GMO foods are not transparently labeled, leaving consumers who want to avoid them without much choice in the matter. Although few fresh foods are GMO, about 80% of the packaged foods sold in US supermarkets are likely to contain one or more GMO ingredients.[22]

The lack of labeling transparency is the result of a decision by the FDA when it first approved GMOs for marketing in the early 1990s. The FDA viewed GMO foods as safe and, therefore, no different from foods developed through conventional genetics. On that basis, and under intense pressure from Monsanto, an early owner of GMO crop seeds and glyphosate, the FDA decided against labeling foods as GMO—a big mistake in our view. If the FDA had required GMO labeling from the start, consumers would have had a choice, and the transparency might have promoted greater trust and fewer objections to GMOs, a point that takes us right to the Non-GMO Project.[23]

The NON GMO seal

Two natural food retailers founded the Non-GMO Project in 2006 in direct response to the nonlabeling of GMO foods. It has proved immensely effective in certifying products free of GMO ingredients. Companies submit products for an independent third-party review of each ingredient, including review of the manufacturing process and testing of high-risk ingredients (such as corn, sugar, and the like). By the early 2020s, the Non-GMO Project Verified seal appeared on more than 60,000 products from 3,000 manufacturers (Figure 22i in Chapter 10). The Non-GMO Project labels are easy to spot. They depict a monarch butterfly, a reminder of how the herbicides used on GMO crops destroy the milkweed habitats of these insects.[24]

In part to counter the project's extraordinary success, Congress passed the National Bioengineered Food Disclosure Law in 2016. This act required the USDA to set standards for labeling GMO products and ingredients, which it did in ways that seem deliberately obfuscating. It substituted the term *bioengineered* (*BE*) for *GMO* and provided so many loopholes for using its sunshine-on-a-farm seal that finding one in a supermarket is a game of "Where's Waldo?" Side panels of cereal boxes say "contains bioengineered food ingredients" or, in the case of Kellogg's Raisin Bran, "contains a bioengineered food ingredient." You have to guess which ingredient that might be. If anything, the USDA's use of *BE* rather than *GMO* and the hard-to-find labeling has sparked the proliferation of NON GMO seals.

In 2025, the Non-GMO Project was among the largest and most trusted third-party verification programs in use. Companies pay a fee to display the seal on qualified products. In 2023, the program reported $6.8 million in revenue. Its revenue growth is likely to continue; more than half of American adults report looking for non-GMO certification when they shop.[25] Like the USDA ORGANIC seal, the NON GMO seal has an "excellent" rating from *Consumer Reports*; it considers the verification system highly trustworthy and effective.

The Non-GMO Project website lists original Cheerios as a participant, although its boxes were not displaying the seal in 2026. But the NON GMO widget is permitted on 6 varieties of Post's Grape Nuts and Shredded Wheat, 18 varieties of Quaker oatmeal, and many of the Big Four "natural" brands like Annie's, Cascadian Farm, Kashi, and Barbara's, along with 200 or so brands from smaller niche cereal companies.[26]

Together, Non-GMO Project Verified products generated $45 billion in sales in 2023. Most impressively, sales of cereals displaying the seal grew nearly 16% from 2021 to 2023, compared with just 6.5% for cereals making other label claims. Cereals labeled both NON GMO and USDA ORGANIC do even better. General Mills says on its website, "In the spirit of transparency, we've enrolled several products—especially our organic products—in the U.S. Non-GMO Project." Its organic products, of course, are already non-GMO by regulation. We speculate that General Mills is not using the NON GMO seal on Cheerios because of the company's overall philosophy: "Ensuring safe and effective food production, while conserving precious natural resources, is a longstanding commitment for General Mills. We believe biotechnology can help."[27]

Ongoing GMO concerns

One reason for persistent distrust of GMOs is the presence in some cereals of glyphosate, the potentially carcinogenic weed killer sprayed on crops engineered to resist it. Oats, used to make Cheerios, are not GMO and should be free of this herbicide, but no such luck; glyphosate is routinely used to dry oats before harvest. In 2018, the Environmental Working Group (EWG) tested for glyphosate in 28 samples of kids' cereals made with conventionally grown oats. It found glyphosate in all of them. Worse, only 2 had levels of glyphosate considered "reasonably safe for children." The 26 high-glyphosate oat cereals included several varieties of Cheerios (but, reassuringly, not the non-GMO original), oatmeal, and other breakfast cereals. The EWG reported the highest glyphosate level—18 times higher than the benchmark—in Quaker Oatmeal Squares cereal. The EWG report must have generated some action. By 2023, the group reported significant declines in the amounts of glyphosate in oat cereals, although it judged them still higher than they should be.[28]

Despite the relative absence of glyphosate in the original Cheerios, General Mills was still faced with a class action lawsuit for failure to disclose trace amounts of glyphosate in it and Honey Nut Cheerios. A judge eventually dismissed the case on the basis that the complaint had "no allegation that the cereal purchased even contains glyphosate, never mind harmful levels of it."[29]

But GMOs in cereals continue to elicit protest. In 2024, the Organic Consumers Association organized a campaign: "Tell General Mills to reject GMO wheat." The USDA had—for the first time—authorized farmers to grow GMO wheat engineered to resist glufosinate, an herbicide raising enough health concerns to have been banned in the European Union since 2013. And in 2025, Moms Across America, which advocates for healthy communities, did its own testing of glyphosate in cereals, finding 90% to test positive, even those labeled organic. But the highest level—less than 30 parts per billion—was very low: 1,000 times below the action level set by the Environmental Protection Agency.[30]

The moral: if you do not want any GMOs, glyphosate, or glufosinate in your cereals, look for the NON GMO icon or organic labels. Organic cereals will always be GMO-free.

PART III

MARKETING

CHAPTER 13

MARKETING TO KIDS

IT'S GR-R-REAT!

CEREAL COMPANIES spend lots of money and time marketing to children. It's true kids can't drive to the store or purchase cereal on their own, but they can and do beg parents to buy things for them, a tactic marketers call "pester power" or the "nag factor." The Big Four cereal companies were among the first to target marketing directly to young children, using cartoon characters, toys, and prizes as enticements. Child-health advocates are especially concerned about these strategies because they so often promote consumption of the least nutritious cereals. Marketing appeals to kids' tastes and desires, and aims to establish lifetime emotional connections to specific brands.[1] Cereal companies are especially good at all this.

While we were writing this book, we were contacted by Kate Foster-Anderson, who asked if we could help her find the Kellogg cereal that offered a prize—a Schwinn bicycle—won by her husband, Trent, in a contest when he was a young boy. We could. In 1980, Kellogg advertised its "Stick up for breakfast and win a Schwinn" contest, inviting kids to draw a poster of their favorite Kellogg character eating a nutritious breakfast.[2] Nearly half a century later, Trent Anderson still treasures the letter from Kellogg announcing his win. He had drawn a picture of Toucan Sam hanging upside down from the branch of a tree, saying something like "No matter how you look at it, Kellogg's is a great start to your day!" Nostalgia and brand loyalty? You bet. In this chapter, we describe some of the tactics used by cereal companies to attract young consumers, even the very youngest.

Enticing kids with mascots

Cereal companies attract kids with brightly colored boxes, mascots (cartoon characters), and prizes. You know immediately that a cereal is for kids when you see the bright blue Frosted Flakes box with Tony the Tiger, or the red Trix box with its silly rabbit. And for decades these cereals have been advertised to kids on television and through other channels. Kids instantly recognize a cereal by its name, box color, or mascot, and grab it off the shelf—or pester their parents for it. Surely, the best-known cereal cartoon mascot is Tony the Tiger, who stares happily at kids from cereal shelves with its tag line "Frosted Flakes, They're GR-R-REAT!" Big Four companies view mascots as advertising ambassadors, brand icons, and trade characters. Kellogg has Toucan Sam (Froot Loops) and Snap, Crackle, and Pop (Rice Krispies). General Mills uses Trix the Rabbit and Sonny (Cocoa Puffs). Quaker has Cap'n Crunch. Mascots appeal to children through emotional connection and storytelling, creating brand loyalty that lasts long into adulthood. Their use dates back to the Quaker man, who appeared on the Quaker Oats cylinder-shaped oatmeal canisters in 1922. Despite occasional facelifts, he remains much the same, a rare mascot targeted to adults; most are aimed at kids.

When Post introduced Sugar Crisp's three bears—Dandy, Handy, and Candy—along with a catchy jingle in 1949, Kellogg wanted its own memorable mascot. The company turned to its advertising agency, Leo Burnett, for help. Burnett had created brand characters like the Jolly Green Giant, Pillsbury Doughboy, and the Marlboro Man. For cereals, it suggested research. When Sugar Frosted Flakes hit shelves in 1952, shoppers could choose between two mascots: Tony the Tiger and Katy Kangaroo.[3] The kangaroo didn't sell, but the tiger boxes flew off the shelves. Kellogg sent Katy to the mascot vault and focused on Tony. Marketers created a commercial slogan. With a deep, friendly voice, Tony gently roared, "Sugar Frosted Flakes, They're GR-R-REAT!" Frosted Flakes remains one of Kellogg's top-selling cereals.

Impressively, several mascots introduced more than half a century ago are still in use. Post launched Sugar Bear for Sugar (now Golden) Crisp in 1960; General Mills introduced Trix Rabbit in 1959, Lucky the Leprechaun for Lucky Charms in 1964, and Sonny the Cuckoo for Cocoa Puffs in 1965; and in 1963, Quaker Oats would bring to life the only mascot that has the same name as its cereal—Cap'n Crunch. Following Tony the Tiger, Kellogg released Froot Loops with Toucan Sam in 1963, and Dig 'Em Frog for Honey Smacks in 1972.

By the 1970s, the cereal aisle was full of wide-eyed, smiling cartoon characters, and companies paid slotting fees to place the cereals at kids' eye level. Cornell researchers discovered that if stores slotted mascot-illustrated cereals on shelves visible to small children, they sold better. Although the researchers noted that mascots appeared to make "incidental eye contact" with kids in the cereal aisle, General Mills said this was "absurd."[4]

Whether mascots really look at or reach out to kids, they surely sell cereal. We are not the only researchers to study cereal boxes. An analysis of the designs of more than 150 boxes found mascots to be one of the two most common features. Most telling, mascots were much more likely to appear on cereal boxes with the highest sugar content. Other groups have also reported mascot-illustrated boxes to provide more calories, sugar, and sodium, but less fiber and protein, than cereals targeted to adults. Studies report that kids think cereals with a character on the box taste better than cereals without one.[5] Except for the Quaker man, we do not see mascots on adult cereals like All-Bran, Shredded Wheat, or Total. Trix, as they say, are for kids.

Targeting babies and toddlers

We knew about cereal boxes featuring characters from television shows aimed at young children, such as *Sesame Street*, *Clifford the Big Red Dog*, and *Bluey*. But having grown children, we had not even heard of the kids' hand-movement dance song "Baby Shark" until reading about the Kellogg cereal aimed at devotees of what had become an anthem for toddlers (see Figure 28). Starting in summer camps in the 1990s, the song was recorded in several versions, but it did not take off until Pinkfong, a Korean entertainment company, posted its video version to YouTube in 2016. In

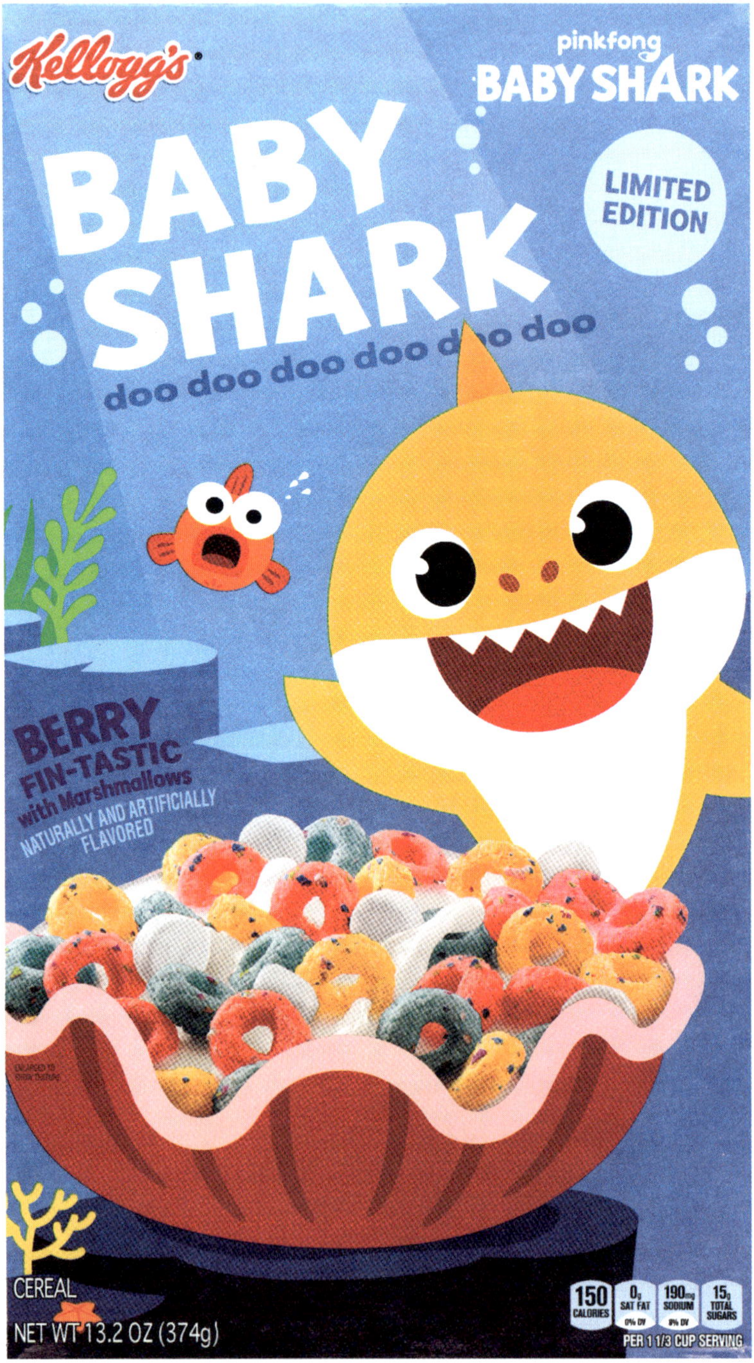

FIGURE 28 Kellogg issued this reversible (the back is illustrated with Mommy & Daddy Shark) limited-edition cereal box in 2019, remarkable for the exceptionally young age of its target customers: toddlers exposed to a Billboard Hot 100 tune, the Korean earworm "Baby Shark."

January 2019, the song reached an impressive 20.8 million streams per week and was number 32 on the Billboard Hot 100. By 2025, it had logged 16.2 *billion* views on YouTube.[6]

The "Baby Shark" song and movements are "wildly popular, wildly catchy, and ridiculously addictive," at least to adoring young children. Parents, we gather, listen to it at their peril; by some reports, it makes them want to cut their ears off, van Gogh style.[7]

In 2019, Kellogg teamed up with Pinkfong to launch the sugary cereal featuring berry-flavored loops and shark fin marshmallows, available only at Walmart and Sam's Club, but since discontinued it. Its ingredient list had sugars in four places, adding up to 15 grams per serving and 40% of calories. The especially complicated ingredient list, which came with brackets inside parentheses, showed this cereal to be decidedly ultra-processed; it contained four synthetic food dyes. Its marshmallows may have been "fin-tastic," but they were still candy. Do you really want your toddler eating candy for breakfast? And do cereal companies really market to babies? Apparently, they doo doo doo doo.

Targeting preschoolers: Before they can read

We love the colorful Froot Loops box promoting breakfast and literacy through its Feeding Reading program, shown in Figure 29. *The Very Hungry Caterpillar*, written by Eric Carle in 1969, is an award-winning book meant to be read to prekindergarten children. In this book, the caterpillar eats its way through increasing numbers of healthy fruits during a week, counting them along the way. But on the weekend, the caterpillar eats junk food and gets a bellyache—uh-oh.

In this new, giveaway version from Kellogg, the caterpillar conveniently eats its way through breakfast foods, including "two bowls of yummy cereal." It asks, "What kind of cereal do you like?" Froot Loops promotes the book, but the cereal on the book's cover looks more like Corn Flakes, and with strawberries—a much better choice. Junk food may give the caterpillar a bellyache, but Froot Loops appears to be exempt from that pejorative, despite its 12 grams of sugar per serving and artificial colors. In this classic cereal marketing strategy, parents are to submit their grocery receipts online for a free book. And this starts before kids can even read—this you can count on.

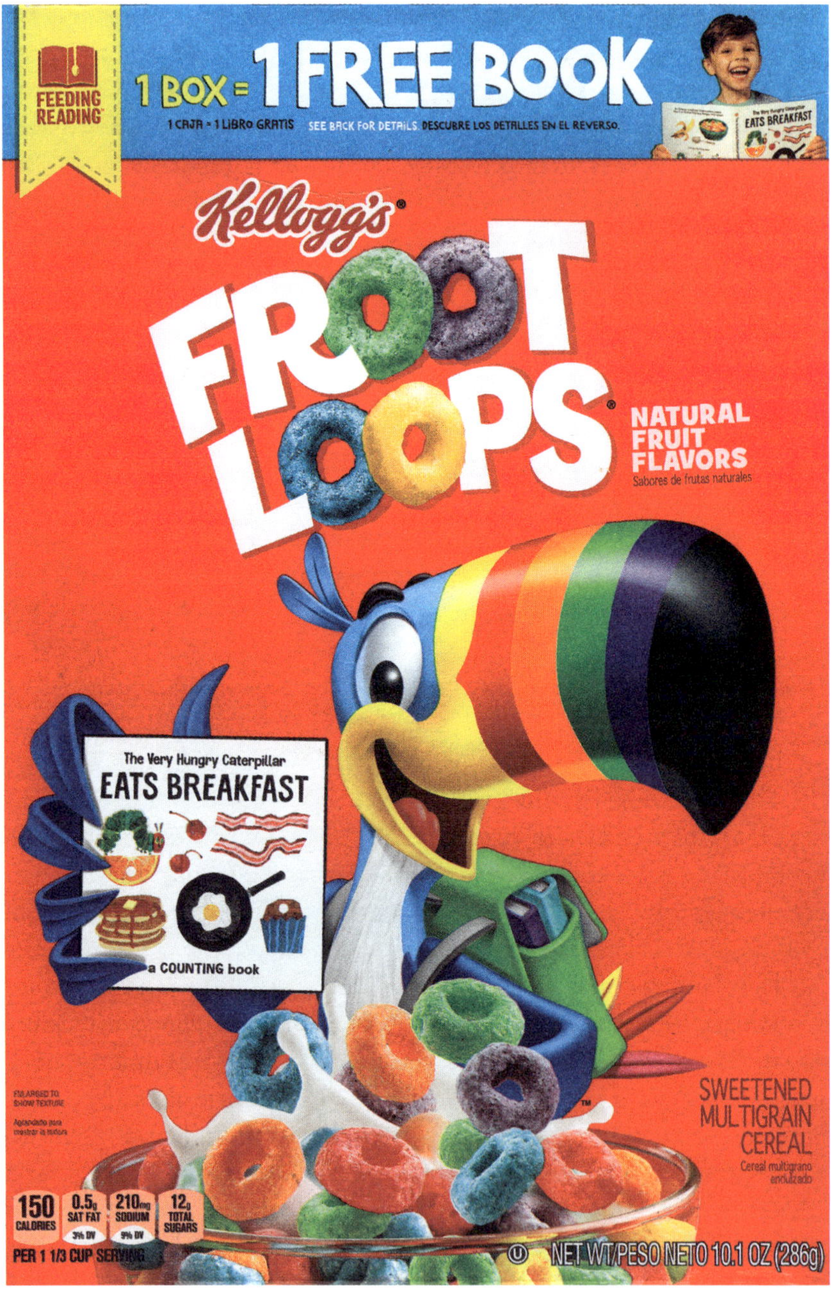

FIGURE 29 Kellogg promoted reading and breakfast with this 2023 Froot Loops box and *The Very Hungry Caterpillar* book giveaway to attract preschool kids.

Targeting kids of any age: Toys and prizes

One of us (LS) was a kid in the 1970s and could think of nothing more fun than a box of sugary cereal with a toy inside, and watching Saturday morning cartoons with cereal ads. Those days are gone; cereals now seem less entertaining and rarely contain collectible toys. Saturday morning ads have toned down. Advocates that we are for child health, we must count this as a win.

Toys, like the collectible globes illustrated on the Cap'n Crunch's Crunch Berries box in Figure 30, were coveted by children, who love free (with purchase) premiums, prizes, games, and toys. For this promotion, all boxes contained a globe, but only 1,000 boxes had a gold one. Kids lucky enough to get one of the gold ones could mail away for a $50 cash prize. Some prizes like these are only promoted on the back of the box, where that Kellogg bicycle contest might have been announced, but others are packed with the cereal.

This "fun globe" box enticed kids to "collect all 3," a sure way to promote multiple cereal purchases. Cracker Jack may have been first to put prizes in the boxes, but cereal companies quickly caught on. By the 1930s, General Mills was adding toys to its kid cereals, and Wheaties offered sports trading cards. Most cereal companies did this, almost always in their most sugary kids' favorites.[8] The in-the-box toys tend to be kitschy items like spy rings, decoders, peel-and-stick tattoos, model cars, balls and jacks, and this globe. They cost the companies pennies but are all that's needed to get kids to beg for the pricey boxes.

Although cereal boxes continued to offer toys until the early 2000s, the move to get rid of them as hazards and lures started much earlier. In 1987, General Mills had to recall 10 million "powerball" toys from Cheerios; a year later, Kellogg recalled 30 million toy "cool flutes" from Corn Pops, and binoculars from Rice and Cocoa Krispies; these toys presented choking hazards, violating the Consumer Product Safety Commission's small parts regulations.[9] Consumer advocates filed lawsuits. By 2010, the toys and prizes were largely gone from the boxes. At that point, advocacy efforts to curb marketing to kids mainly focused on television advertising.

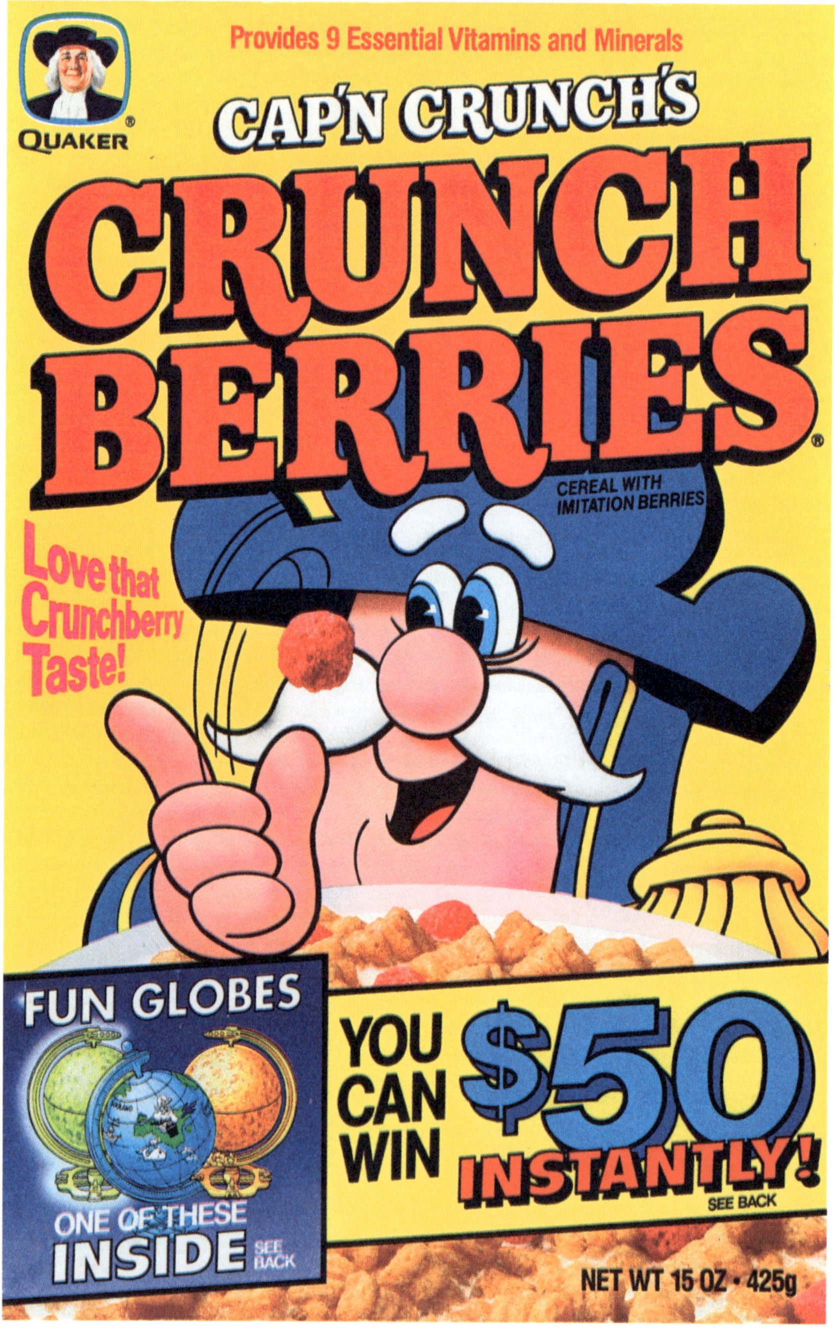

FIGURE 30 This 1987 Cap'n Crunch's Crunch Berries box from the Quaker Oats Company entices kids with one of three free collectible "FUN GLOBES" inside and a chance to "WIN $50 INSTANTLY!"

Restricting kids' marketing: Early attempts

Once upon a time in the late 1960s, Quaker Oats spent 80% of its advertising budget on Cap'n Crunch, helping it to become the number two presweetened kids' cereal. The Big Four had created television commercials featuring beloved cartoon mascot characters—Tony the Tiger, the Trix Rabbit, Cap'n Crunch—to run during Saturday morning cartoon programs for kids. But research in the 1970s found that young children could not distinguish television programming from advertising.[10] This cognitive limitation made them an ideal target group for food marketers, and it greatly concerned child-health advocates.

Alarmed by evidence that advertising to young children promoted sugary foods, that the prevalence of dental caries was rising, and that kids did not understand they were watching commercial messages, three advocacy groups—Action for Children's Television, Center for Science in the Public Interest, and Consumers Union—filed a petition imploring the Federal Trade Commission (FTC) to take action. The FTC attempted to do just that. Its efforts resulted in the ambitious but ill-fated 1978 initiative called "KidVid." Under Chairman Michael Pertschuk, the FTC proposed restrictions that would limit television advertising directed at children under age 8, particularly for foods high in sugar.[11]

Companies, including cereal companies, pushed back hard. They mobilized lobbying efforts, warned that children's television would collapse without advertising revenues, and convinced Congress that the FTC was dangerously overstepping its authority. The Association of National Advertisers (ANA) sued the FTC, saying that Pertschuk had prejudged issues involved in the rulemaking and called for his disqualification. Kellogg also filed suit and provided evidence supporting the ANA's case. Within 2 months, KidVid was over. The backlash was so effective that in 1980, Congress passed the FTC Improvements Act, removing the agency's authority to regulate children's advertising on television. By 1981, Pertschuk had been fired, and the FTC abandoned the effort.[12]

Instead, KidVid inspired self-regulation, the industry-sponsored Children's Advertising Review Unit of the Better Business Bureau, whose role is to promote responsible children's advertising (surely an oxymoron). To Congress, protecting industry profits mattered more than protecting children's health. Even more disheartening, the Federal Communications

Commission (FCC) dropped commercial guidelines for children's programming in 1984. Cereal companies could continue to market directly to children. Quaker could run commercials for Cap'n Crunch, which appeared as 5-minute mini programs, hardly distinguishable from regular programming.

Only with the Children's Television Act (CTA) of 1990 did Congress finally place some limits on advertising, and only during programming for children under age 12. Its guidelines were generous: no more than 10.5 minutes per hour on weekdays and 12 minutes on the weekends, hardly a serious limitation.[13] The FCC also required TV networks to implement 5-second program-commercial separations, or "bumpers," such as "we'll be right back after these messages" to signal to children when a show was ending and advertising was beginning. None of these measures really protected kids against the effects of advertising.

A decade later, health officials were increasingly alarmed by the rise in childhood obesity and the appearance of obesity-related adult diseases, such as type 2 diabetes, among school-age children. In 2001, the US Surgeon General issued a call to action to reverse obesity trends.[14]

In 2006, the Institute of Medicine (IOM) released a landmark report on food marketing to children. Its unambiguous conclusions: companies spent $11 billion a year to reach kids; television advertising influences kids' food preferences and intake and induces them to pester their parents for advertised products. The IOM warned companies that if they did not voluntarily stop marketing unhealthy products to kids, Congress should consider legislation.[15] The food industry response? Self-regulation, of course.

Cereal company self-regulation

In that same year, in response to the IOM report, a group of leading food and beverage companies, including General Mills and Kellogg, joined with the Better Business Bureau to form the Children's Food and Beverage Advertising Initiative (CFBAI). The member companies pledged to advertise products only to children older than 12 (later raised to 13) and only those products that met established nutrition criteria—which they set for themselves. General Mills and Kellogg agreed not to advertise products with more than 12 grams of sugars per serving, leaving most of their sugary kids' cereals as fair game.[16]

Because voluntary marketing restrictions were not particularly restrictive, the Obama administration wanted more rigorous ones. In 2009, Congress called on four federal agencies—the FTC, Food and Drug Administration (FDA), Centers for Disease Control and Prevention, and US Department of Agriculture—to form an Interagency Working Group (IWG) tasked with setting nutrition standards for marketing foods to children. Although the standards were meant to be voluntary, cereal companies objected to them from the start. When the IWG released its draft standards in 2011, we thought they were remarkably generous, but Kellogg and General Mills viewed them as far too restrictive. They submitted extensive comments, arguing that the standards would devastate the economy, destroy jobs, and violate commercial free speech.[17]

Kellogg's vice president of government affairs led food companies in creating the Sensible Food Policy Coalition to lobby for replacing the proposed IWG standards with those created by the CFBAI. The companies reportedly spent more than $60 million on lobbying, which included meetings with elected officials, letter campaigns, educational briefings, and media campaigns. Company officials, including those from Kellogg and General Mills, met with Valerie Jarrett, a senior advisor to President Obama, to express their staunch disapproval of the IWG and its proposed standards.[18]

This worked splendidly for the Big Four. Congress required the IWG to conduct a cost-benefit analysis, something impossible to do and not legally required because the guidelines were voluntary.[19] By late 2011, the IWG's work was finished; its standards were never finalized, and cereal companies returned to setting their own nutrition standards through self-regulation. The CFBAI released uniform criteria in 2014 and issued revisions in 2020. These now say that to be advertised to children, a serving of cereal must contain less than 200 calories and no more than 12 grams of sugars (no change) and contain 8 grams of whole grain or 10% or more of a nutrient of concern (vitamin D, calcium, potassium, or fiber). In 2021, cereal was the most-advertised children's food category, representing 43% of food ads viewed by children on kids' television programs.[20]

That same year, nearly 80% of food ads seen by children on kids' television programming were for CFBAI-approved items. Cereal companies view this as progress, but much of their advertising is for products hardly anyone might consider healthful. Researchers find the nutritional quality of foods marketed to children on TV—even those meeting CFBAI's criteria—to be relatively poor.[21] Cereal companies use 12 grams of sugars as the acceptable cutoff for what they can advertise, permitting most kids' cereals to qualify.

Even so, CFBAI's scope mainly applied to traditional media like TV. While kids' exposure to television advertising dropped by about half from 2009 to 2022, advertising is not disappearing; it is simply migrating to other media.[22] Although the CFBAI core principles now also apply to digital media and product placements, it is not clear how they are implemented or enforced. The World Health Organization has moved to fill this gap; it issued a report in 2023, *Restricting Digital Marketing*, in which it firmly recommended setting standards and enforcing them.

General Mills and Kellogg still advertise sugary cereals to children age 7 to 13; both companies have pledged not to advertise to children under the age of 6 (so much for Baby Shark). Post eventually joined CFBAI; it lists kids' cereals Fruity and Cocoa Pebbles as meeting CFBAI criteria. WK Kellogg created its own Nourishing Food Criteria; these allow up to 25% of the Daily Value for added sugars, conveniently the usual 12 grams per serving. In the wake of its acquisition by Ferrero, WK Kellogg must have withdrawn from CFBAI; it was no longer listed as a member in 2025.

Where does this leave us? CFBAI is a textbook example of industry self-regulation: well-intentioned on paper, modest in impact, and riddled with loopholes. Cereal companies will continue to market and advertise their best-selling sugary cereals to kids. As a food company executive once explained to one of us (MN), they have to. Their shareholders insist on it.

CHAPTER 14

TARGETING ADULTS AND FAMILIES

COMPANIES MARKET all cereals to adults in some way; adults do the buying. Adults are targeted with nutrition and health claims, diet trends, green claims, and the philanthropic tie-ins we discuss in Chapter 16. As we keep saying, cereal boxes reflect American culture like no other food product. Companies market cereals by drawing on the full range of pop culture elements: social media influencers, celebrities, music, art, holidays, and good old-fashioned nostalgia. Using these approaches, cereal companies aim campaigns at specific consumer segments (as marketers call them) identified by gender but also by age: baby boomers (born 1946 to 1964), Gen X (1965 to 1980), millennials (1981 to 1996), and Gen Z (1997 to 2012). Gen Alpha (2013 to 2025 or so) is still too young to control much spending, but at the older end surely influences family purchasing.

These groups have different experiences with breakfast cereals. Millennials are known for eating sugary cereals for snacks, dinner, and dessert. We love the Kellogg tagline "Whatever Froots your Loops," from a campaign to promote eating cereals outside of breakfast. Gen Z buys the most cereal—nearly 70% say they eat cereal once or twice a week—whereas only 45% of boomers do.[1] But even that smaller percentage is high enough to capture the attention of cereal marketers. Here, we present a few examples of how the Big Four use popular culture and nostalgia to sell cereal to specific demographic groups.

Boomer consumers

Cereal companies particularly target boomers for two reasons: they are a big demographic (about 68 million) and strongly brand loyal; they also happen to control more than $76 trillion of American wealth. Baby boomers grew up in an era when cereals were the breakfast of choice, and they view cereals as nostalgic and comforting; nearly half say they still love the same cereals they loved as children.[2]

But as boomers age, they become more conscious of their health. To cereal companies, the mix of nostalgia and health presents multiple marketing opportunities. Tapping into nostalgia, General Mills occasionally brings "retro" boxes back into circulation. In 2014, when cereal sales were declining, the company reintroduced five retro cereal boxes, among them Cheerios from 1954 and Lucky Charms from 1964. These were aimed at boomers to allow them to "be transported back to the time when these five cereals were introduced."[3]

In 2020, General Mills announced it would bring back the 1980s formulations for Trix, Cocoa Puffs, Cookie Crisp, and Golden Grahams. Each box declared its retro characteristics: Cocoa Puffs said, "more chocolatey taste," and Golden Grahams said, "Retro honey is back!" A Big G cereal representative explained, "Our fans crave a taste of nostalgia—and, while these four cereals have always remained popular, we've answered their requests and brought back the taste they remember from childhood."[4] But a cereal blogger (such people exist) observed that the "taste comeback needs to go back to square one," rating Cocoa Puffs "4 clinically sedated cuckoo birds out of 10."[5] Online reviews compared the retro cereals to cardboard and described them as "bland and flavorless."

General Mills, it seems, had not completely reverted to the 1980s formulas. The old Cocoa Puffs, for example, listed sugar as the first ingredient and cocoa third and contained partially hydrogenated oils (trans fats), artificial flavor, and 14 grams of sugars per serving. In the new "more chocolatey" retro version, whole grains came first on the ingredient list, and there were "only" 12 grams of sugars. The trans fats were gone (they had to be disclosed on food labels in 2006 and were essentially banned in 2015); the artificial flavors were also gone, and the puffs were smaller and denser. No wonder the cereal failed to evoke nostalgia.

Cereal companies perform better when they market health to this demographic. Boomers are living longer than previous generations and want to reduce their risk of age-related diseases. In 2010, as the oldest boomers were turning 65, cereal companies took notice. General Mills introduced the heart-shaped Cheerios "hearts matter" campaign wherein Honey Nut Cheerios "make heart health enjoyable." It ramped up marketing of its healthiest cereals, such as Fiber One, hitting all the right buttons for aging boomers: "with whole grain," "65% of daily value of fiber," and "0 grams added sugar." The company highlighted a "boomers pantry" in its 2010 annual report to focus on groups that drive sales. In 2019, a company representative explained this focus: "For people over 55, cereal is attractive because it offers certain nutritional benefits, like fiber" and the company would be "doubling-down . . . to clearly communicate [its] health benefits" to this segment.[6]

Kellogg also caters to the health concerns of boomers. It markets Raisin Bran as a source of fiber and potassium for heart health, All-Bran for promoting regularity and digestive health, and Smart Start's Antioxidants (see Figure 11 in Chapter 6) for better immunity and overall health.[7]

Looking ahead, the United States is expected to have more older adults than children by 2035. In 2025, WK Kellogg raised an alarm about declining cereal sales. Its CEO emphasized that customers are looking for cereal brands that focus on health and nutrition—and are willing to pay more for them.[8] Cereal companies are banking on this generation to keep cereal sales afloat.

Targeting women

Marketing aimed at women dates back to the earliest introductions of cereals. In 1914, Kellogg appealed to the women's suffrage movement with "Votes for Women" on boxes of Toasted Corn Flakes.[9] In later years, messages aimed at women featured empowerment, wellness, weight loss (Chapter 11), and convenience.

Kellogg is the king (or queen) of marketing to women with its billion-dollar Special K brand. In 2024, the company released a Special K limited-edition cereal targeted to millennial and pregnant women (limited editions are only available for a short time). The box, shown in Figure 31, displayed the 39-weeks-pregnant social media influencer and cookbook author Molly Baz, an all-time first for a cereal company. Older generations seeing this box would surely be reminded of the August 1991 *Vanity Fair* cover displaying Annie Leibovitz's then-scandalous photograph of pregnant actress Demi Moore covered by only a "handbra."

Baz was part of Kellogg's "Special for a Reason" marketing campaign, displaying photographs of inspiring individuals on boxes to "celebrate and empower women everywhere"—and to help make Special K more relevant to younger consumers at a time of declining sales. Baz proclaimed her love for cereal on the back of the box: "If you know me, you know I am a freak for cereal. Cereal got me through pregnancy in a very real way."[10] It also paid; she disclosed #paidpartnership to her 816,000 Instagram followers. Kellogg advertised this box only through social media channels and only sold it online. Non-millennials as we are, we snapped one up for a special reason—to write about it here.

Cereal marketers are particularly eager to reach Gen Z women, "on the forefront of music, art, design, fashion, gaming."[11] In 2023, Post produced one of our favorite examples of cereals targeted to younger women: Berry Pebbles. This limited-edition, bright purple box, with tricolored cereal, featured the women of Bedrock—Wilma and Pebbles Flintstone and Betty Rubble—with the slogan "Celebrating women who rock." The back of the box celebrated four groundbreaking women, among them Sally Ride, the first American woman in space, and Sara Christian, the first woman NASCAR driver.

Post recruited Susan Alexandra, a New York City fashion designer, to create this and other box designs as well as a Pebbles-inspired fashion collection. The company said it helped attract millennials and Gen Z: "Not only does this bring new consumers into the fold, but also reminds old fans of a nostalgic time in their childhood enjoying a bowl of Pebbles while watching Saturday morning cartoons." Nostalgia, indeed; 50% of Fruity Pebbles purchases comes from households without kids.[12]

Targeting sports lovers

Companies know the research: cereals with endorsements by celebrity athletes are more likely to be purchased than those without.[13] The marketing is aimed at specific groups. In Figure 32, we show a particularly

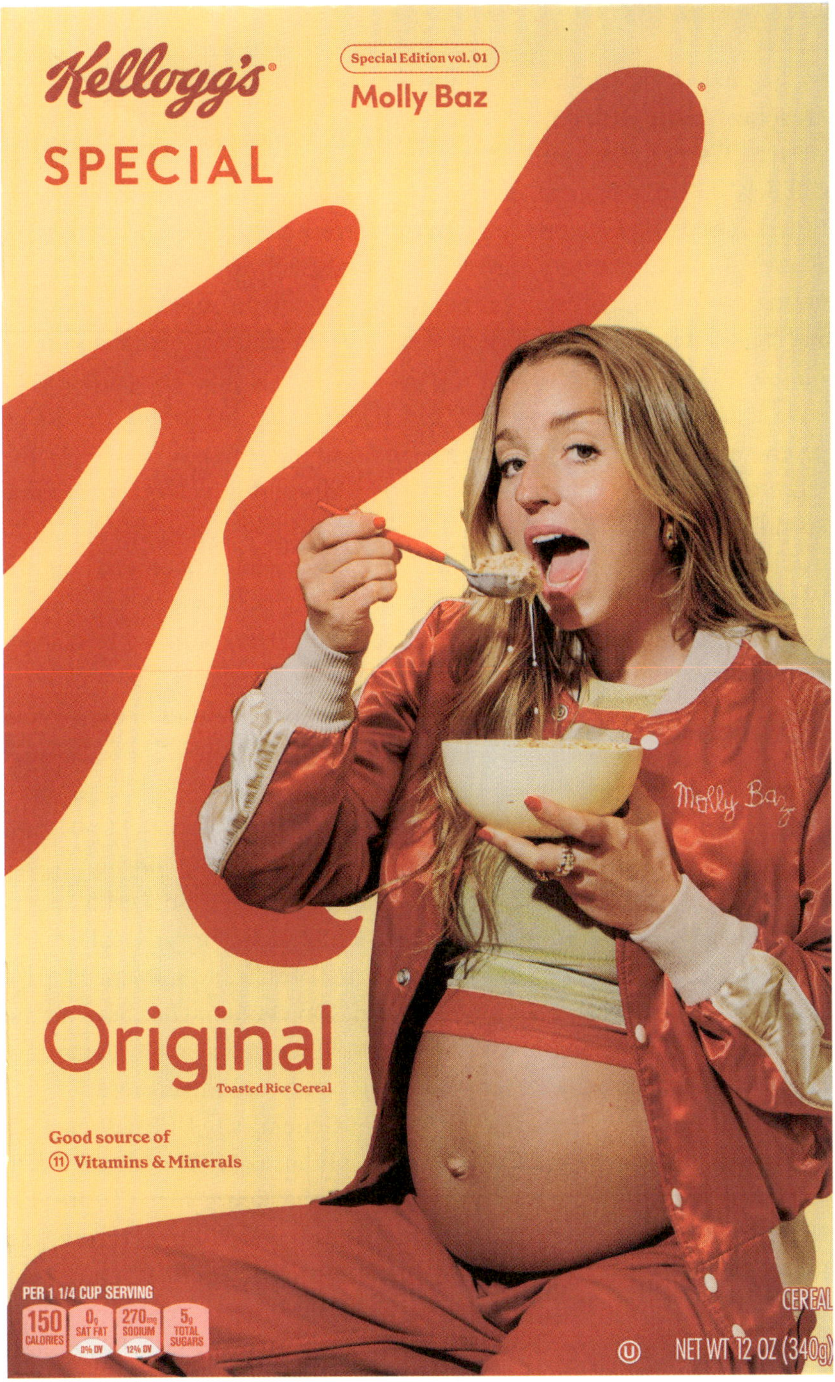

FIGURE 31 In 2024, social media influencer Molly Baz became the first pregnant woman to appear on a cereal box, this one from Kellogg. The message: "Special for a Reason." What reason? Selling cereal to women.

well-timed example, a box targeting Gen Z, all sports fans—and "Swifties." General Mills partnered with National Football League (NFL) football players Travis Kelce and now-retired Jason Kelce, just when Travis was publicly dating megastar pop singer Taylor Swift (they got engaged in 2025). Kelce Mix is a combination of the brothers' three favorite cereals—Reese's Puffs, Cinnamon Toast Crunch, and Lucky Charms—with a marketing campaign that went far beyond the box. It featured a cereal training camp attended by the Kelces, along with merchandise and ads on TV, online, and on social media; a 15-part video series (the Reese's Puffs episode logged 2.1 million views); and podcasts during which the Kelce brothers promoted their new cereal. To do all this, thereby "reigniting the culture of demand generation," General Mills had increased advertising spending by 43% between 2019 and 2024.[14]

That same year, General Mills also announced a partnership with Women's National Basketball Association star and fashion icon Angel Reese. Using a play on her name, Angel Reese's Puffs, the company released a series of four limited-edition boxes, explaining that "Angel's talents in basketball and fashion are an ode to the brand's classic dualities like chocolate and peanut butter, and cereal and milk." The box featured Reese holding a basketball while wearing an emoji cartoon crown.

Earlier that year, 18.9 million viewers watched the National Collegiate Athletic Association Division I women's basketball championship. It was the most-viewed game, men's or women's, ever, on the ESPN cable sports channel, and it made Angel Reese a household name for girls, college students, and basketball fans. Reese was the first athlete, ever, to appear on a Reese's Puffs box. She posted on Instagram, "Don't put me in a box, put me on one."[15] Her financial deal with General Mills was not disclosed, but using her star power makes sense for selling this candy-branded cereal.

These campaigns were a new venture for General Mills. Its past partnerships with athletes had mainly shown up on boxes of Wheaties, a lower-sugar cereal marketed to mostly male adults (see Figure 35 in Chapter 15). Using famous and culturally relevant athletes to market kids' cereals like Reese's Puffs and Lucky Charms was an innovative attempt to compensate for the declining sales of Wheaties—and target younger consumers.[16]

Usually, the appearance of an athlete on a cereal box is an honor and career booster, but sometimes there's an unexpected twist. One example is

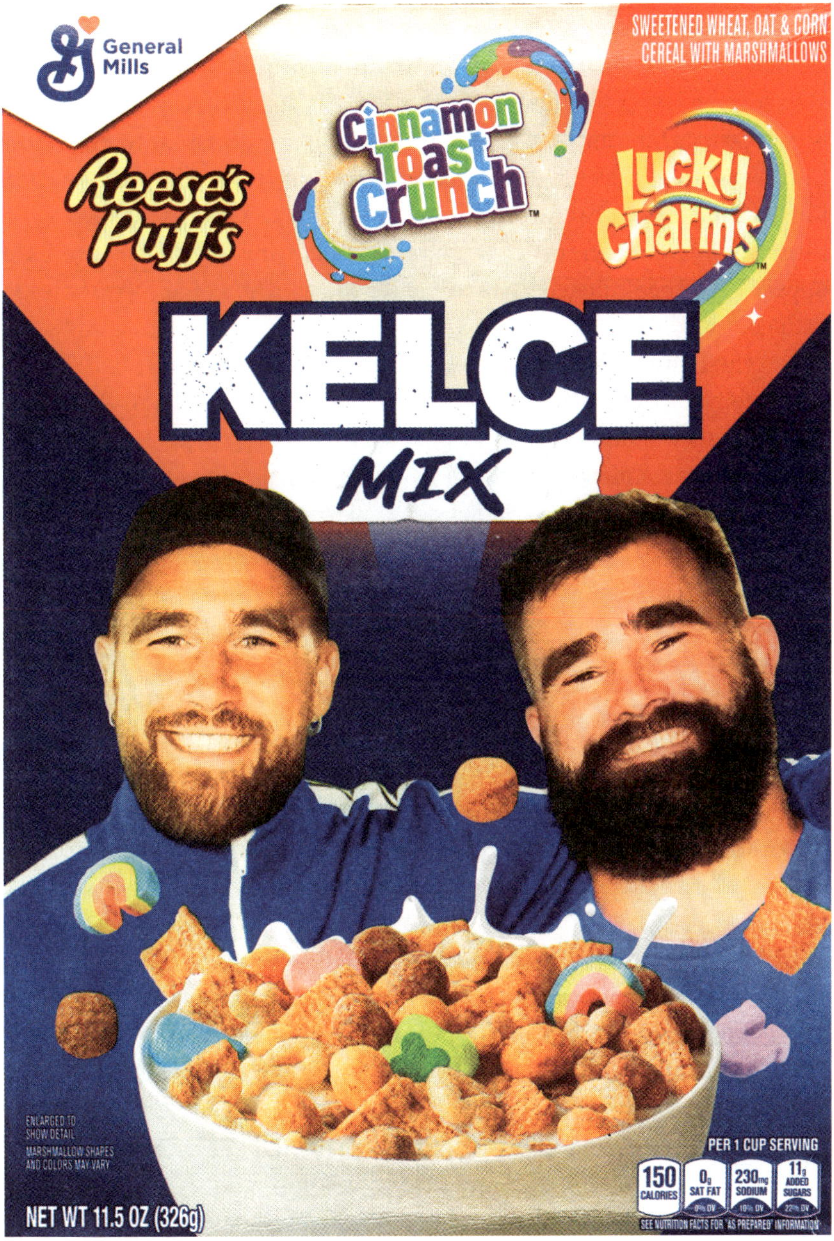

FIGURE 32 In 2024, General Mills featured National Football League players and brothers Travis and Jason Kelce, who picked their three favorite cereals for this limited-edition Kelce Mix.

the partnership between Kellogg and Olympic swimming champion Michael Phelps. He had been prominently featured on a General Mills' Wheaties box after winning six gold medals at the 2004 Olympics. But in 2008, Kellogg one-upped General Mills and signed the rights to Phelps for Corn Flakes and Frosted Flakes.[17] The partnership especially paid off when Phelps shattered world records in the 2008 Olympics, winning eight gold medals, more than any other Olympic athlete in any sport at the time. He appeared on the Kellogg's Frosted Flakes box with Tony the Tiger, holding up a gold medal.

But then things got not so GR-R-REAT! In early 2009, a British tabloid published a picture of Phelps with marijuana paraphernalia. At that point, Kellogg logged another first—the first company to drop a sponsorship agreement: "Michael's most recent behavior is not consistent with the image of Kellogg." Although Phelps apologized publicly, Kellogg did not forgive him, but its competitor, General Mills, did. It put Phelps on a Wheaties box in 2012 and yet again on its Lifetime Achievement box cover in 2016.[18] We love a good comeback story in America; General Mills cashed in on this one.

Marketing to all generations: Music

One way to reach consumers is through music. In 2024, General Mills announced a collaboration with TOMORROW X TOGETHER (TXT), a Korean K-pop boy band popular with Gen Z (the capital letters seem essential for such groups). Each of the five band members appears alone on a box of sugary kids' cereal—Cinnamon Toast Crunch, Cookie Crisp, Lucky Charms, Honey Nut Cheerios, or Trix. SOOBIN, for example, is paired with the rabbit mascot on boxes of Trix, as we show in Figure 33. In a Walmart exclusive, a TXT group photo also appeared on a sixth box, Reese's Puffs. General Mills said this collaboration constituted "a harmonious partnership to bring the refreshing energy of Gen Z's most iconic band to your breakfast table." Walmart also offered an exclusive TXT box of Cinnamon Toast Crunch with photo cards that could only be purchased online for $9. "Refreshing energy" indeed; the box sold out in minutes, leaving fans begging for more.[19]

Cereal and music for breakfast appeals to all generations and is not new. The most famous example is surely how a Kellogg's Corn Flakes commercial

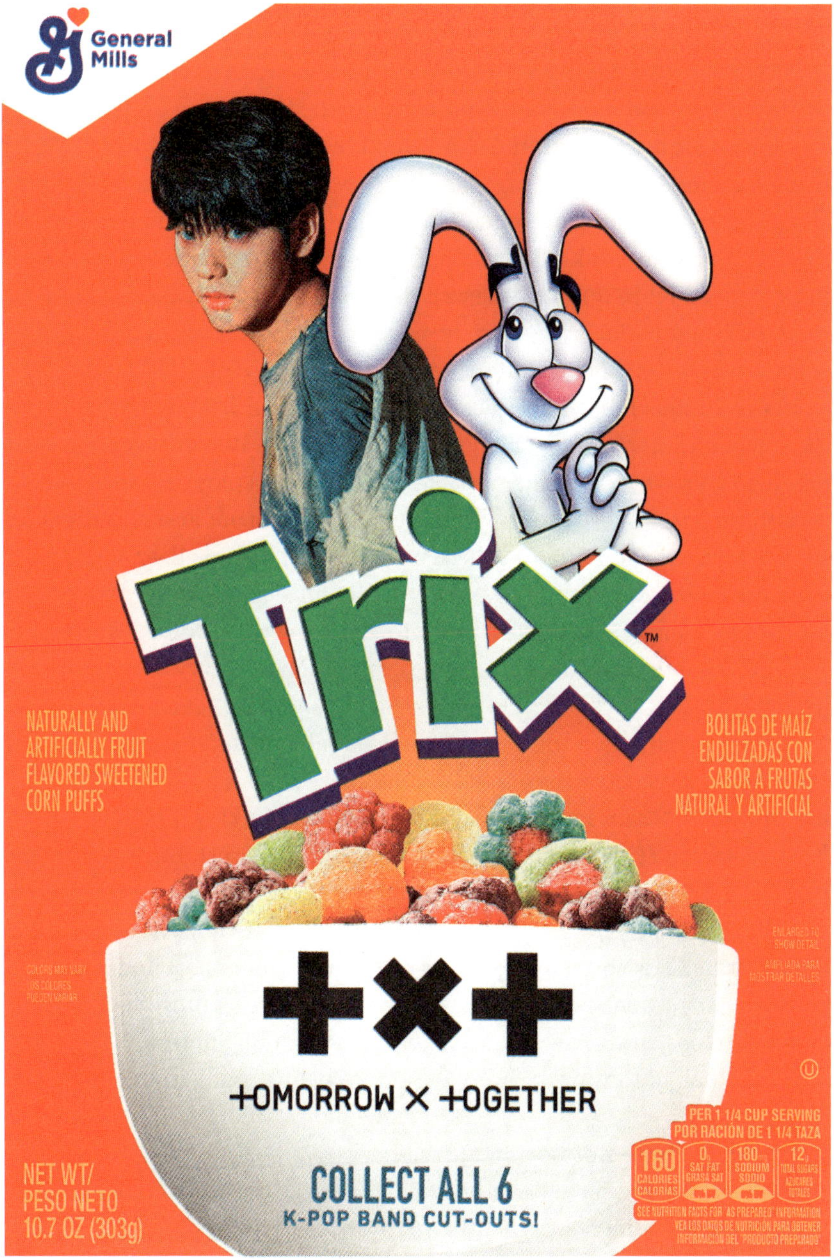

FIGURE 33 General Mills partnered with the Korean K-pop band TXT on a limited-edition series of five cereal boxes, each featuring a different band member, plus a sixth box featuring the group. This Trix box features band member SOOBIN, and it gives fans a stand-alone cutout figure of him on the back of the box.

influenced the Beatles' John Lennon. While writing songs with the television on in the background and repeatedly hearing the 1967 Corn Flakes jingle lyrics "Good morning, good morning, the best to you each morning," Lennon wrote a song with the title "Good Morning, Good Morning." The Beatles included the song on the *Sgt. Pepper's Lonely Hearts Club Band* album released that same year. The album starts with the crowing of a rooster. We like to think this was a nod to Cornelius, the Corn Flakes rooster mascot (see Figure 3 in Chapter 2). But "Good Morning, Good Morning" was not Lennon's favorite song; he called it "a throwaway, a piece of garbage."[20] Even Kellogg's marketers could not have scripted this story.

Using famous musicians in cereal marketing campaigns dates back to 1954, when General Mills partnered with Rainbow Records to print cardboard 45 rpm records on the backs of cereal boxes, a ploy said to have sold 30 million boxes of Wheaties.[21] Kids could cut these out and play them on a record player, and for many, these were the first records they would own. In an era before MTV, YouTube, and TikTok, musicians could release their new songs using cereal boxes ubiquitous in American homes and reach millions. That the music encouraged consumption of sugary cereals seemed irrelevant.

Post especially used music to market cereal, putting "Sugar, Sugar" by the Archies on Sugar Crisp, "ABC" by the Jackson Five on Alpha-Bits, and the Monkees' "I'm a Believer" on Frosted Rice Krinkles. The heartthrob Bobby Sherman (look him up) was the king of the cereal music box in the 1970s. He released four albums and more than 24 new songs with Post cereals, including "Hey, Mr. Sun" and "I Think I'm Gonna Be Alright" on Raisin Bran. Kids could mail away for a poster of him in exchange for two box tops and 50 cents. One fan recalled, "I remember owning 'Sugar, Sugar' by the Archies, and 'Easy Come, Easy Go' by Bobby Sherman. The hard part was having to wait to finish the cereal before being able to play the record."[22]

Musicians have not been featured on cereal boxes nearly as often as athletes, but some have been notable. Even before TXT, General Mills teamed up with the heavy metal and hip-hop artist Ice-T (Tracy Lauren Marrow), who was the controversial 1992 Original Gangster (OG) frontman for the song "Cop Killer." Ice-T later turned to acting, with a star role in TV's *Law & Order: SVU*. In 2022, at the age of 64, he became a Cheerios

Coach (presumably to reach boomers) and appeared on the back of heart-shaped Cheerios varieties to encourage Americans "to get their bodies moving and hearts thumping" (and, of course, to eat a bowl of Cheerios every morning).[23]

Other rappers have also helped market cereals. In 2024, Lil Yachty (Miles Parks McCollum) and Travis Scott promoted General Mills' Reese's Puffs, appearing on four collectible boxes in partial image. These, when cut out and put together, made up a complete picture, requiring the purchase of all four boxes. The Lil Yachty collaboration could not have been better; he released the song "Reese's Puffs Rap."

Marketing to art lovers—and gamers

General Mills and the former street artist turned pop culture art icon KAWS (Brian Donnelly) teamed up in 2021 to release two limited-edition Reese's Puffs boxes with KAWS signature "X" eyes and KAWS COMPANION character hands reaching out of the bowl (yes, more capital letters).[24] General Mills promoted this box to art fans and fashion lovers, but also to younger video gamers. Buyers could scan a QR code on the back of the box to download the KAWSPUFFS app and play an augmented reality (AR) game such as Pokémon GO or Angry Birds. Gamers competed for exclusive prizes, including a KAWS-signed cereal box. General Mills produced the box in the original orange color for stores but also issued a special-edition blue box to mimic the nighttime mode of the AR game. These were only sold online, and for $49.99—augmented cereal reality indeed.

In 2025, General Mills was a $1 million sponsor of the KAWS exhibit at the Crystal Bridges Museum of American Art in Bentonville, Arkansas, the home of Walmart. The museum devoted an entire wing to the cereal company, featuring its KAWSPUFFs and KAWS cereal boxes, artwork, sketches, and life-size collectibles on display.[25] Sometimes, art really does imitate life.

Marketing to families: The holidays

Sugar and spice and everything nice—gingerbread, pumpkin spice, magic clovers, monsters, elves, and Peeps chicks—are all found throughout the cereal aisle at every possible holiday opportunity. Cereal companies lock up retailer shelf space for such "limited-time offers" months in advance and view them as "big bets" to boost sales by reeling in nostalgia seekers, holiday lovers, cereal fans, families, and kids.[26]

One example is what cereal makers do for Halloween, an otherwise seemingly minor holiday. In 1970, General Mills issued a trio of Monster Cereals: Franken Berry (strawberry) and Count Chocula followed by Boo Berry, the first blueberry-flavored cereal. The boxes featured popular monsters, had prizes inside, and quickly became kids' favorites. Over the years, the company added new monsters and flavors such as Frute Brute and Fruity Yummy Mummy. Monster cereals were sold year-round until 2009, when General Mills made them available only at Halloween "to inspire nostalgic joy and spread the spooky spirit," appealing directly to Gen X and families.[27] Today, the Big Four temporarily turn cereal aisles into games of trick or treat: Kellogg with Spooky Froot Loops, Post with Halloween Fruity Pebbles, General Mills with family-size Monster cereals as well as Haunted Chocolate Lucky Charms, and Quaker with Halloween (Cap'n) Crunch.

But Halloween is nothing compared with Christmas. Imitating what candymakers had done for decades, Quaker began its celebration of this major holiday in 1988 with limited-edition Cap'n Crunch's Christmas Crunch cereals containing green and red Crunch Berries. By 1994, this one holiday cereal accounted for up to 18% of the brand's total annual sales. As a Quaker official explained, "We want to make our cereal more fun."[28]

Limited-edition holiday-themed cereals come and go with the seasons, but one brand has been featured at every holiday since the 1950s: Chex party mix. The Ralston Purina Company created Shredded Ralston in 1936, renamed it Chex in the 1950s, and put the first party mix recipe on the back of boxes in 1953. Its purpose: to expand cereal-eating occasions beyond breakfast (this is not a new phenomenon). As the company put it, the Chex party mix recipe "has allowed us to make it more of a social event rather than an isolated consumption occasion." Cleverly, the mix requires not one, but three boxes—one each of Rice Chex, Corn Chex, and Wheat Chex. During the holidays, these cereals are in high demand; nearly half of Chex sales occur during the last 3 months of the year. Party Chex is the gift that keeps on giving—to General Mills, which bought Ralston cereals in 1997.[29]

Not to be outdone, Kellogg's Ho Ho Holiday Rice Krispies hit shelves in 1994 with red and green oven-toasted rice, turning Snap, Crackle, and Pop

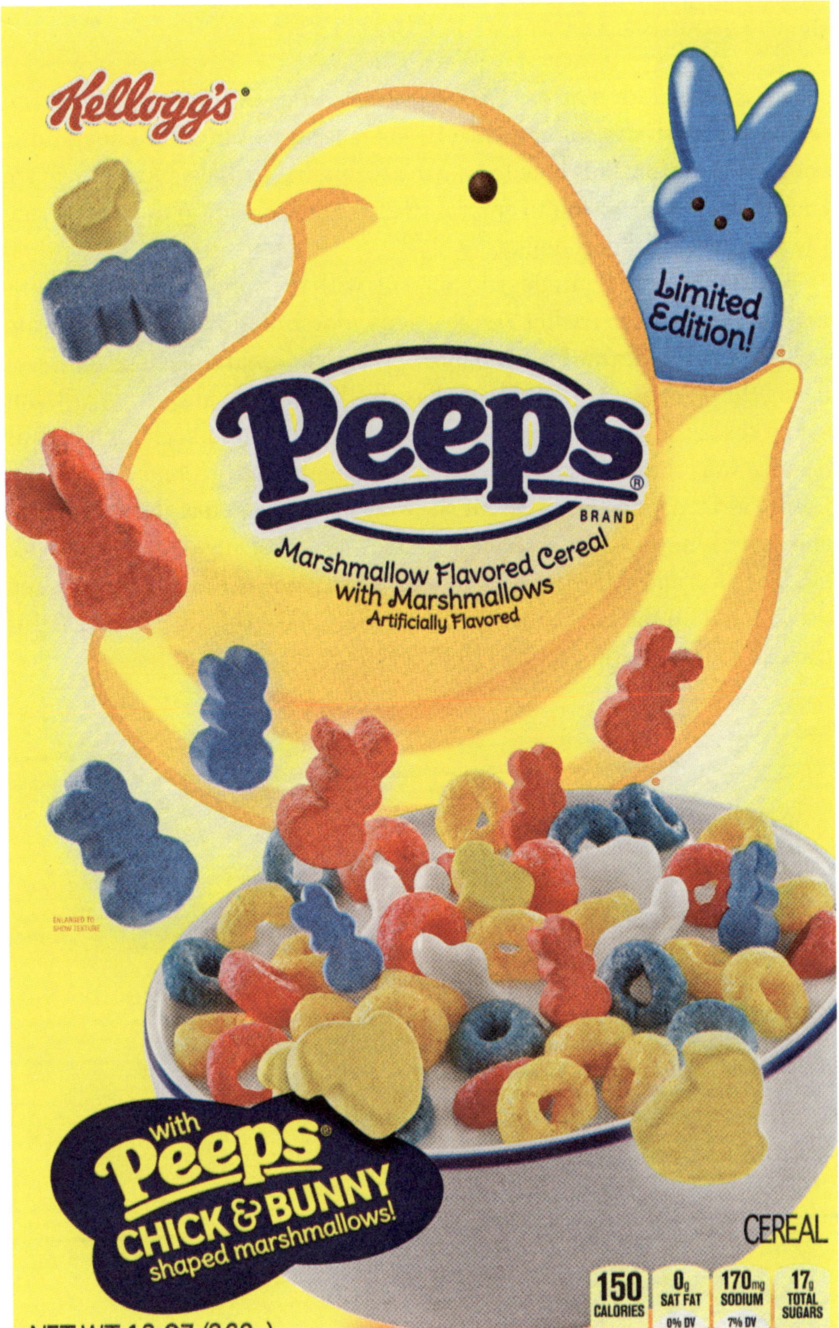

FIGURE 34 Cereal companies release holiday-themed cereals throughout the year. Kellogg's Peeps box, released for Easter of 2025, promoted chick and bunny marshmallows, a typical sugary way to celebrate major and minor holidays.

mascots into Santa's elves. The box said, "same taste in fun colors" and featured Christmas-colored Rice Krispies treats. In 2022, Kellogg ran a contest prompting kids to tell Santa to ask families to make him homemade Rice Krispies treats, and to enter a sweepstakes to win up to $2000 from the company—a sweet holiday deal.[30]

Beginning in 2019, Kellogg teamed up with the confectionery company making the Easter basket staple Peeps marshmallow chicks to create Kellogg's Peeps Brand Marshmallow Flavored Cereal—perhaps foreshadowing the company's eventual purchase by the Ferrero candy company. But at the time, the partnership seemed so outlandish that social media was deluged with comments from people who thought candy cereal was a joke.[31] Candy indeed: the Peeps cereal shown in Figure 34 has three colors of chicks and bunnies marshmallows and 17 grams of sugars per serving (a full teaspoon above the usual 12 grams), and a game of Candyland-inspired Peeps Land on the back of the box (you can't make this up). In 2025, this cereal hit supermarket shelves right on cue.

CHAPTER 15

CEREAL FOR ALL

TARGETING DIVERSITY, EQUITY, AND INCLUSION

As CEREAL COMPANIES began to understand the spending power of historically underrepresented groups—most notably Black, Hispanic, and LGBTQ+ (Lesbian, Gay, Bisexual, Transgender, Queer, and other gender identities) consumers—they aimed box designs, messages, and advertising campaigns specifically for these groups. The cereal industry sometimes refers to this targeting as multicultural or inclusive marketing. Companies use cultural symbols and celebrities to make cereals seem more relatable, appeal to new consumer demographics, and give brands a competitive advantage. More recently, the increased visibility and economic power of the LGBTQ+ community have prompted cereal companies to create brands celebrating Pride Month. These efforts are sometimes thoughtfully inclusive, but can look to us as just what they are—marketing.

Marketing to Black consumers

For decades, cereal companies overlooked Black consumers as a core marketing segment, even though they used images of Black individuals in advertising. The troubling history of racial representation in food marketing dates back to the early twentieth century, when the chef "Rastus"—

a pejorative racial caricature—was first depicted on Cream of Wheat cereal boxes. In one 1921 advertisement, he appeared as a smiling chef holding up a sign that perpetuated stereotypes of illiteracy. Reportedly, Cream of Wheat acquired the chef image when a company executive paid $5 to photograph a railcar waiter.[1]

Nabisco bought Cream of Wheat in 1961; Kraft bought Nabisco in 2000; the current owner, B & G Foods, bought Nabisco in 2007. All continued to use the chef image as late as 2020, when Black Lives Matter calls to end systemic racism induced food companies to remove such depictions.[2]

In the way some academics explain such societal changes, World War II and the Civil Rights movement "delegitimized discourse that disparages the racial other." The use of images of Black people in derogatory ways was finally becoming socially unacceptable.[3] We would argue such uses were never acceptable, but marketers found an even more important reason to make this transition: Black celebrities sell food, and not only to Black consumers; they have broad influence and appeal across diverse consumer groups.

Black households comprise about 14% of the US population, but their spending power represents less than 10%, leading many companies to undervalue them. According to the global consulting firm McKinsey & Company, Black households spent $835 billion on goods and services in 2019 but have increased their spending by 5% annually for the past 20 years and are expected to have $1.7 trillion in purchasing power by 2030. Companies are paying attention.[4]

The rationale for using the names, images, and likenesses of famous Black individuals in marketing extends beyond demographics. Despite societal discrimination, they are major influencers, representing "all of the iconic cultural markers of our society: business, music, entertainment, fashion, sports, government, education." Marketers know that if they design campaigns targeted to "niche multicultural consumers," they will win with the masses.[5]

Advertisers use Blackness representations in two ways: to help them demonstrate a product's role as a cultural resource, and as a metaphor for shared social values of racial equality and cultural diversity. From the perspective of *Advertising Age*, the Black consumer market is a "major brand-building opportunity that's in plain sight." As a spokesperson for General

Mills put it, "We believe that if you root yourself in the African-American culture and understand and value those rituals, customs, and institutions, you can use that knowledge to help tell your brand story and engage consumers."[6]

Wheaties boxes perfectly illustrate how long it took cereal companies to feature famous Black athletes. Although General Mills began using athletes to advertise Wheaties as "the breakfast of champions" in 1934 (Lou Gehrig), the first Black champion, Roy Campanella, appeared only in 1952, on the side of the box. And although no athletes appeared on the fronts of Wheaties boxes until 1958 (Lou Gehrig had been on the back), it took 28 more years to feature a Black athlete on the front of a box: Walter Payton, the Chicago Bears running back, in 1986. The tennis star Althea Gibson was the first Black woman to be featured—in 2001, more than 40 years after winning 11 major tennis titles between 1956 and 1958. As we show in Figure 35, Wheaties commemorated Negro League baseball players in 1996, for their 75th anniversary. But eventually, cereal companies caught on. Basketball legend Michael Jordan, one of the greatest athletes of all time, holds the record for the most appearances on the front of a Wheaties box—19.[7]

Wheaties is a reasonably healthy cereal marketed primarily to adults ("supporting a champion requires a wholesome breakfast"). But most products targeting Black consumers are higher in sugar, fat, and salt; these products are also more available in convenience stores, come with volume discounts (2 for 1), and are advertised on social media timed to coincide with the distribution of food assistance benefits. Twice as many television advertisements target Black consumers as are aimed at white consumers, with more than 80% promoting less healthful brands. Such observations also apply to cereals. Whereas kids' overall exposure to cereal advertisements declined from 2008 to 2011, the exposure of child-targeted brands to Black kids increased by 88% for Kellogg's Froot Loops, and by 72% for General Mills' Reese's Puffs.[8]

People who grew up in the 1990s are sure to remember Ralston's Urkel-O's cereal, named after the nerdy Black teenager Steve Urkel, played by Jaleel White on the ABC hit show *Family Matters*. In 1991, Ralston launched the strawberry-and-banana-flavor sugary loops cereal, and in 1992 it released a box that promoted "Urkel for President." Kids could enter

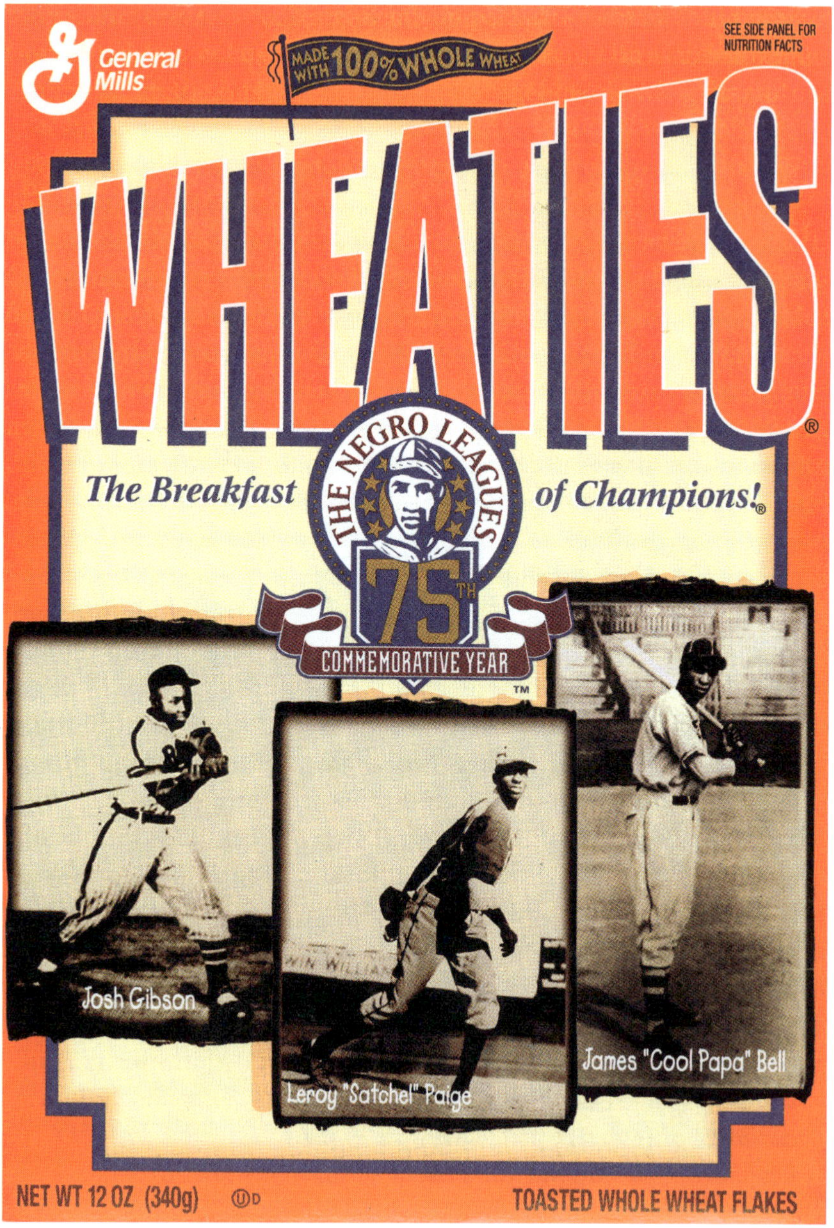

FIGURE 35 This 1996 General Mills' Wheaties box commemorates the 75th anniversary of the Negro League baseball teams, more than half a century after the height of their flourishing. Major League Baseball officially recognized these leagues as members only in 2020.

a contest to win a trip to Washington, DC.[9] Although the TV show lasted until 1997, this cereal was soon discontinued.

From our perspective, cereal companies' marketing aimed at minority groups is complex, although the motive is always the same: to sell more cereal. Occasionally, as a result of oversight or, perhaps, racial insensitivity, a cereal company blunders badly, as we discuss next.

The Corn Pops fiasco

Ah, the power of social media. On October 24, 2017, Saladin Ahmed, who identified himself as a writer, posted on Twitter (now X): "Hey @KelloggsUS why is literally the only brown corn pop on the whole cereal box the janitor? This is teaching kids racism."[10] We show the offending illustration in Figure 36.

The ensuing Twitter storm dropped right into the ongoing American culture wars: Do Corn Pops have a race? Do Corn Pops have a gender? Why are there no female characters in this game? Should parents be concerned about the wild behavior of the Corn Pops in the shopping arcade?[11]

The then-host of the *Daily Show*, comedian Trevor Noah, viewed this incident in its cultural context: "Racist or not racist? Not racist because there's nothing wrong with being a janitor. But maybe it is. There's no such thing as a brown Corn Pop. So they basically added one to give him the job of janitor on the box."[12]

Within just a few hours of Ahmed's tweet, Kellogg responded: "Kellogg is committed to diversity & inclusion. We did not intend to offend—we apologize. The artwork is updated & will be in stores soon."

The Washington Post described Ahmed as a thoughtful, award-nominated writer of science fiction and fantasy, including Marvel's Black Bolt series, and quoted him as exulting in his "tiny victories . . . I used the computer in my pocket to get a cereal company to make their boxes less racist." Perhaps, but it did pressure Kellogg to revise the box design.

Black-owned cereal companies

Over the past two decades, Black entrepreneurs have brought culturally relevant products to the highly competitive cereal market. In 2007, at the

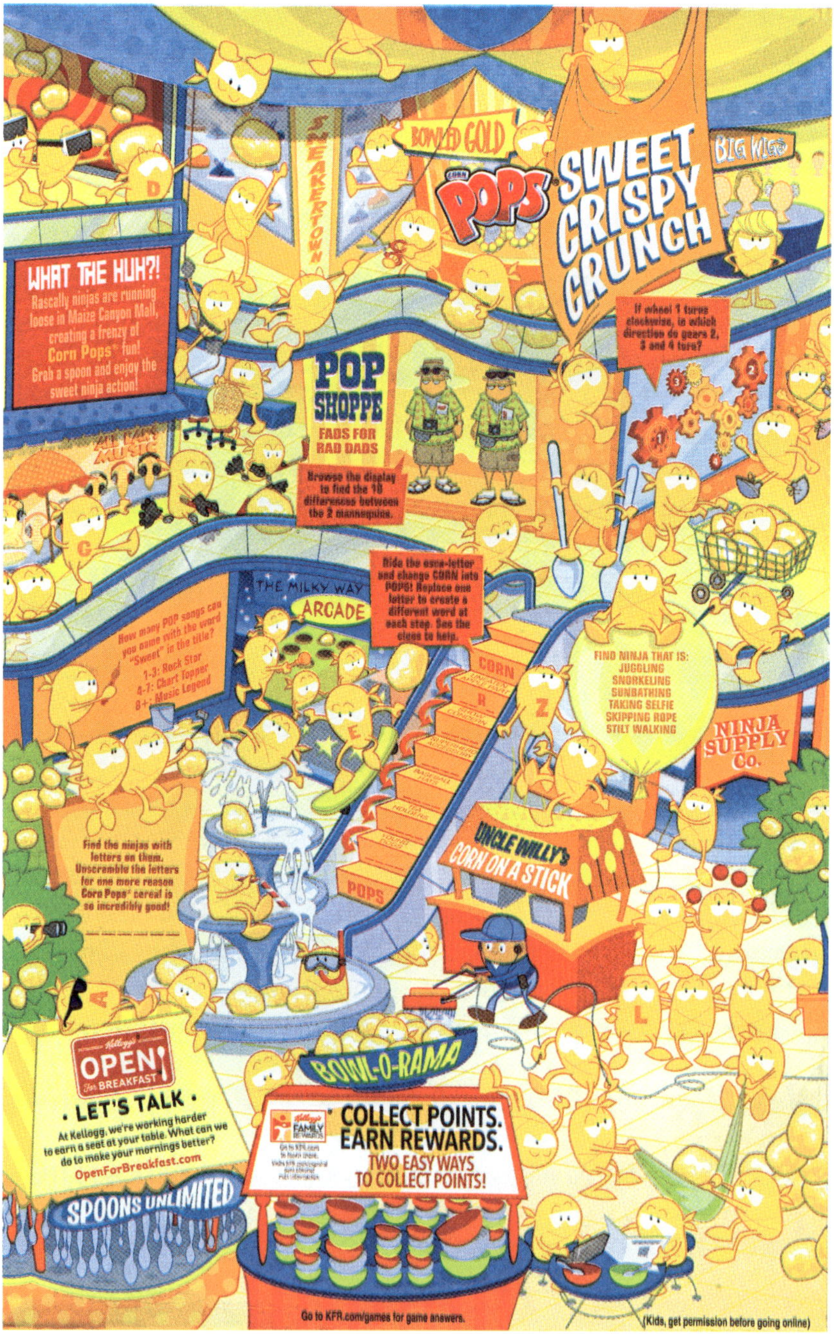

FIGURE 36 The kids' game on the back of this 2017 Kellogg's Corn Pops box depicted a large number of yellow Corn Pop characters frolicking in a shopping arcade. Only one, the janitor cleaning up, was brown.

age of 74, legendary R&B artist and Rock & Roll Hall of Famer Lloyd Price launched a line of food products under the brand Lawdy Miss Clawdy—named for his hit song. The brand included four varieties of Make Momma Proud cereal, each featuring a "trailblazing icon" of the National Black & Entertainment Hall of Fame: Dorothy Dandridge, Lloyd Price, Louis Armstrong, and Sugar Ray Robinson. The company said it would donate proceeds from the sale of these cereals to a new Hall of Fame building in Harlem, New York, and three universities in Louisiana. The cereals were to be sold at a Soul Food Museum in Chicago.[13] If they were, it was not for long. In 2014, the cereal trademark was canceled, and we cannot find evidence of sales or donations.

In 2020, a Black-founded and -owned company, Legacy Cereal, set out to produce Proud Puffs—a chocolate-flavored, vegan cereal in the shape of a fist. The box featured a Black family on the front. The back had a word search game for kids, who could circle affirmative words such as *powerful*, *kind*, *proud*, *unstoppable*, and *blessed*. Owner Nic King said he wanted to "make cereal for the culture" with a goal to "uplift the Black and brown community. I needed to make sure I was putting something healthy and that had nutritional value back inside my community. I didn't want to push another sugary cereal."[14] If this cereal ever made it to market, we missed it. Too bad; we liked its mission.

Most famously, rappers Snoop Dogg (Calvin Cordozar Broadus Jr.) and Master P (Percy Robert Miller) introduced a line of kids' cereals in 2023. Although they were originally branded Snoop Loopz, Kellogg complained of brand infringement, and the rappers renamed the cereal line Snoop Cereal. The boxes boast of "more marshmallows" and list sugar as the first ingredient; the cereals are colored with artificial dyes and are artificially flavored. Their virtue? "With every purchase, you are making a difference. We are proud to support Future Bosses through education and sports. Our mission is to help tackle homelessness and feed needy families." But the Environmental Working Group ranks Snoop Cereal varieties as close to the worst because of their additives and high sugar content (14 grams per serving).

After initially making an offer to buy the company (which Snoop declined), Post agreed to manufacture, package, sell, and distribute the product in exchange for 50% of the profits. Post said it would treat Snoop

Cereal like its other brands and ensure wide distribution to major retailers such as Target and Walmart. The cereals were available from online sources but never gained the in-store traction critical for building brands and sales. In 2024, the rapper duo sued Walmart and Post for conspiring to keep their cereals off the shelves.[15] We have yet to see them at Walmart or any store we frequent. We cannot tell whether this is an example of systemic racism or whether Post refused to pay enough in slotting fees to get the cereals on shelves. Regardless of the outcome of their lawsuit, we wish Snoop Dogg and Master P had developed a healthier product to market to kids. Maybe next time.

Marketing to Hispanic/Latino consumers

For American Heart Month in 2024 and again in 2025, General Mills released heart-shaped Honey Nut Cheerios with the front (or back) of the box in English and the opposite face in Spanish, in versions such as Mamá, Abuelo, Mi Amigo, Mi Amor. These were all followed by the tagline, in English, "MAKES MY HEART HAPPY" as we show in Figure 37. These boxes directly targeted the burgeoning Spanish-speaking population in the United States, 65 million strong, one out of every five Americans, increasing by more than 600% since 1970 and by more than 20% just since 2010.[16]

These consumers have plenty of spending power, estimated at $2.8 trillion by 2026. Hispanics are said to drive 16% of the growth in consumer-packaged goods (which cereals are part of) and to prioritize spending in categories for their families' needs (which cereals want to be part of).[17]

By 1991, Hispanic spending had reached $191 billion. General Mills created a "special markets group" to address this growing demographic. In 1993, the company introduced Buñuelitos, puffed corn balls (like Kix), coated with honey, sugar, and cinnamon, supposedly tasting like the fried Mexican buñuelo pastry, typically eaten dipped in syrup or honey. General Mills launched Buñuelitos in major Hispanic markets in Texas, California, South Florida, Chicago, and New York City.[18] The cereal had 14 grams of sugar per serving (43% of calories), came in a fiesta-colored box, and was meant to appeal to both kids and adults. A Mexican chef offered his opinion. "I don't want to be rude," he said. "It's a nice, cinnamon cereal. But it's no buñuelo." Others must have agreed. It was discontinued a year later.

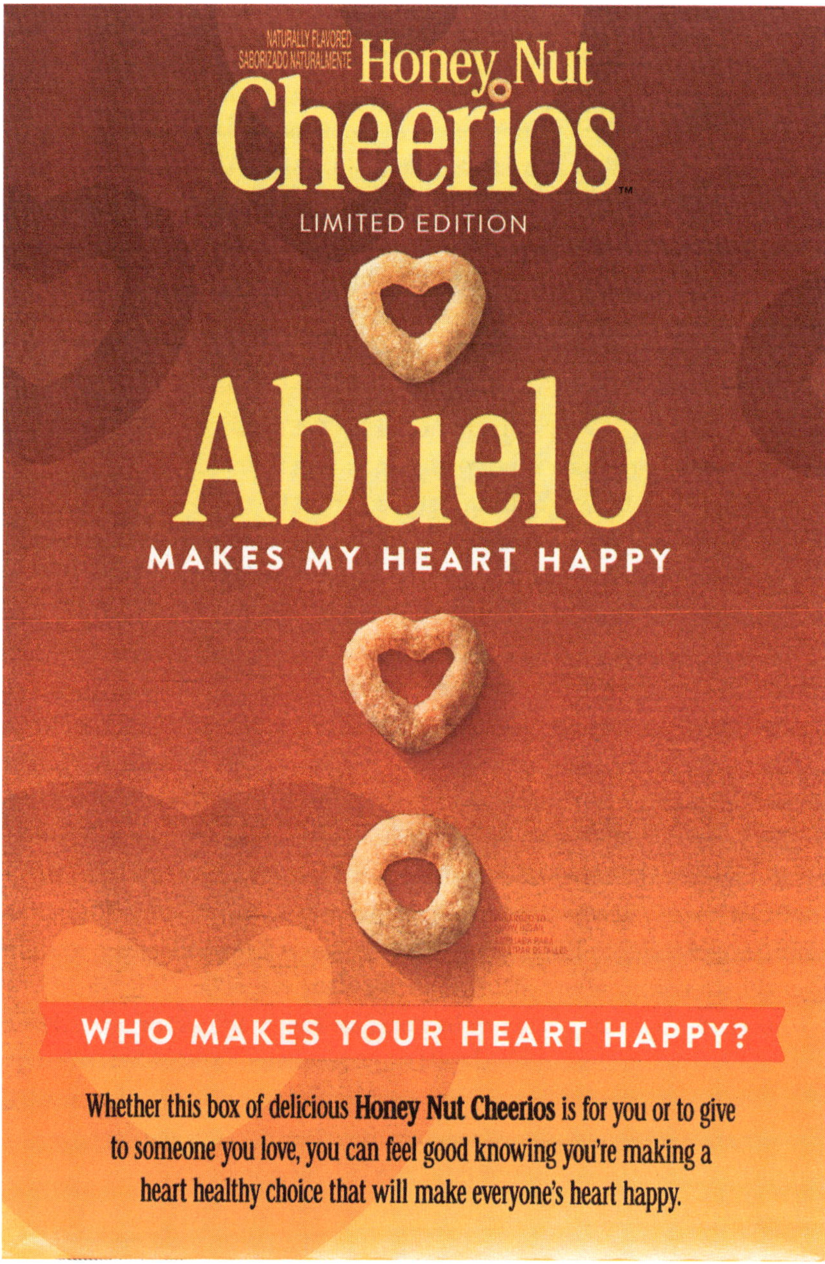

FIGURE 37 General Mills' 2024 campaign targeted the increasingly large and powerful Hispanic market with heart-shaped cereals for various family members, in this case Abuelo (grandfather).

General Mills tried again in 2006, this time importing its La Lechera Flakes, cornflakes sweetened with Nestlé brand La Lechera condensed milk, from Mexico—a cereal also later discontinued. In addition that year, it introduced Dora the Explorer cereal in partnership with the Nickelodeon children's television program featuring Dora, an animated Latina heroine who switches between English and Spanish as she travels to solve mysteries. The cereal box included elements in Spanish as well as in English and was aimed at Latin American women and children enrolled in the federally funded Women, Infants, and Children (WIC) program. We discussed Dora cereal and its discontinuation in Chapter 3.

Within the next few years, the Big Four expanded efforts to reach Hispanic consumers even more. Between 2009 and 2010, Post and General Mills each doubled their advertising spending to the Spanish-speaking population. Post, for example, invested nearly $10 million to advertise its Honey Bunches of Oats cereal to Hispanic shoppers. It recruited the advertising agency LatinWorks to lead its Hispanic-targeted marketing strategies. As Post put it, "We are incredibly proud that Honey Bunches of Oats is the #1 ready-to-eat cereal brand among Hispanics in the United States and are continuing our commitment to support and engage with this growing audience through culturally-relevant content and meaningful experiences."[19] In 2025, Post was still claiming its cereals as first among Hispanic households.

Kellogg also launched cereals to appeal to the US Hispanic market. In 2011, it introduced Zucaritas (see Figure 44 in Chapter 17) and Zucaritas Chocolate, sold throughout Latin America. Zucaritas, which translates to "little sugary things" in English (and Frosted Flakes in cereal-speak), was the #1 selling cereal brand in Mexico, and chocolate was its most popular flavor. One Mexican-born blogger said she got that "feeling of nostalgia and tinge of excitement to be able to buy in the U.S. a cereal we had eaten in Mexico."[20] Although that reaction was just what Kellogg wanted, the cereal appeared to cut into sales of Frosted Flakes. Kellogg discontinued selling it in the United States and shifted to other kinds of targeted marketing.

Between 2018 and 2021 Kellogg increased its Hispanic media budget by 40% and won the 2022 Hispanic Marketing Council's Marketer of the Year award. Later in 2022, the company launched a digital and in-store cereal advertising campaign—On Mom's tables Aquí y Allá ("here and there")—featuring Special K, Corn Flakes, Frosted Flakes, Froot Loops, and Apple Jacks. The campaign's goal was to "authentically capture the emotional relationship that bicultural Latina moms have had with our brands throughout their lives."[21] Kellogg must have realized that this group already liked its existing brands and considered them more prestigious; it could just promote them without having to introduce anything new.

Cereal companies also have more subtle ways of appealing to Spanish-speaking audiences, such as showing front-of-package and side-panel elements in Spanish as well as English. The Food and Drug Administration (FDA) requires box labels to be in English, but it makes an exception for products sold in Puerto Rico or US territories. General Mills uses the right-side panel for the English elements and the left-side panel for the Spanish elements on some brands; for other brands, it presents both together, as in Total Sugars/Azúcares Totales.

Kellogg's cereals also use both languages on some of its brands—presumably those most popular with Hispanic households. When asked, a representative explained, "Kellogg offers a selection of products in bilingual packaging to welcome our ever-growing Hispanic population with their favorites here in the United States. Because our packages communicate important nutrition information, it is important to provide key elements in Spanish for these consumers. By offering the Nutrition Facts in Spanish and English, the nutrient value of the products is easily understood."[22] Bravo! We are all for more nutrition information in a format that people can understand and use to make informed choices, and we wish all companies were doing this.

Although diversity, equity, and inclusion (DEI) efforts were becoming targets of political opposition in 2025, cereal makers continued to use multicultural marketing efforts to attract new consumers and create new brand loyalists. As a Kellogg official put it, cereal companies needed to be "future-proofing" their businesses to continue growing and remain relevant.[23] If nothing else, this made good business sense.

LGBTQ+ marketing

Gender identity rights are highly controversial and politically fraught in the United States. Yet, in 2016, Kellogg partnered with GLAAD (Gay and

Lesbian Alliance Against Defamation), one of the world's largest advocacy nonprofit media organizations working on behalf of people who identify as LGBTQ+. Melania Trump had promised to make combating cyberbullying one of her key issues, and bullying was in the news.[24]

In 2018, Kellogg announced its All Together Cereal, combining all of its kids' cereal mascots on one box. Visitors to Kellogg's pop-up café in New York City could get a special edition "All Together Cereal" box and make their own "All Together" cereal by mixing Kellogg's varieties. Kellogg released the box to support GLAAD's annual Spirit Day in support of inclusivity and against bullying.[25]

Kellogg's All Together Cereal was available online only in 2019 and 2020. In May 2021, Kellogg rebranded it as Together with Pride, releasing it to celebrate Pride Month, again in partnership with GLAAD. As shown in Figure 38, the cereal was in Pride rainbow colors, dusted with edible glitter. A limited edition was available in stores of select major retailers, and the box design turned Kellogg's logo into a Pride rainbow accompanied by the full cast of cartoon characters, with Mini (the Frosted Mini Wheat) holding the Pride flag. The top of the box provided a tear-out wristband for kids to "proudly share and wear their pronouns." A media campaign offered fans the opportunity to join the #BoxesAreForCerealChallenge via TikTok. When customers sent in proof of purchase, Kellogg donated $3 per box to GLAAD—up to a maximum of $140,000 (in fine print).[26]

The Together box stated, "Leave boxes for cereal—and let people be who they were meant to be. . . . Boxes are for cereal, not people." Kellogg explained all this as "the embodiment and celebration of Kellogg Company's commitment to diversity, equity, and inclusion, not just within Kellogg Company, but also at the tables of our cereal fans coast to coast. As Kellogg has grown its multiyear allyship with GLAAD, the company hopes to spread the word on allyship and show its support for the transgender and gender nonconforming communities."[27] One reason why Kellogg did this must surely be that LGBTQ+ consumers have more than $5 trillion in spending power globally, and Gen Z customers (born 1997 to 2012) are more likely to buy brands that support their values of diversity and social justice.[28]

As should have been expected, this cereal and media campaign brought on immediate pushback. Critics pointed out that the cereal company's founder, Dr. John Harvey Kellogg, had been a Seventh-day Adventist who

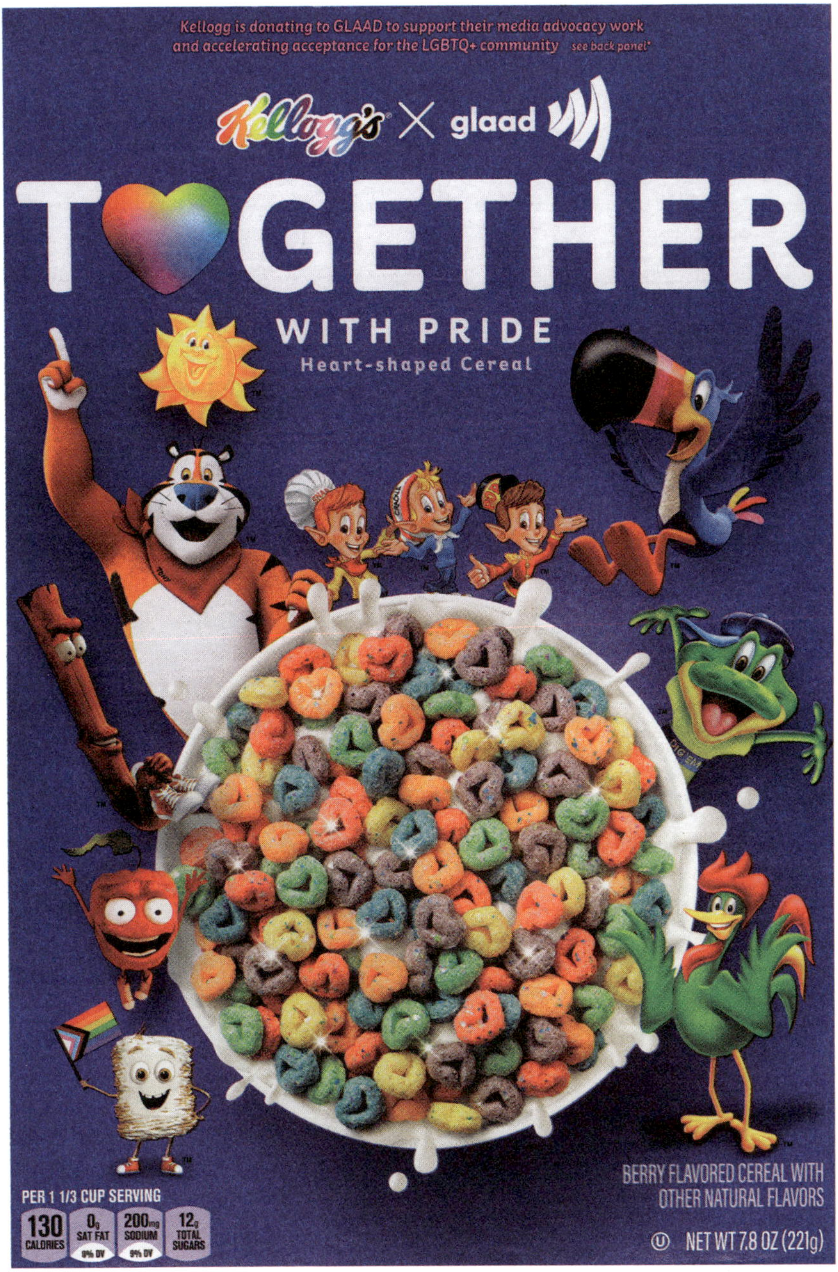

FIGURE 38 For Pride Month in 2021, Kellogg partnered with the LGBTQ+ advocacy organization GLAAD to produce a Pride-colored box and cereal with the company's iconic cartoon mascots promoting acceptance and a stance against bullying.

had invented cornflakes to curb what he considered to be "unhealthy" sexual behaviors. Dr. Kellogg would not be pleased, argued a group of Catholic journalists.[29]

The America First Legal Foundation (ALF), a conservative legal non-profit run by Stephen Miller, an advisor to President Trump (and in 2025 policy deputy chief of staff), also disapproved of this cereal. The ALF filed a complaint against Kellogg with the Equal Employment Opportunity Commission, alleging that the company promoted diversity and gender parity among its employees and noting that Kellogg was targeting children with its rainbow heart-shaped cereal and mascot holding an LGBTQ flag. Kellogg, the ALF said, "is yet another big corporation that will break the law and hurt its shareholders' interests to serve the twisted woke ideology of its officers and directors." ALF complained to the company that it had abandoned its fiduciary responsibility: "Management has hijacked the brand to advance an extreme political and social agenda . . . and discarded the Company's long-held family-friendly marketing approach to politicize and sexualize its products." In response, a Kellogg official said, "At Kellogg, our aspiration is to better reflect the diversity of our consumers and to strengthen our inclusive culture."[30] Perhaps because of the Trump administration's fierce opposition to DEI in any form, the company has not reissued the cereal.

Who would have ever thought a rainbow-colored sugary cereal and a message of togetherness would incite such controversy? Like the happy-go-lucky mascots on the front of the cereal box—can't we all just get along?

CHAPTER 16

MARKETING PHILANTHROPY

DO GOOD, FEEL GOOD

As part of their corporate social responsibility commitments, cereal companies engage in philanthropy. They do this mainly in two ways: donations and cause marketing. Companies directly donate cereal or money to nonprofit groups engaged in worthy causes. More often, they partner with a social or environmental cause and use their cereal brands to generate support or funds for that cause. In these campaigns, customers are encouraged to buy cereals and engage with the brand, thereby triggering the company's donation of cereal or cash to the cause. In-house company marketing and brand teams often lead these "do good, feel good" consumer-focused campaigns as part of their mission to build brand loyalty and increase market share.

In both scenarios, the recipient partners get money and resources to help them address important societal or environmental challenges. But the donating companies also benefit—a lot. Philanthropic campaigns improve public image, enhance consumer loyalty, and, not least, provide substantial tax advantages. Often, the benefits to donor companies far outweigh whatever contributions they make, as has been demonstrated for soft-drink philanthropic partnerships.[1] Here, we present some of our favorite examples of cereal company campaigns created to support five worthy causes: education, environmental sustainability, endangered species, military families, and antihunger efforts.

Supporting schools: Box Tops for Education

Box Tops for Education is arguably the most popular cause marketing program ever created in its peer category of philanthropy campaigns. Its widget is shown in Figure 22j (Chapter 10), and earlier versions appear at the tops of boxes shown here in Figures 40 and 41. Launched in 1996 by General Mills, the program provides funding to schools serving kids age 5 to 13 as an "easy way to earn cash for your school." All you have to do is buy participating cereals and then cut out the coupons and mail them in (or, these days, submit them electronically). Each coupon is worth 10 cents. General Mills adds them up and sends a check to your designated school.

Since its inception, the Box Tops program has generated nearly $1 billion in donations to schools. This sounds impressive, but it means that people had to buy a lot of cereal. We love the economics of this system. You buy a box of cereal (roughly $6 in early 2026), and your school gets a 10-cent donation. The average return to a school is $750.[2] This amount is either a little or a lot, depending on your viewpoint. For a small school in a low-income area, it could mean the welcome addition of new books and basic school supplies.

Occasionally, a celebrity will get involved and help a lucky school score a big win. In 2024, for example, General Mills teamed up with Grammy Award–winning musician John Legend, who endorsed the company's Legendary Teachers campaign. Legend helped the Box Tops program award $30,000 to a low-income Los Angeles school; he also encouraged families to download the Box Tops app so they could buy even more General Mills products to support schools.[3]

The Box Tops website lists the cereals that carry the redeemable coupon. In 2026, more than 100 cereals participated in the program, including top-selling Big G brands such as Lucky Charms, Cocoa Puffs, and Kix, as well as smaller co-branded cereals like KitKat, Hershey's Kisses, and Hot Wheels.

Of the participating cereals, less than a third meet the USDA's nutrition criteria for healthier Smart Snacks. General Mills has never claimed the program is about health or nutrition. But to us, given its focus on funding schools and serving young children, the lack of concern about nutrition seems like a missed opportunity. We view the program as a sophisticated marketing tool. The company, however, firmly denies this: "Box Tops for Education is NOT a brand marketing program. It is a fundraising program for parents and a way for General Mills to support local communities and schools."[4]

Although General Mills denies its marketing intent, it admits its business purpose: "While giving back to communities and schools may be considered a philanthropy to some, Box Tops for Education payments to schools are treated as a corporate business expense."[5] General Mills gets to deduct donations to Box Tops for Education from its taxes. But the company reaps even more reward: it scores product sales, brand loyalty, access to school-age children, and community goodwill.

The program benefits General Mills in one other critical way: it provides a whole lot of personal data that can be used for targeted marketing. In 2019, the company went electronic and introduced the Box Tops for Education app. In 2023, it eliminated the need to mail in the box top coupons. You can simply scan your grocery store receipt and supply your name, date of birth, and zip code. When you do this, the company knows where you shopped and what you purchased—just what it needs for targeted marketing. It gets all that for a donation of 10 cents. During the back-to-school season in 2025, you could connect your Box Top and Walmart accounts for double coupon value (20 cents); then, Walmart also had your purchasing data. Box Tops for Education is a classic example of a "do good, feel good" program—more on your dime than General Mills'.

Supporting environmental sustainability

In 2019, the Union of Concerned Scientists (UCS) called on cereal makers to channel their purchasing power and leverage their supply chains to encourage farmers to grow grains more sustainably and do a better job of conserving soil and water. Cereal companies, the UCS said, ought to do more to overcome the ways industrial grain production pollutes water supplies, erodes and depletes soil, reduces biodiversity, and emits heat-trapping greenhouse gases. General Mills took on that challenge and devoted a website to its regenerative agriculture commitment "to advance regenerative agriculture on 1 million acres of farmland by 2030." As General Mills defines it, regenerative agriculture is "a holistic, principles-based approach to farming and ranching that delivers positive environmental, social, and economic outcomes."[6] Whatever this means in practice, it would largely be accomplished by the company's small organic and health-focused brands—like Cascadian Farm Organic.

Although you would never know it from the boxes, the Cascadian Farm brand is owned by General Mills and is the poster child for the company's regenerative mission. The website explains that Cascadian Farm intends to make "a world of difference" by using organic methods to promote ecological balance, regenerate soil health, reduce chemical pollution, and cultivate pollinator habitats. In 2019, the brand committed to "the conversion of 50K acres to regenerative agriculture by 2030" as part of its Northern Plains Regenerative Oats Project. This commitment accounts for 5% of the total General Mills goal, covers a small amount of land, and only applies to oats. Cascadian Farm is a small brand, and most of its cereals are made from wheat and corn—like the corn-based Honey Vanilla Crunch shown in Figure 39. According to one source, total Cascadian Farm cereal sales were around $12 million in the early 2020s compared with $450 million for oat-based Cheerios.[7]

In 2021, Cascadian Farm boxes appeared with a banner: "(heart icon) THE FARMLAND. JOIN US IN RESTORING 25 MILLION SQ.FT." This referred to a separate 2-year partnership and $750,000 gift to The Nature Conservancy to rebuild wildlife habitat and regenerate groundwater on 25 million square feet of farmland in the Sacramento Valley. Cascadian Farm explained its partnership with The Nature Conservancy as a means "to protect natural resources like wildlife habitat and groundwater to help farms become more resilient. . . . By supporting Cascadian Farm, you help enable our commitments to projects like these—in this case, helping to build resilience across more than 600 acres, 1 sq ft at a time. Join us in Cascading Change." The environmental advocate Anna Lappé pointed out that 25 million square feet comes to 68% of the area of New York City's Central Park, making this effort another small contribution to General Mills' million-acre commitment.[8]

In 2024, Cascadian Farm introduced a limited-edition cereal "made with Climate Smart Kernza Grain, which can help improve soil health and

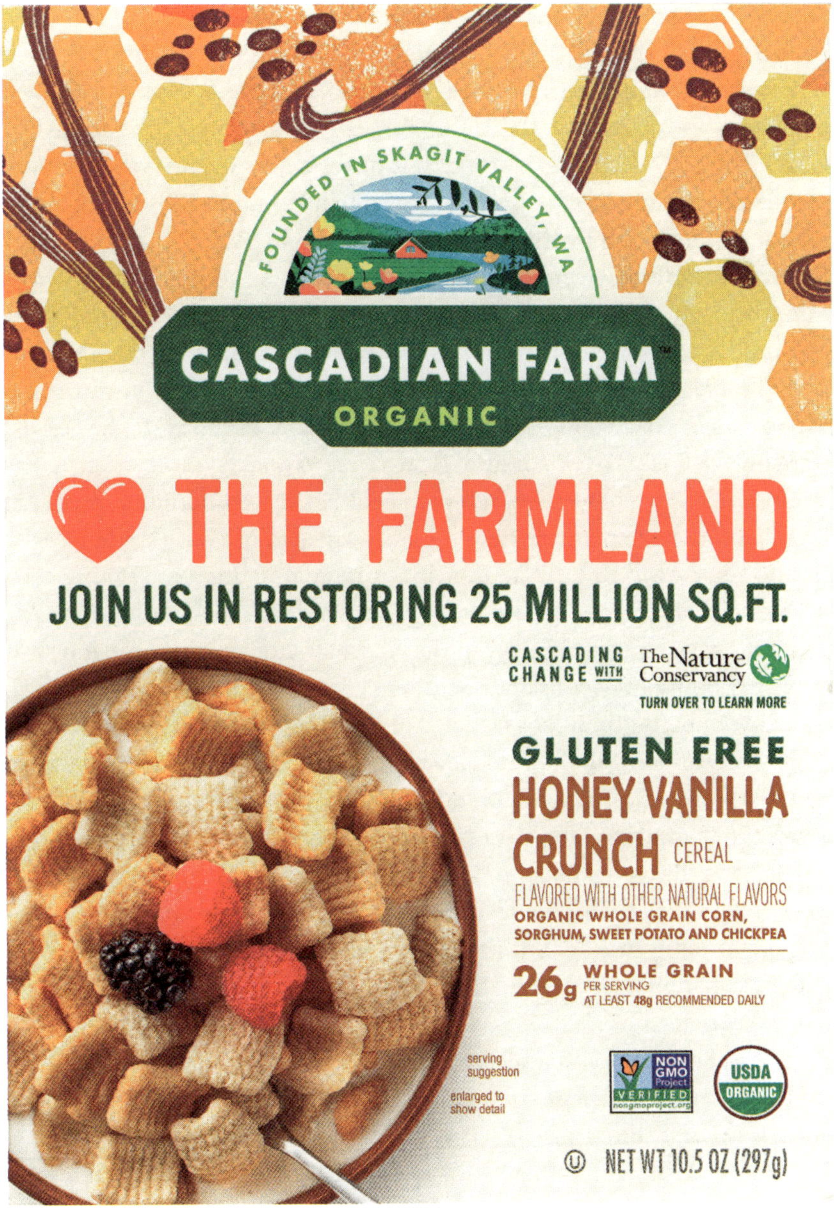

FIGURE 39 Consistent with its commitment to the environmental benefits of organic farming methods and land restoration efforts, Cascadian Farm supports "CASCADING CHANGE WITH The Nature Conservancy," as shown on this box from 2023. General Mills has owned Cascadian Farm since 1999 when it bought the brand from Small Planet Foods.

reduce water pollution." As the box explains, Kernza—the registered name owned by The Land Institute—is a perennial wheatgrass grain with a deep root system that holds soil, stores carbon, and prevents erosion. The box bears two seals: USDA ORGANIC (certified by Oregon Tilth) and NON GMO Project VERIFIED. Although it has 9 grams of sugars from three sources, everything in it (except for sea salt and vitamin E) is impressively organic as indicated by the asterisks: "Ingredients: Whole Grain Wheat*, Kernza Perennial Grains*, Cane Sugar*, Rice*, Whole Grain Oats*, Sunflower Oil*, Honey*, Molasses*, Crisp Rice*, Sea Salt, Rice Flour*, Natural Flavor.* Vitamin E (mixed tocopherols)." Late in 2025, the company launched four new "1% Kernza Initiative cereals, committing to expand its Kernza commitment and quadrupling grain use." The cereals were only available at the natural food stores Whole Foods and Sprouts.

Organic, as we have seen, refers to codified crop production methods. From a marketer's point of view, it makes sense to use farmland preservation to sell cereal. But unlike the USDA-regulated organic farming standards, no such standards have been established for regenerative methods. This puts regenerative farming in the crosshairs. Its unverified claims can apply to nonorganic foods and suggest to consumers that the products are the same or better than those labeled organic, when they do not have to be and mostly are not. To fill this void, more than 10 third-party regenerative certification and verification organizations have popped up, each with its own set of standards and processes for regenerative farming, further contributing to the confusion and skepticism. Critics view regenerative claims as nothing more than "greenwashing" by large multinational companies. Understandably, they call for a common definition, certification bodies with transparent and credible standards, and third-party oversight of foods labeled regenerative.[9]

Cascadian Farm was founded in 1972 by Gene Kahn, an idealistic pioneer in the organic movement. He merged Cascadian Farm into Small Planet Foods—the distributor listed on Cascadian Farm boxes—but sold the brand to General Mills in 1999. The Cascadian Farm website only mentions General Mills in the context of the company's donation of the Cascadian Home Farm to the Rodale Institute in 2022.

For further details of the origins of Cascadian Farm, you must go to the General Mills website. It describes how Cascadian Farm has partnered with

The Xerces Society (for conservation of bees and other invertebrates) and The Land Institute (regenerative agriculture) and helped make General Mills "the largest producer of natural and organic foods in North America." General Mills named Kahn its vice president of sustainable development in 2003, and he remained with the company until 2010. A business school case study explains why Cascadian Farm downplays its corporate ownership. When focus-group participants learned who owned the company, many no longer trusted the brand's products.[10]

This is unfortunate. We think Cascadian Farm cereals are worth trusting, and we wish General Mills would not put this small, respected organic brand in the awkward position of having to defend the company's regenerative claims as trustworthy. We support organic farming methods for their well-documented benefits to the environment and transitioning farming practices as close to organic as possible—in spirit as well as letter.

But we also wish General Mills and other leading cereal companies would do more to get their suppliers to produce grains more sustainably and organically. We think General Mills should be more explicit about how it defines its suppliers' regenerative practices and how it counts acres as farmed regeneratively. We wish the company would step up and make the same organic commitments for Cheerios and its other top-selling Big G brands as it has for Cascadian Farm.

Supporting endangered species

We are intrigued by the environmental efforts of Nature's Path Organic. This privately held, family-owned company makes the EnviroKidz line of USDA Organic, Non-GMO Project Verified cereals, which include varieties such as Koala Crisp, Choco Chimps, Panda Puffs, and Gorilla Munch. The niche brand aims to attract kids and animal lovers by promoting the protection of the potentially endangered species that correspond to the cereals—and the company donates to those causes.

Our favorite is Turtle Splash, which offers the symbolic adoption of baby turtles as part of the company's commitment to environmental education and animal conservation. You have to take the box apart to read what is printed on its inside. There, you learn about endangered sea turtles and get a secret code that gets you a certificate of adoption. If you donate

$50 or $100, you receive a certificate indicating that you have saved 500 or 1,000 turtles, respectively, along with postcards, stickers, and an activity book. The brand's website says, "When you buy EnviroKidz, you're giving animals hope for a brighter future on Earth. We donate a Portion of sales to organizations around the world that help save vulnerable and endangered animals." The company donates 1% of all sales to its animal partners, which the box says amounted to more than $4.2 million in 2020.[11] In 2026, Walmart was selling the cereal for about $6. This means that for each box sold, the company donates six cents to turtle and other animal protection efforts.

Supporting military families

In a press release announcing a partnership between Cheerios and the United Service Organizations (USO), the nonprofit that supports military service members, General Mills explained that the company "has a longstanding commitment to supporting our troops and their families. The Cheer program lets them know that we recognize them and are grateful for all they give to our country."

Just before Thanksgiving 2011, Cheerios buyers could clip out the Cheer postcard shown in Figure 40, write a cheery note of thanks, stamp it, and mail it to the USO, which then distributed the cards to military families whose loved ones were on active duty. General Mills donated $150,000 to the USO to kick off the program, and it pledged to donate one additional dollar for every postcard received, up to an additional $100,000. The funds would be used to reconnect military families with their deployed service members. The press release quoted the USO president: "We love this campaign because it gives cheerfulness directly to individuals while providing funds to support programs that will reach all of the people we serve." Worthy as it was, the campaign has not been repeated.

Supporting antihunger activities

Each of the Big Four cereal companies has committed to help end hunger—which makes sense for any food company. In 2019, General Mills announced its goal to "enable 30 billion meals for hungry people by 2030,

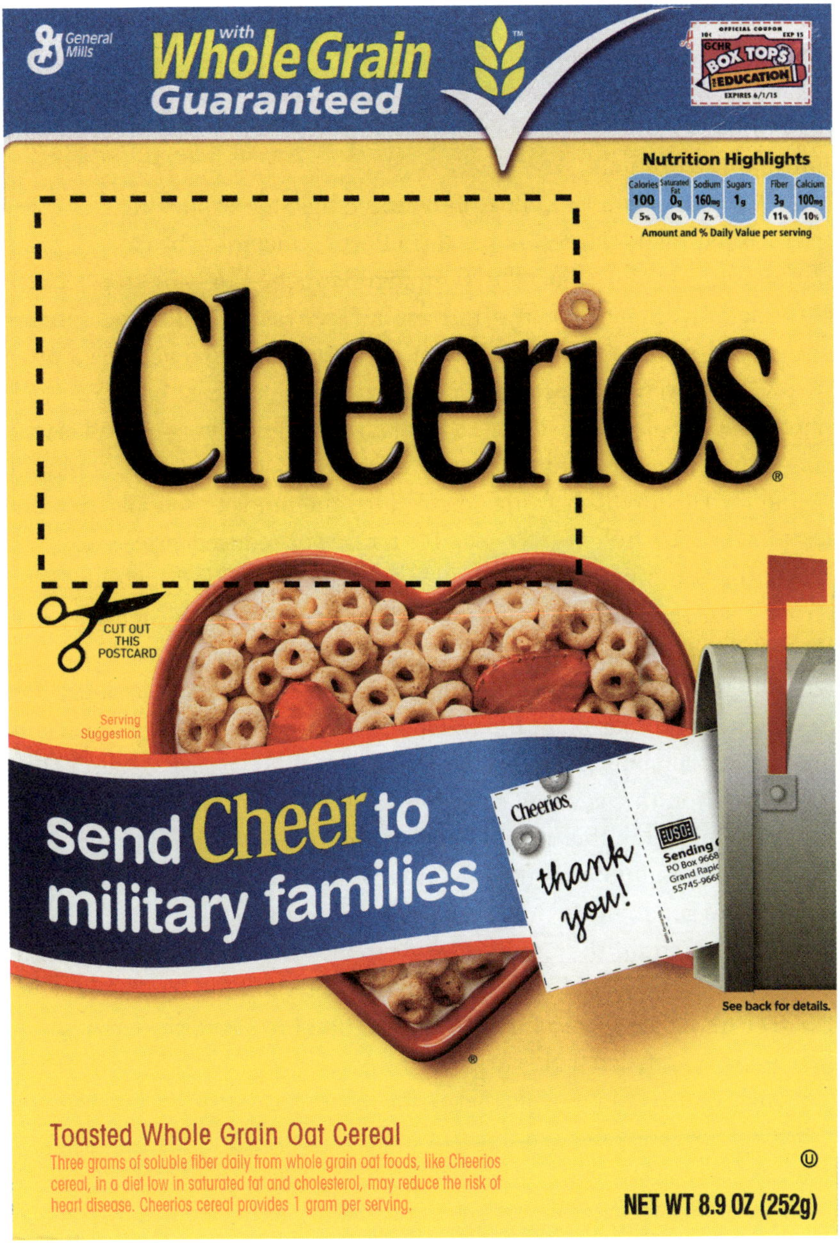

FIGURE 40 For 2 months in 2011, General Mills issued Cheerios boxes with cutout postcards to "send Cheer to military families," support USO programs, and sell Cheerios.

together with our nonprofit impact partners." Five years later, the company reported surpassing this goal by more than 40%.[12] Post reported donating 55 million bowls of cereal in 2023. Each company makes similar commitments and has similar partnerships with local and national antihunger organizations.

In 2011, for example, Kellogg announced the Share Your Breakfast campaign as part of its "largest marketing effort . . . including broadcast, print, digital and social media." The campaign launched in time to celebrate National Breakfast Day and to raise awareness of childhood hunger. Consumers were to photograph their breakfasts and upload the pictures to a Kellogg website, post them on social media, or text them. For each photo, Kellogg pledged to donate a breakfast to a child who might otherwise go without. The company ultimately donated $200,000 to the nonprofit Action for Healthy Kids, which distributed the funds to schools where at least half of the students were eligible for free or reduced-price meals.[13]

Another example: General Mills partnered with Big Machine Label Group (which represents country musicians such as Reba McEntire and Rascal Flatts) on the Outnumber Hunger campaign in 2012 to help raise $2 million for Feeding America, the largest US hunger relief organization (see Figure 41). To explain the collaboration between country musicians and a cereal company, a Big Machine official said, "If you ask General Mills, they'll tell you this is about the moms, and moms also are the country target." Confirming this, a study of cause marketing had found that 80% of shoppers—but 93% of moms—said they would switch to a brand that supported a good cause.[14] Mom campaigns often involve kids. Thus, Rascal Flatts appeared on the Cookie Crisp cereal box with a banner: "HELP FEEDING AMERICA [logo] SECURE 5 MEALS FOR YOUR LOCAL FOOD BANK." The back of the box, noting that 1 in 6 Americans struggles with hunger, instructed kids to go online and enter a unique code number, for which General Mills would make a 65-cent donation to Feeding America. Kids could also download a free song of their choice (in tiny print, "Offer good while supplies last").

In 2019, Post partnered with Walmart to sell cereals in boxes specially marked "Fight Hunger. Spark Change." For each box of the marked cereals (e.g., Oreo O's, Honey Bunches of Oats), Post donated 10 cents (that amount again) to Feeding America. Kellogg and General Mills have also participated in the Walmart program, which includes many kids' sugary cereals.

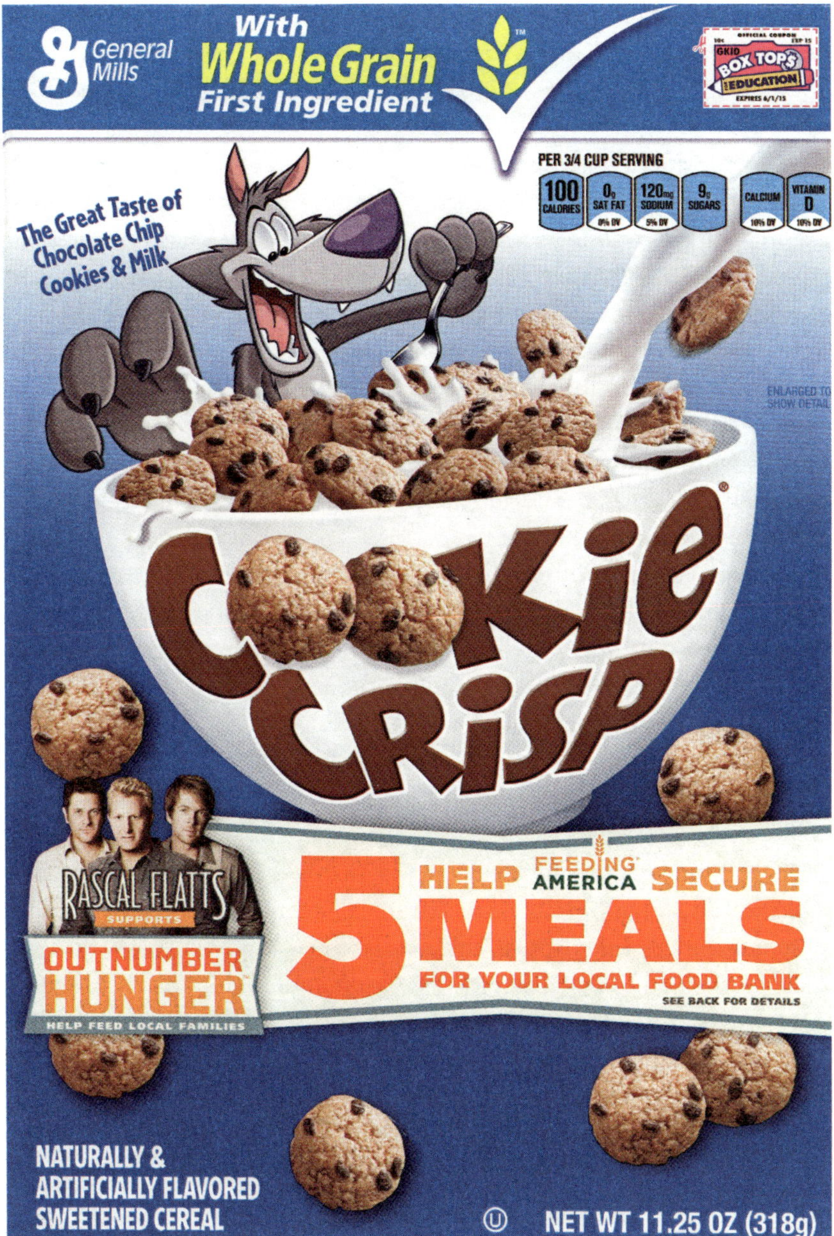

FIGURE 41 General Mills partnered with Feeding America in 2012 and put its logo on the front of this Cookie Crisp box to demonstrate the company's commitment to addressing hunger in America—by buying this cereal, of course.

Walmart benefits from the cereal sales, but customers and suppliers do the donating. Still, the results are notable. Between 2014 and 2024, the Walmart program donated $186 million to Feeding America's food bank network.[15]

General Mills engages in antihunger efforts in other creative ways. In 2022, its Big G Cereals partnered with the Academy of Nutrition and Dietetics to copromote accessible and affordable breakfasts. At the academy's annual meeting and trade exposition, the company provided a giant cereal slide, encouraged dietitians to use social media to help raise hunger awareness, and hosted a competition to test dietitians' knowledge of the benefits of cereal for breakfast. More concretely, it donated $250,000 to Share Our Strength's No Kid Hungry campaign, to which it has contributed more than $9 million since 2012.[16] Share Our Strength is an antihunger nonprofit; it launched No Kid Hungry in 2010 to make sure kids are fed at school and during summers.

In 2023, General Mills again committed to donate $250,000 to No Kid Hungry during the academy's annual meeting. It also pledged to donate $5 any time a dietitian posted a photo of the Big G Cereals booth on social media with #BigG4Good; the company's total donation was $255,000. That same year, in collaboration with Kellogg, Post, and Quaker, General Mills further supported No Kid Hungry by, among other actions, providing cereal breakfasts at meetings with legislators in Washington, DC, on National Cereal Day.[17]

Kellogg engages in similar campaigns. In 2022, the company partnered with No Kid Hungry for its Breakfast for All campaign. Consumers could purchase cereals (like Apple Jacks and Frosted Mini-Wheats) and send their receipts to Kellogg for either a $5-off coupon for another Kellogg purchase or a donation to No Kid Hungry. This campaign resulted in Kellogg donating $250,000 to help hungry kids. In 2025, WK Kellogg partnered with Feeding America for the same campaign, but with one change: customers no longer had to choose between coupons or donations. The company would donate $10 to Feeding America for each proof of purchase of its participating cereals (Frosted Mini-Wheats, Frosted Flakes, and Froot Loops), and the customer would receive a coupon for a future purchase of the same amount. The 90-day campaign included fine print that said, "Maximum donation $250,000." These contributions are deductible from taxes but also achieve one other goal: antihunger organizations are less inclined to say anything publicly about the nutritional quality of the donated products.

As cause marketing antihunger campaigns go, the most fun are cereal box domino challenges. These are competitions to line up the longest possible chain of upright cereal boxes to be toppled over like dominoes. Once toppled, the boxes go to local food banks. To our amazement, a Guinness World Records title exists for "The Most Cereal Boxes Toppled in a Domino Fashion." The 2023 title went to Move For Hunger, an antihunger nonprofit, for the toppling of 12,952 cereal boxes in a Detroit basketball arena. For this particular event, the Michigan-based WK Kellogg Co, along with the retailer Kroger, donated the cereal boxes, and Tony the Tiger set off the domino toppling. More commonly, these contests generate cereal sales. A school that collected 700 boxes one year pledged to collect 7,000 the next.[18]

Efforts to end hunger in America, urgent as they may be, still have a long way to go. Whether a mostly sugary breakfast cereal is the best way to feed people in need is highly debatable. What is not debatable is the benefit of cereal philanthropy to the Big Four in reputation, brand loyalty, goodwill, tax advantages, silence about the sugar, and—the point of all this—ongoing sales.

CHAPTER 17

CEREAL GOES INTERNATIONAL

With cereal sales waning in the United States, analysts advise the Big Four companies to capitalize on the increasing westernization of global markets to boost sales. They tell cereal companies to get busy introducing their products into Asia, Africa, and the Middle East, where low incomes and cultural unfamiliarity with breakfast cereals have long been barriers: "Going forward, the biggest driver of growth in the global breakfast cereal market will be the rising influence of Western dietary patterns in these developing countries."[1]

On a global level, American companies are market leaders; Kellanova (formerly Kellogg) leads sales, followed by General Mills and Nestlé, PepsiCo, and Post, which includes Weetabix, number one in the UK. For a long time, Kellogg dominated the global market, but General Mills began to challenge that dominance in 1990 when it formed the joint venture with Nestlé known as Cereal Partners Worldwide (CPW) to distribute products from both companies. CPW began by selling cereals in France, Spain, and Portugal, and by 2025 it operated 15 international factories, distributing products in 130 countries.[2]

Kellogg's history of international expansion explains its long-term lead. It began overseas production of Corn Flakes in 1924 in Sydney, Australia, followed by the establishment of manufacturing plants in Botany, New South Wales (1928), and England (1938). Fast forward to the early 1990s, when Kellogg took advantage of the Soviet Union's collapse to open plants in Latvia, Belarus, and Russia. It also opened plants in India and China. By 2021, Kellogg operated 21 international manufacturing facilities, producing 23 brands for distribution in 180 countries. But in 2023, Kellogg sold its business in Russia, which included three manufacturing plants, fully exiting that market. Although North America remained Kellogg's largest cereal market, international sales accounted for about 40% of its revenues; the company expected this percentage to increase from sales in Latin America, Africa, the Middle East, and Asia.[3] It remains to be seen how the company's 2023 split into WK Kellogg (domestic cereals) and Kellanova (international), and their 2025 acquisition by Ferrero and Mars, respectively, will affect global market shares.

All cereal companies have faced barriers selling to international populations who did not grow up eating ready-to-eat cold cereals and who typically ate quite different breakfast staples, if they ate breakfast at all. In countries like India, cold milk proved a particularly tricky problem. If people consumed milk, they usually drank it hot. Every country has its own labeling and ingredient regulations, forcing companies to package cereals in country-specific boxes. To the companies dealing with such challenges, the cultural and health implications of replacing traditional breakfasts with sugary cereals were irrelevant; their sole goal was to expand the cereal market. In this, they succeeded, as illustrated by the example of Kellogg's experience in India.

Case study: India

What cereal companies were up against is illustrated by the Indian market. At a New Delhi supermarket in 2007, we bought the box shown in Figure 42. Its back panel said: "Being a mother is quite difficult. . . . Getting your child to eat breakfast can be a struggle. . . . You need a perfect balance of something filling and tasty" and "1 serving of Kellogg's Chocos = fibre of 2 chapattis + calcium of 2 glasses of milk." On the side panel: "Chocos breakfast provides 'SOLID' Nutrition because it has: 'goodness of 2 chapattis, calcium of 2 glasses of milk, 11 essential vitamins and minerals.'"

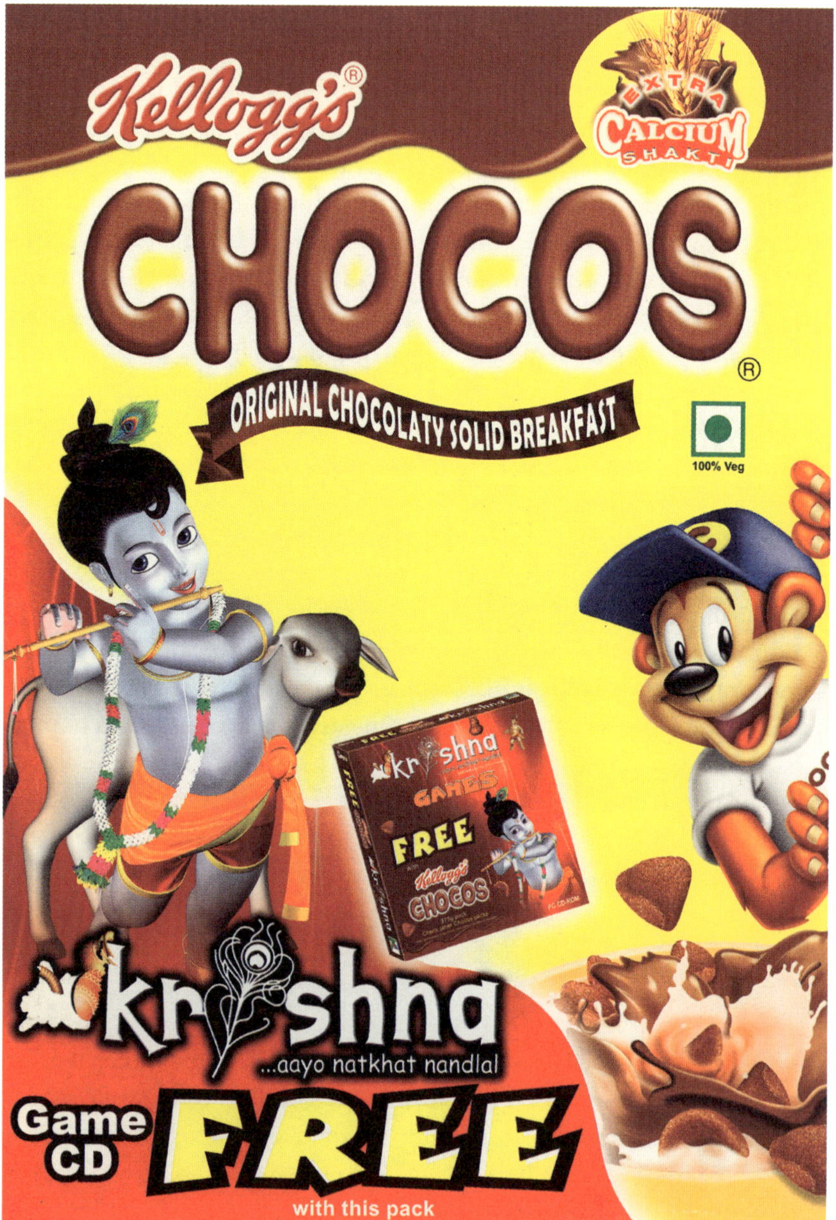

FIGURE 42 Kellogg's challenge in introducing its cereals to India was to convince people to replace traditional breakfast foods with products like this 2007 box of "CHOCOLATY SOLID BREAKFAST." The enticement of a free game CD undoubtedly helped.

It was not just that Kellogg was positioning Chocos as an alternative to chapatis (unleavened flatbreads); it was marketing this chocolate-flavored sugary cereal as nutritionally *better* than traditional Indian foods. CPW used the same strategy. In Turkey, it advertised that its cereals have "as much calcium as two servings of feta cheese, and the iron of four eggs"—not mentioning that these nutrients are added through fortification.[4]

In the early 2000s, typically common Indian breakfasts included a variety of highly flavored, spicy, and hot traditional chapatis, parathas (another flatbread), or vadas (fried snacks). At first, Indian consumers found the cereal flakes to be too bland, cold, and insubstantial, especially because they usually added boiled and sweetened milk, which made the flakes soggy. The cereal's high price was also an issue.

We thought marketing presweetened breakfast flakes as more nutritious than traditional Indian breakfasts seemed condescending and offensive, as did others.[5] The companies' first foray into India's market was by all measures a failure. Consumers purchased cereals one time as a novelty but did not repeat purchases—*the* critical factor in growing market share.

But to Kellogg and General Mills, India seemed ripe for the cereal invasion. Its population was growing rapidly, and younger people are attracted by convenience foods and Western dietary patterns. Kellogg began operations in India in the early 1990s with products such as corn flakes, wheat flakes, and basmati rice flakes. These did not sell well, but when Frosties launched in 1997, it did better, especially when the company reduced prices. Kellogg also replaced the rooster on packages (like the box shown in Figure 3 in Chapter 2) with images more appealing to India's large vegetarian population. It illustrated the boxes with more familiar images such as the Chocos' Krishna, and it used words like *shakti* ("power") on its iron-fortified cereals. In 2023, about 15% of Indian households bought Kellogg breakfast cereals, but the company's immediate goal was 25%, which it considered merely "scratching the surface." Kellogg's spinoff Kellanova had a 75% share of the cold cereal market in India that year.[6]

Food colors, international style

In 2025, artificial colors were still widely used in kids' cereals sold in the United States and in countries throughout Latin America. We have cereal boxes produced in 2024 and 2025 from Bolivia, Colombia, Costa Rica, and Mexico with various combinations of FD&C Red 40, Yellow 5 and 6, and Blue 1. We also have a box of Froot Loops from Canada containing those colors and sweetened with stevia; it comes *avec grimauves*—with marshmallows. As we noted in Chapter 5, US advocates for getting rid of the artificial dyes observed that some American cereals marketed in Australia, New Zealand, and some countries in Europe were able to substitute natural colors for the artificial dyes used in the US versions.[7] We show an example from France in Figure 43.

Indeed, some countries have more stringent rules governing artificial colors. Canada, for example, limits synthetic colors to specified parts per million (ppm). For cereals, Red 40 (known as Allura in Canada) cannot exceed 300 ppm either by itself or when combined with other colors, explaining why its Froot Loops are somewhat less vibrant than those sold in the US.[8]

Although the Food and Drug Administration (FDA) banned Red 3 (erythrosine) in 2025, the European Food Safety Authority (EFSA) essentially banned it in Europe in 2011, allowing it only in maraschino cherries and fruit cocktail. Red 40 is still used in Europe and listed as Allura Red or E129 on labels. But since 2010, the European Union and the United Kingdom require cereals with dyes to be labeled "may have an adverse effect on activity and attention in children."[9] This warning was all it took to prompt some companies to switch to natural color dyes.

Froot Loops sold in Australia and New Zealand are labeled "No artificial flavours or colours" and instead list "natural colours (paprika extract, carmine, curcumin, vegetable carbon, copper chlorophyll)." And as US food safety advocates have pointed out, whereas General Mills' Trix in the US contains Red 40, Yellow 6, and Blue 1, the equivalent box in Australia promotes "no artificial colours," instead listing "chlorophylls, carmine, and carotene."[10] We have a box of Nestlé's Trix from Germany, *mit bunten Farben aus der Natur* ("with bright natural colors") from carotene dyes. Our 2025 box of Canadian Froot Loops (*sans grimauves*) uses concentrated carrot juice, anthocyanin, annatto, turmeric, and concentrated watermelon, blueberry, and huito juices—from huito fruit trees in the Amazon, an indigenous source of a dye called jagua blue.

Also touched on in Chapter 5, concerns about food dyes have typically focused on their effects on childhood hyperactivity. In 2007, EFSA commissioned a study to determine whether hyperactivity was linked to consuming mixtures of food dyes (and the preservative sodium benzoate). Its "Southampton" study, conducted by researchers at Southampton University in the UK, found some evidence for the link, but its results were difficult to interpret. EFSA initially viewed the evidence as too weak and inconsistent to take action, but it eventually interpreted the totality of the evidence as showing a "direction of travel" between the artificial dyes and behavior.[11] It ruled that six specific colors could continue to be used, but only when accompanied by the warning; that mostly ended their use.

Consumers in many countries around the world do not have to make trade-offs when it comes to cereal and artificial colors. The cereal companies managed to find substitutes because they had to. In 2025, Kellogg and General Mills finally announced they would remove colors in the US by the end of 2027—finally catching up with the rest of the world.

Front-of-package labels: Nutri-Score

The Nutri-Score front-of-package labeling system first appeared on products in France in 2017.[12] Created by Sorbonne professor Serge Hercberg, the system is used in France and several other European countries. The logo contains five sections in colors (dark green to red) with letters (A to E). The system assigns the letters on the basis of a complicated algorithm that considers the usual negative nutrients (saturated fatty acid, sugars, salt) as well as several positives (fiber, protein, fruit, vegetables, beans, nuts, and healthy oils) and calories. We show an example, in this case Kellogg's Unicorn Froot Loops with a Nutri-Score of C, in Figure 43.

Nutri-Score's European Scientific Committee has updated the algorithm several times in response to criticism, on one hand that it is too restrictive and penalizes healthy foods, but on the other that it insufficiently penalizes sugars and ultra-processing. Recent changes allow distinctions between cereals with differing amounts of sugar. Hercberg has proposed adding an ultra-processing designation to the logo. But as an indication of the algorithm's complexity, the user guide spans 135 pages.[13]

The strengths and weaknesses of Nutri-Score are exemplified by three cereals, all sold in France in 2024: Kellogg's Trésor with a Nutri-Score of D ("Choco Nut Flavour"); Kellogg's Unicorn Froot Loops (Figure 43) with

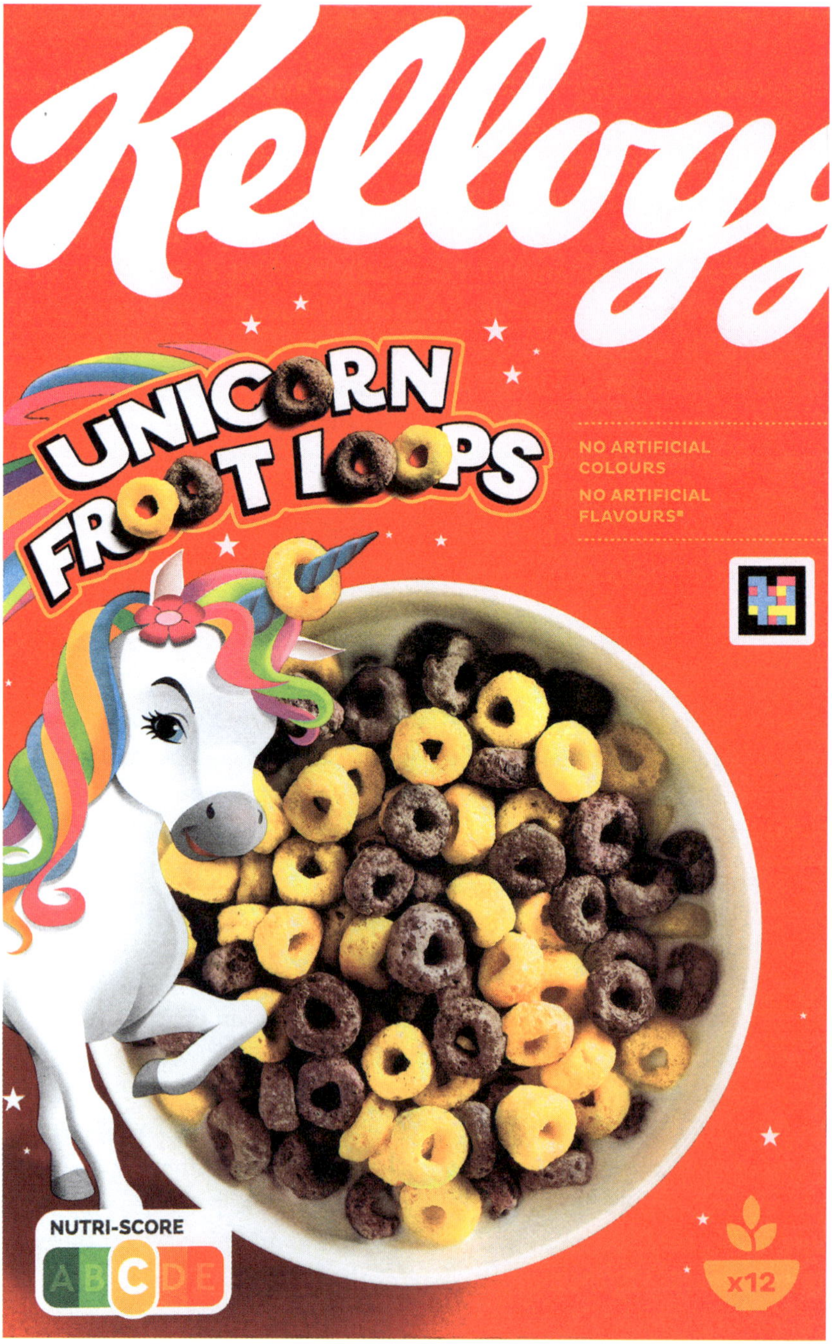

FIGURE 43 This 2024 Kellogg's box, purchased in France, displays a NUTRI-SCORE rating of C, indicating it is a poor (although not terrible) choice based on an algorithm that evaluates a food's overall nutritional value.

a Nutri-Score of C ("No artificial colours, No artificial flavours"); and Nestlé's Bio Chocapic ranked Nutri-Score A ("C'est fort en chocolat!"). The French labels are even harder to read than those in the United States, not least because they are printed in multiple languages and, in the case of Trésor, in a microscopic black font on a barely contrasting dark red background. To try to make sense of why their Nutri-Scores vary so much, here are a few nutrition details, per serving:

Trésor (D): 137 calories, 1.4 g saturated fat, 7.8 g sugar, 1.1 g fiber, 7.1 g protein.

Froot Loops (C): 115 calories, 0.3 g saturated fat, 7.5 g sugar, 1.2 g fiber, 2.5 g protein.

Chocapic (A): 117 calories, 0.5 g saturated fat, 6.7 g sugar, 2.4 g fiber, 2.6 g protein.

We view these cereals as nutritionally much alike, with only minor differences. We are happy the A-scored Chocapic is Bio (organic), and it does have a little less sugar and twice as much fiber per serving as the other two, but it is still a low-fiber, sugary, candy-flavored, ultra-processed choice.

Hercberg defends Nutri-Score as scientifically based and demonstrated to improve food choice, and he cites considerable evidence to support these contentions. The ferocity of food industry opposition to this system suggests that it must be reducing sales of the lower-graded items. Italian agribusiness, for example, has lobbied forcefully for an alternative scheme, NutrInform, backed up by industry-funded studies. To us, the Italian alternative resembles the industry-favored and widely ignored Facts Up Front used on US cereal boxes.[14]

Indeed, food industry lobbying against Nutri-Score has been so blatantly self-serving that it has become the focus of case studies and research. One particularly revealing study examined published research and opinion papers that argue against use of Nutri-Score: study results were 21 times more likely to find flaws with Nutri-Score if the authors had financial ties to food companies or if a food company sponsored the research.[15]

Proponents of Nutri-Score expected it to be adopted by the European Commission as a labeling system throughout the European Union, but some analysts now consider it to be in full retreat. Several countries have dropped its use, leaving Nutri-Score on packages only in France, Spain, Germany, Belgium, Luxembourg, and the Netherlands. In March 2025, the Commission took Nutri-Score off its agenda, leaving its future uncertain.[16]

Front-of-package: Warning labels

A growing number of countries in Latin America, among them Argentina, Brazil, Chile, Colombia, Mexico, Peru, and Uruguay, require foods defined as high in saturated fat, sugar, sodium, or calories (and sometimes artificial sweeteners and caffeine) to display black "high-in" or "excess" warning labels.[17] The labels are part of broader public health efforts aimed at preventing obesity, especially among children. Some countries do not allow packages with warning labels to display cartoons, or be sold or used in schools, or advertised on television.

This movement began in Chile in 2007, led by public health nutrition professor Dr. Ricardo Uauy and Dr. Guido Girardi, a public-health-oriented pediatrician who was a member of the Chilean senate. Despite strong opposition from the food industry, they convinced the legislature to pass the Law of Food Labeling and Advertising in 2012. This law, which took effect in 2016, required black stop-sign warning labels, but it also restricted marketing of foods displaying warning labels on media and in schools to children under the age of 14.[18]

We saw the warning labels for the first time at a meeting in Rome when Dr. Girardi autographed the box of Kellogg's Zucaritas to one of us (MN), shown in Figure 44: *"para Nestle la buena con cariño* [with affection], *Junio 20."* It displayed two warning labels from the Chilean Health Ministry: *ALTO EN AZÚCARES* ("high in sugars") and *ALTO EN CALORÍAS* ("high in calories"). This cereal had the usual 12 grams of sugars per serving.

The law also banned cartoons on cereals with warning labels, but early in 2020, we were in a Santiago supermarket and were surprised to see several kids' cereals illustrated with cartoons. The companies had evaded the warning requirement by replacing the sugars with artificial sweeteners. Mexico, learning from this example, included artificial sweeteners (*edulcorantes*) in its warnings: *Contiene edulcorantes, no recommendable en niños* ("Contains sweeteners, not recommended for children").

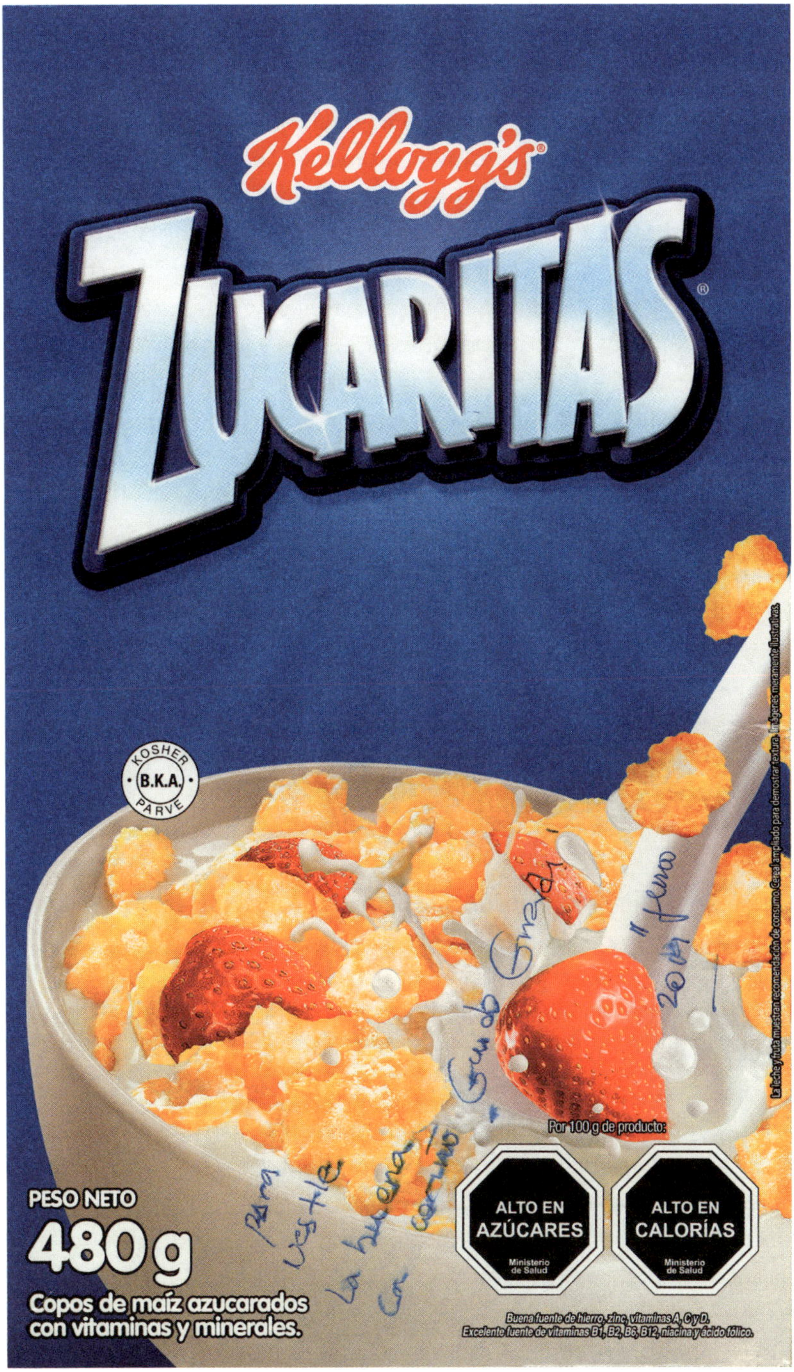

FIGURE 44 In 2016, Chile became the first country to require warning labels on foods high in sugar, salt, saturated fat, or calories. Kellogg's Zucaritas' *ALTO EN AZÚCARES* and *ALTO EN CALORÍAS* meant *adios* to Tony the Tiger.

Food companies did everything they could to oppose the Chilean initiatives, invoking the Latin American equivalent of the First Amendment. They succeeded in delaying implementation of the labeling law for nearly a decade by engaging in the equivalent of "a hard-fought guerrilla war."[19]

In Mexico, food industry lobbying succeeded in getting the largely indigestible sweetener allulose to be considered natural, despite Canada and the UK having banned it as a suspected carcinogen. Because Mexican law did not specifically mention allulose, it did not have to be counted as an artificial sweetener and required no warning label.[20] The Mexican law requires warning labels on cereals with more than 275 calories per 100 grams, more than 10% of calories from sugar, or more than 1 milligram of sodium per calorie. In terms of a 1-ounce serving, this means that warning labels are required on any cereal with more than 83 calories, 2 grams of sugar, or 83 milligrams of sodium. Most cereals exceed these standards.

After the law took effect, Mexican agents surveyed retail stores for monitoring and noncompliance. During one enforcement sweep, they confiscated 380,000 boxes of Kellogg cereals—Froot Loops and Cocoa Krispies—that exceeded the standards but had cartoons on the boxes and no warning labels.[21] In 2023 and again in 2025, we saw cereal boxes with round and square blank stickers covering up cartoons or celebrities on boxes that had violated the rules.

But companies have other ways of evading the law. On our 2025 visit to Mexico, we bought a box of Nestlé's chocolate Letritas (similar to Alpha-Bits) with a cartoon rabbit and no warning labels; its sugar and calories were just below the cut points. A box of Kellogg's Zucaritas displayed Tony the Tiger with a banner proclaiming a 70% reduction in sugar; its sugar was below the cut point, and its *alulosa* ("allulose") did not count.

We snapped up a box of Kellogg's Froot Loops *con deliciosos malvaviscos* ("with delicious marshmallows") with warnings about excess sugar and calories. In accordance with the law, it did not have a cartoon on the front, but it did depict a blowup of a *malvavisco* in the precise shape of the toucan mascot. The box was also illustrated with the black beak and tail of the mascot wrapped around the sides of the box—a work-around, literally. Kellogg offered another kind of Froot Loops, boasting about the addition of a new artificial blue color dye; its back panel taught kids how to use the colors: "yellow plus blue equals green."

It is easy to understand why cereal companies would object to warning labels and do everything they can to evade them. Warning labels reduce sales, and improve public understanding of nutrition. They deter children from wanting the labeled products that cannot be brought to school and are subject to social disapproval. And as happened in Chile and Mexico, they encourage companies to reformulate their products with artificial sweeteners, which we also consider unhealthy, especially in cereals marketed to children.[22]

From a public health standpoint, the replacement of traditional breakfasts by conveniently packaged cold cereals is part of the "nutrition transition," the increasing westernization of diets accompanied by a shift from widespread conditions of undernutrition to population-wide weight gain and obesity-linked chronic diseases.[23] The warning labels on cereal boxes—and the accompanying marketing restrictions—are examples of how public health advocates in Latin America are attempting to counter the potentially serious health consequences of this transition. How cereal companies will continue to fight such measures will be of great interest to us.

CONCLUSION

As we come to the end of this book, we hope we have convinced you that cereal boxes are more than merely packages for sugar-sweetened grains; they are archival treasures revealing a colorful and detailed history of American food politics and culture. The sheer size of the cereal box—most measure 12 by 8 inches—makes it possible for cereal companies to use them as marketing billboards. We could not have recounted the political history of food ingredients, claims, and marketing with such precision, detail, and illustration using canned vegetables or boxed macaroni and cheese—although they also have their own stories. But the cereal aisle, with its brightly colored boxes, cartoon mascots, and promises of nutrition and health, is a source of endless fascination, and not only for us. Breakfast cereal is an iconic American-invented food, ubiquitous in our culture, and a product that has made its way onto millions of tables around the world.

Much of this book focuses on the boxes and antics of the Big Four cereal companies—Kellogg (now WK Kellogg/Ferrero and Kellanova/Mars), General Mills, Post, and PepsiCo/Quaker Oats. These large, aggressive, and competitive companies are in the business of selling processed grains with whatever add-ins will entice shoppers to put the boxes in grocery carts, mostly on the basis of what the boxes say. Today, with cereal sales declining, all the major companies want to revive domestic sales and expand internationally.

We organized this discussion of the politics and culture of cereal into three broad categories: ingredients, claims, and marketing, although the lines between these categories blur; everything is about marketing. But as we look back to the early 1900s when ready-to-eat breakfast cereals were first invented, we find it remarkable how little their ingredients have changed. From the beginning, cereals were based on grains, with sugars, nutrients, colors, and flavors added in as soon as they could be. Kellogg's Rice Krispies in 2026 has the same four ingredients it did in 1928—rice, sugar, malt flavor, and salt. Other ingredients come and go, but the core ingredients have stayed much the same.

A century after their invention, cereal boxes are still making health claims. The companies began by promoting their products for digestive health, then added claims for the benefits of naturally occurring vitamins and minerals almost as soon as the functions of these nutrients were discovered. Recognizing that promoting nutrients sold cereals, the companies pushed for fortification, as much of it as they could get. Once Congress authorized nutrient content and health claims in 1990, the Big Four pressed the Food and Drug Administration (FDA) to permit both kinds, often succeeding—and always to the benefit of sales.

Claims proliferated in the cereal aisle. Those for better digestive health were joined by overt or implied claims for prevention of cancer, heart disease, and osteoporosis, and later by less scientifically supported claims for benefits such as enhancing immunity, childhood attentiveness, or sleep. By the early 2020s, the struggles over the need to substantiate health claims had reached a standoff. In 2026, while we still see nutrient content claims on most cereals, and heart-health claims on some, we haven't seen anything new since the 2023 sleep claim. But we expect cereal companies to dream up new ones any day.

Cereal companies will always look for new ways to sell their products, drawing on public affection for nostalgia, sugar, vitamins, and health and targeting specific demographic and identity-diverse segments of the population. Cereal marketing has kept pace with transitions in media, from print in the early 1900s, to radio in the 1920s, television in the 1950s, cable in the 1980s, and digital social media of the 2000s. In today's era of on-demand media and information, cereal companies have stepped up with branded apps and marketing on YouTube, TikTok, and more. The Big Four now pay to have pop-up ads appear on our phones and computers, delivering targeted messages and promotional offers to kids as well as to adults. And they pay dietitian influencers to share videos on TikTok and Instagram featuring cereal brands, nutrition and health messages, and recipes to reach young adults.

Much of cereal marketing is aimed at kids, beginning with the bright, primary-colored boxes illustrated with cheerful cartoon mascots and continuing to include as much sugar as companies can get away with. When kids grow up, they still feel a strong emotional connection to their favorites—the companies' prized nostalgia effect and intense brand loyalty. Marketing techniques that evoke nostalgia have worked for more than a century. The take-home lesson for the Big Four: the more the market for cereals seems to change, the more it stays pretty much the same. And therein lies the most serious problem for this industry.

Big Cereal appears to be in a financial free fall; sales have been declining for years. In the first quarter of 2025, the WK Kellogg Co reported "weaker than expected consumption trends," which translated to lower sales and a net income drop of more than 45% from the previous year.[1] In 2025, Ferrero, one of the world's largest producers of chocolate and seller of candy and Nutella, bought the company for about $3 billion in order to shore up its business in North America. Ferrero had acquired some of Kellogg's cookie brands in 2019, but cereal had not been part of that deal.[2]

Similarly, the Kellogg Company spun off Kellanova, which retained Kellogg's international cereals but was sold off to Mars in 2025. Mars is a pet care and snack food company, with candy brands such as M&M'S, Snickers, and Skittles. We suspect these will soon turn up in breakfast cereals. Although US regulators approved this $36 billion deal right away, the European Union viewed it as raising antitrust violations and launched an investigation; it eventually approved the sale.[3] Both Ferrero and Mars are private family-owned corporations that are not beholden to public shareholders, Wall Street analysts, or quarterly earnings reports. We don't know yet whether this will make any difference to cereal marketing strategies, but are likely to find out soon.

While Kellogg was disappearing as an iconic cereal company, other cereal companies were also in trouble. General Mills reported a decline in sales of its Big G cereals and announced a restructuring plan that would cost the company an estimated $130 million by the end of 2028. A company representative said, "While this news represents hard choices, they are necessary to fund product innovation . . . and position General Mills' long-term success." PepsiCo's Quaker Oats closed a manufacturing plant in 2024, and a year later—to the day—Post announced the closure of two cereal plants, citing the category decline.[4]

When we walk the supermarket cereal aisles, based on the number of General Mills' cereals occupying shelf space, its Big G brands still appear predominant. But they face increasing competition. Private (or store) brands now account for 9% of the market share for cereals, and this percentage is expected to increase, not least because every popular Big Four brand seems to have its very own store-brand copycat. Walmart, for example, offers Great Value Fruit Spins for Froot Loops, Magic Treasures for Lucky Charms, and Berry Crunch for Cap'n Crunch's Crunch Berries—at greatly reduced prices. We cannot help but mention that store-brand cereals often contain more sugar and less whole grain than those from the Big Four yet have managed to slip below the radar of consumers and health critics.

Competition also comes from smaller start-up cereal companies selling products in Sprout's Farmers Market, Whole Foods, and co-op health food stores. Niche "better-for-you" brands, such as Nature's Path Organic, Lovebird, Catalina Crunch, Seven Sundays, and Purely Elizabeth, are largely unknown to the general public, but they are working their way into national chain grocery stores like Kroger, Target, and Walmart. Most niche brands are certified USDA Organic or display the Non-GMO Project Verified widget, or both. These brands claim higher-quality nutrition. They include novel ingredients such as sorghum and cassava flour as grain replacements, monk fruit sweetener to replace sugar, and pea protein to boost the protein content. In reality, some of these ingredients signal that the products are ultra-processed, despite their aura of health.

These new brands appeal to customers who are focused on health, are tired of the Big Four, want higher quality, and are willing to pay for it. Lovebird, a start-up cereal company created by a former General Mills employee, says it is "made by a father for his daughter." Its tagline: "goodbye fake stuff, hello real cereal." Lovebird advertises that its cereal will "remove inflammatory gut disruptors," free as it is of refined grain, refined sugar, and "inflammatory" oils (in quotes because of the lack of convincing evidence for the harm of seed oils).[5] Its boxes sell for about twice the price of a Big Four cereal, and we cannot yet tell whether products like these will appeal to a mass market or be acquired by a Big Four cereal company attempting to remain relevant to younger consumers.

We mention relevance because we are at an especially interesting moment in cereal politics. The advent of the second Trump administration's movement to Make America Healthy Again (MAHA) has cast a harsh light on the sugar and color additives in breakfast cereals as factors in the declining health of America's children. The movement's focus on child health reminds us of the 1969 White House Conference on Food, Nutrition, and Health and its recommendations to reduce childhood food insecurity. Many of its recommendations were implemented, among them the creation of the Supplemental Nutrition Program for Women, Infants, and Children (WIC) and expansion of the food stamp program (now SNAP), both targets of severe budget cuts in 2025. The MAHA assessment also reminds us of the Obama administration's initiative to end childhood obesity within a generation. Its task force report, with goals similar in many respects to those of MAHA, was strongly criticized as an overreach of government interference with personal choice.[6]

Today, in a changing political landscape, America confronts a perhaps ironic juxtaposition of overweight and malnutrition resulting from overconsumption of low-cost ultra-processed foods of poor nutritional quality, especially by low-income groups. Although many of its breakfast cereals are ultra-processed, Kellogg says "not all 'ultra' processed foods are bad for you."[7] The company insists on the cereal industry's party line: eating breakfast cereals results in better diets and does not promote overweight. We don't disagree—weight gain depends on the entire diet, not just one food—but we view cereal companies as potential change agents to improve the cereal category, if not the entire food industry, and we wish they would do this.

Cereal companies have demonstrated their ability to reformulate for decades, whether by fortifying nutrients, reducing sugar, removing partially hydrogenated oils (trans fats), increasing whole grains and fiber, or promising to remove petroleum-based artificial food dyes. We cannot predict what will come next for cereals. We hope that the MAHA movement will succeed in eliminating artificial colors and other chemicals from the food supply and will induce the FDA to produce a better front-of-package icon for the revised criteria for Healthy (Figure 22e) and a more explicit warning label for ultra-processed products, as well as for foods high in saturated fat, sugar, and salt (Figure 22f).

What will become of the cereal aisle? We wish we had a crystal ball and could tell you. For the sake of cereal enthusiasts like us, we hope this industry continues to reinvent itself—but with better-quality ingredients, less sugar, no artificial colors or flavors, and more organic ingredients in cereals priced so everyone can afford them. We want cereal companies to put excitement about health back into their boxes and cereal aisles. Until then, we will continue to buy—and critically evaluate—the new, outrageous, or entertaining boxes and scrutinize the next moves by the major cereal companies as they navigate today's and tomorrow's marketplace, cultural, and political landscapes. May their next 120 years be as fascinating, entertaining, and instructive as their first.

ACKNOWLEDGMENTS

We have been asked repeatedly what it's been like for the two of us to write this book. To our great pleasure, we turned out to be seamless writing partners, with similar styles, viewpoints, and complementary information to contribute. We each drafted sections and traded them back and forth until we agreed on what they said. Throughout the entire process, we never met in person, although we occasionally used Zoom to work out issues related to chapter content and organization. For both of us, it has been a joy to work together on this book; we couldn't wait to get to it every day.

With that said, we have many people to thank for their advice, information, and support throughout this process: Kate Adamick, Jennifer Berg, Elinor Blake, Ken Castronuevo, Shirin Daly, Leonard Davis, Rebecca Davis, Katherine Diaz, Carolyn Dimitri, Michael Jacobson, Maya Joseph, Johanna Kolodny, Alice Lichtenstein, Jerry Mande, Charles Platkin, Jennifer Pomeranz, Adaire and Mark Putnam, Andrea Thomas, Dana Tupa, and Lisa Young. We particularly want to thank Alicia Estes of NYU's business library, Charlotte Priddle of the NYU Library's Special Collections, and Brooks Johnson of the *Minneapolis Star Tribune* for providing data we could not have obtained any other way.

For gifts of cereal boxes, we especially thank Michaela DeSoucey for lending us the Kellogg's Corn Pops we discuss in Chapter 15 (Figure 36). Friends, family, and colleagues brought us or sent photographs of boxes from their home countries or from their far-flung travels: Gloria Guevara Alvarez, Dr. Dennis Ballwieser, Amy Bentley, Jennifer Berg, Amedeo

Bettauer, Natasha Bernstein Bunzl, Paulina Magaña Carbajal, Lourdes Castro, Earlene Cruz, Jocelyn Harris, Rebecca Nestle, Beth Noveck, Niyati Parekh, Eitan Sasson, Lisa Sasson, Michael Suenkel, Charlotte Vallaey, and Kathleen Wolff.

We are indebted to Anna Soloniuk for creating a figure illustrating trends in cereal fortification; we could not use it in the book but will in talks. For the high-resolution box scans, we are deeply grateful to Niki Kekos, Stevia Ndoe, and Professor Rose DeSiano of NYU Tisch Photography, and especially to Malia Guyer-Stevens of the NYU Library's Special Collections for her patience and help with the David Pollack cereal box collection and our last-minute requests. Thanks to Natalie Holden at Jacksonville University for quickly and precisely recreating high-resolution widget images.

Everlasting thanks to Max Sinsheimer, our literary agent, for his appreciation of the concept of this book and steadfast counsel and support —and even tech help—throughout the process.

For exceptionally thoughtful comments on an early draft of the manuscript, we thank Andrew Smith and Ken Albala, and we can never express enough thanks to UC Irvine sociologist David Meyer for his gratifyingly enthusiastic editorial review. Much appreciation to Rebecca Nestle and Joanne Csete for all the good catches during proofreading.

We are privileged to have had the support of the University of California Press team, with special thanks to Kate Marshall, the best editor anyone could ask for, Natalie Gomez, who patiently shepherded the document and art submission process, and designer Kevin Barrett Kane, who brought this book to life. We so appreciate the sharp-eyed help of copyeditor Lou Doucette in keeping us from errors factual and grammatical, and production manager Julie Van Pelt for moving this project along so seamlessly.

From Marion: Thanks to my NYU Nutrition and Food Studies colleagues and staff, to Dean Jack Knott and Cherrie Short for supporting my late-in-life career, and to Steven Ho, Cliff Rene, and Bill Nesheim for tech support well above the call of duty. I thank my children, Charles and Rebecca Nestle, for letting me talk endlessly about this project in our weekly Zoom meetings, and their partners, Cynthia Mulvihill and Michael Suenkel, for adding to my family. Last, but certainly not least, I thank my partner, Mal Nesheim, for his patience, steadiness, wisdom, and support for so much in my life.

From Lisa: The experiences and knowledge I share would not have existed without my amazingly talented nutrition team and the executive leaders at Kellogg's, with whom I served; I learned the cereal business from the best in the world. You know who you are, and I am forever indebted. And to my students at Jacksonville University, who asked me every day, "Is it done yet?" Yes, you will get your Honors Cereal Seminar. It is done! Endless thanks to my children, Parker and Samantha Sutherland, who served as my personal focus group and ate a lot of cereal growing up. And most of all, to my life partner and husband Hoyt Sutherland, thank you for your endless enthusiasm about this project, for listening to me talk about it endlessly, and for cheering us on every step of the way.

CEREAL BOX ILLUSTRATIONS

NOTES

Many sources of the information we cite in this book are on the internet, some with dates, but some undated. Unattributed quotations are from company websites or cereal box labels. We did not include URLs in part for reasons of space but mostly because they change or disappear so frequently. All online references were available in mid-2025 before the Trump administration revised or eliminated websites dealing with equity and other now-forbidden topics. Sites no longer available are often findable through the Wayback Machine at https://web.archive.org. To search internet sources, use titles or, for academic articles, their digital object identifier (doi) codes. Citations are in a modified *JAMA* reference style that uses standard abbreviations for academic journals; if their titles are not obvious, use the abbreviation to search for them online. The notes abbreviate the names of frequently cited government agencies and nongovernmental groups as shown below. Those listed in the parentheses are the overarching agencies (e.g., ARS is part of USDA).

AHA	American Heart Association
ARS	Agricultural Research Service (USDA)
CDC	Centers for Disease Control and Prevention (HHS)
CFR	Code of Federal Regulations
CSPI	Center for Science in the Public Interest
EFSA	European Food Safety Authority

ERS	Economic Research Service (USDA)
FDA	US Food and Drug Administration (HHS)
FNS	Food and Nutrition Service (USDA)
FTC	Federal Trade Commission
HHS	US Department of Health and Human Services
IARC	International Agency for Research on Cancer (WHO)
IOM	Institute of Medicine (now National Academy of Medicine)
NCHS	National Center for Health Statistics (CDC)
NIH	National Institutes of Health (HHS)
NOP	National Organic Program (USDA)
SNAP	Supplemental Nutrition Assistance Program (USDA)
USDA	US Department of Agriculture
WHO	World Health Organization of the United Nations
WIC	Special Supplemental Nutrition Program for Women, Infants, and Children (USDA)

Chapter 1. Breakfast Cereals: The Basics

1. Johnson IJ, ed. *The History and Manufacture of Breakfast Cereals: Teacher's source book*. Cereal Institute; 1951; Soultana MV, et al. Prehistoric cereal foods of southeastern Europe: an archaeobotanical exploration. *J Archaeol Sci*. 2019;104:97–113. doi:10.1016/j.jas.2018.11.004
2. Kellogg JH. *Plain Facts for Old and Young: Embracing the natural history and hygiene of organic life*. IF Segner; 1887.
3. National Health Association. James C. Jackson, M.D. Dec 29, 2021.
4. Markel H. The secret ingredient in Kellogg's Corn Flakes is Seventh-Day Adventism. *Smithsonian*. Jul 28, 2017; Markel H. *The Kelloggs: The battling brothers of Battle Creek*. Vintage; 2017.
5. Cavendish R. The battle of the corn flakes. *History Today*. Feb 2, 2006.
6. Stolberg SG, Severson K. Kennedy declares "sugar is poison" while announcing ban on food dyes. *New York Times*. Apr 22, 2025.
7. Post CW. *The Road to Wellville*. Postum Cereal Company; 1903.
8. Markel H. *The Kelloggs: The battling brothers of Battle Creek*. Vintage; 2017:135(note 63); Steve. How Battle Creek became the cereal city. Calhoun

County Visitors Bureau, Mar 6, 2020; Braden DR. Kellogg's breakfast revolution. The Henry Ford Archive of Innovation. Aug 21, 2020.

9. Fast RB, Caldwell EF, eds. *Breakfast Cereals and How They Are Made*. American Association of Cereal Chemists; 1990.
10. Kellogg's. *Cereal: The Complete Story*. Kellogg; 2010.
11. Examples: Mattes RD. Ready-to-eat cereal used as a meal replacement promotes weight loss in humans. *J Am Coll Nutr*. 2002;1(6):570–577. doi:10.1080/07315724.2002.10719257; Cho S, et al. The effect of breakfast type on total daily energy intake and body mass index: results from the Third National Health and Nutrition Examination Survey (NHANES III). *J Am Coll Nutr*. 2003;22(4):296–302. doi:10.1080/07315724.2003.10719307
12. Kant AK, Graubard BI. Within-person comparison of eating behaviors, time of eating, and dietary intake on days with and without breakfast: NHANES 2005–2010. *Am J Clin Nutr*. 2015;102:661–670. doi:10.3945/ajcn.115.110262; Adolphus K. The effects of breakfast on behavior and academic performance in children and adolescents. *Front Hum Neurosci*. 2013;7:425. doi:10.3389/fnhum.2013.00425
13. USDA/ERS. *Changes in the Market Structure of the Breakfast Foods Industry*. Rep No 623. 1963; USDA/ERS. *Food Availability (per Capita) Data System: Grains. Flour and cereal products: per capita availability*. Jan 8, 2025.
14. Statista. Consumption of breakfast cereals (cold) in the U.S. 2011–2024. Feb 5, 2024; Zhu Y, et al. Association between ready-to-eat cereal consumption and nutrient intake, nutritional adequacy, and diet quality in adults in the National Health and Nutrition Examination Survey 2015–2016. *Nutrients*. 2019;11(12):2952. doi:10.3390/nu11122952; Terry AL, et al. Breakfast intake among children and adolescents: United States, 2015–2018. *NCHS Data Brief*. 2020;(386):1–8.
15. Ferreday N. The cereal killers. Industry Note #378. Rabobank. Apr 2013; Back A. It's the breakfast of champions no more: cereal is in long-term decline. *Wall Street J*. Sep 15, 2023.
16. Freedonia Focus Reports. *Food Retail: United States*. May 2022; Packaged Facts. *Food Market Outlook 2021: Grocery shopping, home cooking, & food preferences in the waning pandemic period*. Jul 2021.
17. Statista. Breakfast cereals—worldwide. Mar 2025; Barnes Reports. *Breakfast Cereal Manufacturing Industry. 2024 world industry & market outlook*. 2023; Freedonia Focus Reports. *Food Retail: United States*. Jan 2019.
18. Johnson B. As General Mills market lead narrows CEO says company must "behave like a leader." *MN Star Tribune*. Dec 23, 2024; Clapp J, et al. Corporate concentration and power matter for agency in food systems. *Food Policy*. 2025;134:102897. doi:10.1016/j.foodpol.2025.102897
19. Hinds M. U.S. drops 10-year antitrust suit against 3 largest cereal makers. *New York Times*. Jan 16, 1982.

20. Cotterill R, et al. *Harvesting and Tacit Collusion in the Breakfast Cereal Industry: A case study of Nabisco Shredded Wheat and Post Grape Nuts.* U Conn Food Marketing Policy Center; 1994; Barrett J. Two House members seek cereal pricing investigation. *Supermarket News.* Mar 13, 1995.
21. Circana OmniMarket Total Store View. 52-weeks ending Dec 1, 2024.
22. IBIS World. Cereal production in the US. Feb 2024.
23. OpenSecrets. Your home for money in politics.
24. See notes 18 and 21. Pangarkar T. Breakfast cereal market projected to grow at 6.1% CAGR, crossing USD 139.0 billion by 2033. *Market.us News.* Jul 4, 2024.
25. Berning J, Rabinowitz AN. Targeted advertising in the breakfast cereal industry. *J Agric Appl Econ.* 2017;49(3):382–399. doi:10.1017/aae.2017.1
26. Experience the art of J. C. Leyendecker at the Haggin Museum in Stockton, California. Feb 20, 2024.
27. Kellogg Company. What's in the power of a name. *Kellogg News.* Jan 1949.
28. Quaker Oats Co. v. General Mills, 134 F.2d 429 (7th Cir. 1943). Justia U.S. Law. 2024; Miller J. The brand naming strategy behind Cheerios. *Branding Strategy Insider.* Dec. 4, 2019.
29. Wunch NG. Kellogg's Froot Loops brand profile in the United States in 2024. Statista. Jun 18, 2024.

Chapter 2. The Cereal Box: An Overview

1. FDA. *Guidance for Industry: A Food Labeling Guide.* Jan 2013; Food product labeling and packaging 101. *Trustwell.* Mar 15, 2022.
2. 21 CFR, Chapter 1, Subchapter B, Part 101—Food labeling.
3. FDA. Food labeling: general provisions; nutrition labeling; label format; nutrient content claims; health claims; ingredient labeling; state and local requirements; and exemptions; final rules. *Fed Regist.* 1993;58:2066–2294; FDA. *Changes to the Nutrition Facts Panel.* Mar 28, 2024.
4. FDA. *Guidance for Industry: Reference Amounts Customarily Consumed (List of Products for Each Product Category).* Mar 2018; FDA. *Guidance for Industry: Serving Sizes of Foods That Can Reasonably Be Consumed at One Eating Occasion.* Mar 2018.
5. Cereal portion control matters: you could be taking in a lot more calories than you think. *Consumer Reports.* Dec 11, 2014; Rolls BJ, et al. Variations in cereal volume affect the amount selected and eaten for breakfast. *J Acad Nutr Diet.* 2014;114(9):1411–1416. doi:10.1016/j.jand.2014.01.014
6. FDA. *Daily Value on the Nutrition and Supplement Facts Labels.* Mar 5, 2024.
7. FDA. Food allergies. Sep 17, 2024; FDA. *Guidance for Industry: Questions and Answers Regarding Food Allergen Labeling.* 5th ed. Jan 6, 2025.

Chapter 3. Sugars: Ingredient #1 or #2

1. Kellogg JH. *The New Dietetics: What to eat and how: A guide to scientific feeding in health and disease.* Modern Medicine Publishing Co; 1921.
2. USDA/ERS. *Changes in the Market Structure of the Breakfast Foods Industry.* Rep No 623. 1963; Kolhmeier L. Snap, crackle and divestiture. *New York Times.* Apr 25, 1976; Gaine C. Where do kids get their added sugars? Sugar Association. Jul 2019.
3. US Senate. *Hearings before the Consumer Subcommittee of the Committee on Commerce United States Senate Ninety-First Congress, Second Session on Dry Cereals.* July 23, August 4 and 5, 1970. [Quote: p. 12].
4. MeTV Staff. 6 cereals from our childhood that got rid of the word "sugar." MeTV. Apr 21, 2016.
5. 9 surprising facts about Smacks cereal. *Cereal Guru.* June 21, 2019.
6. Environmental Working Group. Children's cereals: sugar by the pound. May 2014.
7. Post Consumer Brands. Post Consumer Brands brings back beloved 90s OREO O's cereal. *PR Newswire.* Jul 6, 2017; Saletta E. Oreo fans left devastated as popular product is axed just before Christmas. *Daily Mail.* Dec 12, 2024.
8. Licensing International. Sweetening the cereal aisle. Jan 22, 2020.
9. Zhang J. New Hershey's/General Mills collaboration is cereal the '90s way: breakfast candy. *Eater.* Jan 6, 2020; Canady R. Do you eat Reese's Puffs daily or are you miserable? *Medium.* Dec 23, 2023; Post Consumer Brands. Calling all Twinkie fans: it's official! New Post Hostess Twinkie cereal is coming soon. *PR Newswire.* Nov 13, 2019; Painter, K. New leader at Post finds cereal lovers still love the sweet stuff. *MN Star Tribune.* Oct 12, 2019.
10. Barboza D. Kraft plans to rethink some products to fight obesity. *New York Times.* Jul 2, 2003; Warner M. Altering Alpha-Bits: not as simple as A B C. *New York Times.* Aug 11, 2005.
11. Some breakfast cereals marketed to kids are more than 50 percent sugar. *Consumer Reports.* Oct 1, 2008.
12. Glaberson H. General Mills achieves further sugar reduction in its cereals. *Bakery&Snacks.* Dec 10, 2010.
13. Jargon J. General Mills to reduce sugar in cereals. *Wall Street J.* Dec 9, 2011.
14. Geller M. General Mills steps down sugar in kids' cereals. Reuters. Dec 9, 2010; Jargon J. Success is only so sweet in remaking cereals. *Wall Street J.* Oct 11, 2011.
15. Monteiro CA, et al. Ultra-processed foods, diet quality, and health using the NOVA classification system. FAO. 2019.
16. Bray GA, et al. Consumption of high-fructose corn syrup in beverages may play a role in the epidemic of obesity. *Am J Clin Nutr.* 2004;79(4):537–543. doi:10.1093/ajcn/79.4.537; Bocarsly ME, et al. High-fructose corn syrup causes characteristics of obesity in rats: increased body weight, body fat

and triglyceride levels. *Pharmacol Biochem Behav.* 2010;97(1):101–106. doi:10.1016/j.pbb.2010.02.012

17. Heller L. CSPI, CRA campaign in favor of controversial sweetener. *Food Navigator-USA.* Sep 8, 2007.
18. Watson E. Senators: HFCS is being “significantly mischaracterized.” *Food Navigator-USA.* Aug 9, 2011; Watson E. FDA denies corn sugar petition: “We are not persuaded by the argument.” *Food Navigator-USA.* May 30, 2012.
19. Truxel et al. v. General Mills Sales, Inc, No. 4:16-cv-04957-JSW (N.D. Cal. Aug. 29, 2016); Watson E. General Mills prevails in false ad lawsuit over sugar in cereals . . . after three-year battle. *Food Navigator-USA.* Aug 14, 2019; Schroeder E. Post agrees to settle cereals labeling lawsuit. *Food and Business News.* Mar 5, 2012.
20. Luna A (FL-13). H.R. 8688—Stop Spoonfuls of Fake Sugar Act 2024. Congress.gov. Jun 11, 2024; Weisman E. Kennedy’s war on corn syrup brings a health crusade to Trump country. *New York Times.* Dec 10, 2024.
21. Hadley v. Kellogg Sales Co., No. 16-CV-04955-LHK (N.D. Cal. Aug. 29, 2016); Hadley v. Kellogg Sales Co., No. 16-CV-04955-LHK (N.D. Cal. Aug. 10, 2017); Hadley v. Kellogg Sales Co., No. 16-CV-04955-LHK (N.D. Cal. Nov. 23, 2021).
22. Plaintiffs v. General Mills Sales Inc., No. 4:16-CV-04957-JWS (N.D. Cal. Aug 29, 2016); Siegner C. Can cereal be sugary and “healthy”? Judge dismisses lawsuit against General Mills. *Food Dive.* Sep 9, 2019.
23. USDA/FNS. National level annual summary: WIC data tables. Aug 2025.
24. Oliveira V, Frazão E. *The WIC Program: Background, trends, and economic issues*, 2009 edition. USDA/ERS (ERR-73). Apr 2009.
25. WIC, 7 C.F.R. Pt. 246. Revisions, reorganization, republication. Final rule. *Fed Regist.* 1977;42–166:43211.
26. WIC, 7 C.F.R. Pt. 246. Revisions, reorganization, republication. Final rule. *Fed Regist.* 1980;45–220:74854.
27. Franklin G. *Raisin Bran and Other Cereal Wars.* iUniverse; 2014; Minnesota WIC Office. WIC foods—questions. Minnesota Department of Health. Aug 3, 2023.
28. WIC, 7 C.F.R. Pt. 246. Revisions in the WIC Food Packages. Final Rule. *Fed Regist.* 2024;89–76:28488.
29. New York Department of Health, WIC Program. State WIC APL—cereal. May 9, 2024; Dong D, et al. *WIC Household Food Purchases Using WIC Benefits or Paying Out of Pocket: A case study of cold cereal purchases.* USDA/ERS (ERR-207). May 2016.
30. Texas Health and Human Services WIC Program. Discontinuation by General Mills of Dora the Explorer cereal. Aug 22, 2018.

Chapter 4. Grains and Fiber: The Whole Point

1. Benisi-Kohansal S, et al. Whole-grain intake and mortality from all causes, cardiovascular disease, and cancer: a systematic review and dose-response meta-analysis of prospective cohort studies. *Adv Nutr.* 2016;7(6):1052–1065. doi:10.3945/an.115.011635
2. General Mills. *General Mills 1997 Annual Report.* 1997.
3. FDA. Health claim notification for whole grain foods. Jul 1999; General Mills. A whole new way to defend yourself. *New York Times.* Jul 12, 1999.
4. General Mills. *General Mills Annual Report: 2000.* 2000.
5. Oldways Whole Grains Council. *Our history. The Whole Grain Stamp.*
6. General Mills goes whole grain. *Food Navigator-USA.* Oct 5, 2004.
7. Krasny LT. FDA denies petition on whole grain descriptors. *Food Processing.* Feb 23, 2006.
8. FDA. Draft guidance for industry and FDA staff: whole grain label statements. Feb 2006.
9. Jacobson M, et al. Letter to Dr. Margaret Hamburg, FDA Commissioner. Feb 3, 2012.
10. Satchi & Satchi. Video: *General Mills—"Whole Grain Nation."* Adforum.com. 2006.
11. General Mills. Letter to Dietary Guidelines Advisory Committee. Oct 12, 2009: Appendix E.
12. Harris J, et al. Nutrition-related claims on children's cereals: what do they mean to parents and do they influence willingness to buy? *Public Health Nutr.* 2011;14(12):2207–2212. doi:10.1017/S1368980011001741
13. Olson E. And down this aisle, many whole grain options. *New York Times.* Feb 3, 2011; Wilking C. General Mills uses whole grain claims to distract from sugar content. Public Health Advocacy Institute. Dec 14, 2011.
14. Lin BH, et al. Trends in whole grain intakes 1994–2018: The roles of age, food source, and school food. USDA/ERS. Apr 12, 2023.
15. General Mills. *Annual Report 2008 Continuous Growth.* 2008.
16. Kellogg adds fiber, hoping to bowl cereal consumers over. ABC News. Jun 4, 2009.
17. Kellogg Company. Q1 2010 earnings call transcript. Roic.ai. Apr 29, 2010.
18. FDA. *Guidance for Industry: The Declaration of Certain Isolated or Synthetic Non-Digestible Carbohydrates as Dietary Fiber on Nutrition and Supplement Facts Labels.* Jun 2018.
19. See note 13. General Mills achieves record-level results in fiscal 2010. Jun 29, 2010; General Mills, Inc. Q2 2011 earnings call transcript. Dec 16, 2010.
20. Kellogg's boosts America's fiber intake with cereals that offer fiber and whole grains. *PR Newswire.* Feb 7, 2012.

Chapter 5. Flavors and Colors: Natural and Artificial

1. 21 CFR § 101.22. Foods; labeling of spices, flavorings, colorings and chemical preservatives.
2. Goodman MJ. The "Natural" vs. "natural flavors" conflict in food labeling. *Food Drug Law J.* 2017;72(1):78–102.
3. Yet another lawsuit about the lack of fruit in "Froot Loops." *Lowering the Bar.* Apr 29, 2010; Videtto v. Kellogg USA, No. 2:08-cv-01324-MCE-DAD (E.D. Cal. May 20, 2009); Reasonable consumer would know "Crunchberries" are not real, judge rules. *Lowering the Bar.* Jun 2, 2009.
4. Boboltz S. Sorry, but turns out your favorite blueberries may be entirely fake. *Huffington Post.* Oct 29, 2014; Dvora v. Gen. Mills Inc., No. 11-1074 (U.S. Dist. Ct., C.D. Cal., dismissed May 16, 2011); Hardy S, et al. False advertising case against cereal maker dismissed with leave to amend. Lexology. May 23, 2011.
5. Kellogg. Kellogg brands celebrate the season with delicious fall flavors. *PR Newswire.* Aug 26, 2015.
6. Chasan A. Pumpkin spice season kicks off earlier each year. Here's a look at the history of America's enduring love for the pie-inspired flavor. CBS News. Aug 22, 2024.
7. Casey C. Hundreds protest food dyes in cereals outside Kellogg headquarters. *Food Dive.* Oct 16, 2024.
8. Hari V. Kellogg's: Remove artificial food dyes and BHT from your cereals! *Food Babe.* Apr 22, 2024; Hyslop G. W.K. Kellogg's under fire for chemicals in US cereals: key takeaways for other producers. *Bakery&Snacks.* Sep 27, 2024.
9. Newman J. How Froot Loops landed at the center of U.S. food politics. *Wall Street J.* Nov 21, 2024; Shankar D. RFK Jr. and Gavin Newsom agree: ban artificial food dyes. *Forbes.* Nov 4, 2024.
10. FDA. HHS, FDA to phase out petroleum-based synthetic dyes in nation's food supply. Apr 22, 2025; The President's Make America Healthy Again Commission. *The MAHA Report: Making our children healthy again (assessment).* The White House. May 13, 2025; Spence C. On the psychological impact of food colour. *Flavour.* 2015;4:21; General Mills. *General Mills Annual Report 1996.* Aug 14, 1996.
11. FDA. Color additives in food. Jul 6, 2023.
12. FDA. Color certification reports. Apr 17, 2025.
13. Miller MD, et al. Potential impacts of synthetic food dyes on activity and attention in children: a review of the human and animal evidence. *Environ Health.* 2022;21(1):45. doi:10.1186/s12940-022-00849-9; CSPI. Synthetic food dyes: health risks, history, and policy. Undated; Weiss B, et al. Behavioral responses to artificial colors. *Science.* 1980;207(4438):1487–1489. doi:10.1126/science.7361103

14. FDA. Color additives. Apr 26, 2024; FDA. Color additive history. Nov 3, 2017; CSPI. CSPI urges FDA to ban artificial food dyes linked to behavior problems. Jun 22, 2008; Kobylewski S, Jacobson MF. *Food Dyes: A rainbow of risks.* CSPI; 2010; FDA. Nutrition Food Advisory Committee, transcript of minutes. Mar 30, 2011; FDA Science Board. Advisory Committee Meeting. Oct 7, 2019; FDA. Color additives questions and answers for consumers. Dec 14, 2023.
15. FDA. FDA is finally addressing requests for a definition of "Natural." Nov 14, 2015.
16. General Mills to eliminate artificial colors, flavors from entire cereal line. ABC News. Jun 22, 2015; Ramakrishnan S. Kellogg to stop using artificial products in cereals and snacks. Reuters. Aug 4, 2015; Watrous M. Kellogg to remove artificial colors, flavors from cereal. *Food Business News.* Aug 4, 2015.
17. Banford V. General Mills: 75% of our cereals now free from artificial colors and flavors. *Bakery&Snacks.* Jan 20, 2016; Poinski M. Big Food hit pause on switching to natural colors. What will it take to make the shift? *Food Dive.* Jun 3, 2021.
18. Office of Environmental Health Hazard Assessment. *Health Effects Assessment: Potential neurobehavioral effects of synthetic food dyes in children.* California Environmental Protection Agency. Apr 2021; International Association of Color Manufacturers. IACM statement on final OEHHA report. Apr 16, 2021; Doering C. FDA bans red dye no. 3 over link to cancer in rats. *Food Dive.* Jan 15, 2025.
19. CSPI. FDA moves to eliminate carcinogenic Red 3 from foods. Updated Jan 15, 2025; FDA. FDA to revoke authorization for the use of Red No. 3 in food and ingested drugs. Jan 15, 2025; FDA. HHS, FDA to phase out petroleum-based synthetic dyes in nation's food supply. Apr 22, 2025.
20. Ettinger J. No more artificial colors in colorful General Mills' breakfast cereals. Organic Authority. Sep 10, 2024; Newman J. Silly rabbit! Food activists come for General Mills. *Wall Street J.* Nov 19, 2024; Hyslop G. Levelling the playing field: Kellogg's feels the brunt of social media to remove chemicals from its kiddies' cereals sold in the US. *Bakery&Snacks.* Apr 23, 2024.
21. Crawford E. California bans common food dyes in schools days after FDA, stakeholders discuss proposed systematic post-market review process for chemicals in foods. *Food Navigator-USA.* Oct 1, 2024; Severson K. Kennedy plans to phase out 8 commonly used food dyes. *New York Times.* Apr 21, 2025; Hyslop G. General Mills boycott reflects rising tide of consumer discontent. *Bakery&Snacks.* Apr 22, 2025; Hyslop G. General Mills under fire for "healthy" claims as dye controversy heats up. *Bakery&Snacks.* May 15, 2025.
22. Creswell J. No more food dyes in Froot Loops? Not so fast. *New York Times.* Apr 25, 2025.

23. Johnson B. Take two: General Mills taking artificial colors out of its food. *MN Star Tribune*. Jun 17, 2025; Doering C. Froot Loops maker WK Kellogg to remove artificial colors by 2027. *Food Dive*. Jul 21, 2025; Hyslop G. The snackdown: MAHA throws a Froot Loop at Kellogg's. *Bakery&Snacks*. Sep 2, 2025.
24. HHS & USDA. *The Scientific Foundation for the Dietary Guidelines for Americans*. Dec 2025; HHS & USDA. *Dietary Guidelines for Americans, 2025–2030*. Jan 7, 2026.

Chapter 6. Nutrients: The More, the Better

1. Kellogg Company. The greatest packages for the greatest name in cereal. *Kellogg News*, 1952 Mar;XV(3).
2. Miller WJ, Neathery MW. Newly recognized trace mineral elements and their role in animal nutrition. *BioScience*. 1977;27(10):674–679. doi:10.2307/1297552
3. Rosenfeld L. Vitamine—vitamin. The early years of discovery. *Clin Chem*. 1997;43(4):680–685. doi:10.1093/clinchem/43.4.680; Semba RD. The discovery of the vitamins. *Int J Vitam Nutr Res*. 2012;82(5):310–315. doi:10.1024/0300-9831/a000124; Kellogg's. Food fortification in focus. Kelanova. 2023.
4. National Nutrition Conference for Defense. *JAMA*. 1941;116(23):2598–2599. doi:10.1001/jama.1941.02820230042013
5. FDA. Standards of identity. Mar 14, 2024; Backstrand JP. The history and future of food fortification in the United States: a public health perspective. *Nutr Rev*. 2002:60(1):15–26. doi:10.1301/002966402760240390
6. FDA. Vitamin and mineral-fortified foods. *Fed Regist*. 1966;31–118:8526.
7. USDA. *Food and Nutrient Intake of Individuals in the United States, Spring 1965. Household Food Consumption Survey, 1965–66*, Rep No 11, 1972; CBS Reports. *Hunger in America*. May 1968.
8. *White House Conference on Food, Nutrition, and Health: Final report*. 1970.
9. Martin D. R. B. Choate Jr., food lobbyist, dies at 84. *New York Times*. May 12, 2009. US Senate. *Hearings before the Consumer Subcommittee of the Committee on Commerce United States Senate Ninety-First Congress, Second Session on Dry Cereals*. July 23, Aug 4 and 5, 1970: 31, 6, 14.
10. IOM. *Dietary Reference Intakes: Guiding principles for nutrition labeling and fortification. Overview of food fortification in the United States and Canada*. National Academies Press; 2003; FDA. General principles governing the addition of nutrients to foods notice of proposed rule making. *Fed Regist*. 1974;39–116:20900.
11. FDA. Food additives permitted for direct addition to food for human consumption; Folic acid. *Fed Regist*. 2016;81–73:22176.

12. General Mills, Inc. *2024 Global Responsibility Report.* 2024; CDC. *CDC's Second Nutrition Report.* May 14, 2024.
13. FDA. Questions and answers on FDA's fortification policy guidance for industry. Nov 2015.
14. FDA. *Guidance for Industry: Reference Amounts Customarily Consumed: List of products for each product category.* Feb 2018; Amidor T. Why are cereal companies changing their fortified nutrients? *US News.* Mar 16, 2020.
15. Lobo V, et al. Free radicals, antioxidants and functional foods: impact on human health. *Pharmacogn Rev.* 2010 Jul;4(8):118–126. doi:10.4103/0973-7847.70902
16. Pruthi S, et al. Vitamin E supplementation in the prevention of coronary heart disease. *Mayo Clinic Proc.* 2001;76(11):1131–1136. doi:10.4065/76.11.1131; Fortmann SP, et al. Vitamin and mineral supplements in the primary prevention of cardiovascular disease and cancer: an updated systematic evidence review for the U.S. Preventive Services Task Force. *Ann Intern Med.* 2013;159(12):824–834. doi:10.7326/0003-4819-159-12-201312170-00729; Bjelakovic G, et al. Mortality in randomized trials of antioxidant supplements for primary and secondary prevention: systematic review and meta-analysis. *JAMA.* 2007;297:842–857. doi:10.1001/jama.297.8.842; National Center for Complementary and Integrative Health. Antioxidant supplements: what you need to know. Jul 2023.
17. Lempert P. The top 10 food predictions for 2013. *Supermarket News.* Dec 3, 2012.
18. Big Food marketing LIES. *Food Babe.* Aug 23, 2022; Kuster E. The calories and nutrition in one baby carrot. Livestrong.com. Oct 7, 2021.
19. O'Keefe J Jr, Harris W. From Inuit to implementation: omega-3 fatty acids come of age. *Mayo Clin Proc.* 2000 Jun;75(6):607–614. doi:10.4065/75.6.607
20. NIH. Omega-3 fatty acids. NIH Office of Dietary Supplements. Dec 17, 2024.
21. Fries W. Omega-3s as a functional food: fatty acids in cereal and more. WebMd.com. Mar 29, 2011; Schroeder E. General Mills launches Total Plus Omega-3s cereal. BakingBusiness.com. Jun 22, 2020.
22. McKeon G, Hallman W. Characterization and comparative analysis of foods with front-of-package protein claims. *Curr Dev Nutr.* 2019;3(Suppl 1):nzz051.P04-149-19. doi:10.1093/cdn/nzz051.P04-149-19
23. Van Allen J. Protein: Why it's so popular right now. *Washington Post.* Jul 22, 2014; Nunes K. The power of protein will be tested in 2014. *Food Business News.* Feb 28, 2014.
24. Wu G. Dietary protein intake and human health. *Food & Function.* 2016 Mar;7(3):1251–1265. doi:10.1039/c5fo01530h; Hoy MK, et al. Protein intake of adults: What We Eat in America, NHANES 2015–2016. Jan 2021.

25. Weiler M, et al. Is it time to reconsider the U.S. recommendations for dietary protein and amino acid intake? *Nutrients.* 2023;15(4):838. doi:10.3390/nu15040838; Gunnars K. 10 science-backed reasons to eat more protein. Healthline. Feb 9, 2023; HHS & USDA. *The Scientific Foundation for the Dietary Guidelines, 2025–2030.* 2025; HHS & USDA. *Dietary Guidelines for Americans, 2025–2030.* Jan 7, 2026.
26. Delimaris I. Adverse effects associated with protein intake above the recommended dietary allowance for adults. *ISRN Nutr.* 2013:126929. doi:10.5402/2013/126929; Antonio J, et al. A high protein diet has no harmful effects: A one-year crossover study in resistance-trained males. *J Nutr Metab.* 2016:9104792. doi:10.1155/2016/9104792.
27. CSPI. "Cheerios Protein" has negligibly more protein, but far more sugar, than Original Cheerios. Nov 9, 2015; CSPI. General Mills: Cheerios Protein. October 8, 2021.
28. Casey C. General Mills packs protein into Ghost cereal. *Food Dive.* Apr 10, 2024; Casey C. General Mills powers up portfolio with Wheaties Protein. *Food Dive.* Apr 16, 2024.
29. Walansky A. Cheerios sneaks vegetables into our breakfast. Food Network. Dec 19, 2023.

Chapter 7. Overcoming the Claims Barrier: Cancer and Heart Disease

1. Geiger C. Health claims: history, current regulatory status, and consumer research. *J Am Diet Assoc.* 1998;98(11):1312–24. doi:10.1016/S0002-8223(98)00294-6; Wartella E, et al., eds. *Front-of-Package Nutrition Rating Systems and Symbols: Phase I report.* National Academies Press; 2010.
2. Burkitt D. Possible relationships between bowel cancer and dietary habits. *Proc R Soc Med* 1971;64:964–965; Graham S, et al. Diet in the epidemiology of cancer of the colon and rectum. *JNCI.* 1978;61:709–714; Brandt supports Kellogg All-Bran cancer education efforts. *Food Chem News.* Nov 5, 1984.
3. Burros M. Health claims on food put F.D.A. in a corner. *New York Times.* Feb 19, 1986.
4. FDA Center for Food Safety and Applied Nutrition. 1999. Letter to M. Nestle from Alan Levy. College Park, MD: FDA.
5. All-Bran anti-cancer message is not a health claim, Kellogg's Costley says. *Food Chem News.* May 6, 1985:28–29; Ippolito P, Mathios A. *Health Claims in Advertising and Labeling: A study of the cereal market.* FTC; Aug 1989; Levy AS, Stokes RC. Effects of a health promotion advertising campaign on sales of ready-to-eat cereals. *Public Health Rep.* 1987;102:398–403.
6. Kellogg Company. *A Citizen's Petition: The relationship between diet and health.* Kellogg Company; 1985.

7. Sugarman C. Political skirmish over FDA proposal: debate persists on issue of product health claims. *Washington Post.* Feb 17, 1988.
8. Mitchell P. Making health claims: controversy over an FDA proposal. *Washington Post.* Aug 12, 1987; Hilts P. Panel says White House delayed effort to curb food health claims. *New York Times.* Nov 15, 1990; Hilts P. In reversal, White House backs curbs on health claims for food. *New York Times.* Feb 9, 1990.
9. Sugarman C. The new chow hounds: states join forces to monitor product claims. *Washington Post.* Sep 21, 1988; Burros M. The "food police" keep busy with health claims. *New York Times.* Feb 27, 1991; Associated Press. Kellogg sues Texas official for slander. *Washington Post.* Apr 1, 1991; Iowa sues Kellogg over disputed ads. *Rochester Post Bulletin.* Oct 11, 1990:28–29; Kellogg settles lawsuit over Special K ad claims. United Press International. Oct 3, 1991.
10. Hilts P. In reversal, White House backs curbs on health claims for food. *New York Times.* Feb 9, 1990; FDA. Food labeling: health messages and label statements; reproposed rule. *Fed Regist.* 1990;55:5176–5192; Burros M. U.S. agency seeks uniform labeling: in a reversal, Sullivan says federal standards should pre-empt local laws. *New York Times.* June 28, 1990.
11. Nutrition Labeling and Education Act of 1990. Public Law 101-535. 104 Stat 2353 (1990).
12. FDA. Dietary supplements: general requirements for nutrition labeling: proposed rules. *Fed Regist.* 1993;58:33690–33751; Burros M. In switch, F.D.A. offers looser rules on labels. *New York Times.* Feb 11, 1992.
13. Gladwell M. Food label agreement reached: White House ends agencies' feud over nutrition information. *Washington Post.* Dec 3, 1992; FDA. Food labeling: general provisions; nutrition labeling; label format; nutrient content claims; health claims; ingredient labeling; state and local requirements; and exemptions; final rules. *Fed Regist.* 1993;58:2066–2941 [Quote p. 2503].
14. Pitts P. Gauging the strength of F.D.A. regulation. *New York Times.* Jul 6, 2003; Kaufman M. FDA eases rules on touting food as healthful. *Washington Post.* Jul 11, 2003.
15. FDA. Authorized health claims that meet the significant scientific agreement (SSA) standard. Mar 28, 2024.
16. FDA. Label claims for conventional foods and dietary supplements. Mar 28, 2024; FDA. A food labeling guide for industry. Jan 2013.
17. CDC. Heart disease facts. Oct 24, 2024.
18. Keys A. Prediction and possible prevention of coronary artery disease. *Am. J. Public Health.* 1953;43:1399–1407. doi:10.2105/AJPH.43.11.1399
19. Azcuenaga M. A high-fiber, low-cholesterol approach to health claims: The Federal Trade Commission's "Reasonable Basis" standard. FTC Comments. Sep 10, 1990.

20. FDA. § 101.75 Health claims: dietary saturated fat and cholesterol and risk of coronary heart disease. *Fed Regist.* 1993;58 (Jan 6):2758.
21. FDA. § 101.77 Health claims: fruits, vegetables, and grain products, particularly soluble fiber, and risk of coronary heart disease.
22. AHA. Heart-check digital grocery list. www.heart.org. 2025.
23. Day K. The power of institutional endorsement. *Washington Post.* Jan 31, 1997.
24. Best D. US: Kellogg puts "heart-healthy" logo on cereals. Just Food. Feb 10, 2012.
25. Hadley v. Kellogg Sales Co. 273 F Supp 3d 1052 (ND Cal, Aug 10, 2017).
26. Watson E. Kellogg agrees to settle sugary cereal class action with $20m fund. *Food Navigator-USA.* Oct 23, 2019; Schroeder E. Post agrees to settle cereals labeling lawsuit. *Food Business News.* Mar 5, 2021.
27. Wiener-Bonner D. Millennials abandoned cereal: General Mills is betting that kids and older people will bring it back. CNN. July 20, 2019; Stockton S. General Mills brings back heart-shaped Cheerios, new packaging. *Shelby Report.* Jan 27, 2024.
28. Brody J. Beware food companies' health claims. *New York Times.* Sep 21, 2004.

Chapter 8. More Heart-Health Claims: Ingredient Petitions

1. Fitzsimmons R. Oh, what those oats can do. Quaker Oats, the Food and Drug Administration, and the market value of scientific evidence 1984 to 2010. *Comp Rev Food Sci Food Safety.* 2011;11(1):56–99. doi:10.1111/j.1541-4337.2011.00170.x
2. Tipton T. Oats: researchers say that oat products can have the same positive impact as oat bran for those interested in reducing their risk for heart disease. *Los Angeles Times.* Nov 3, 1988; Anderson JW, Gustafson NJ. Hypocholesterolemic effects of oat and bean products. *Am J Clin Nutr.* 1988;48(3):749–753; Kinosian B, Eisenberg J. Cutting into cholesterol: cost-effective alternatives for treating hypercholesterolemia. *JAMA.* 1988;259(15):2249–2254; Confusing array of oat bran cereals fill grocery shelves to help. *Chicago Tribune.* Sep 21, 1989.
3. Anderson JW, et al. Oat-bran cereal lowers serum total and LDL cholesterol in hypercholesterolemic men. *Am J Clin Nutr.* 1990;52(3):495–499. doi:10.1093/ajcn/52.3.495
4. Sugarman C. Knowing your oats: big business cashes in on the little kernel that fights cholesterol. *Washington Post,* Oct 12, 1988; Moser PW. How I made $812 in the oat bran craze. *Fortune,* Oct 9, 1989; USDA, ERS. Food Availability (Per Capita) Data System. Grains. Oats; Saturday Night Live. *Colon Blow.* YouTube. Nov 11, 1989.
5. *Cheerios Wake Up to the One with Oat Bran.* Video, 1989. YouTube. Jul 1, 2018; Deutsche J. Has Kellogg's lost its snap? *New York Times.* Sep 24, 1989;

La Ganga ML. Kellogg to fire new salvo in oat bran war: cereal giant's second new product to debut. *Los Angeles Times*. Aug 30, 1989.

6. Swain JF, et al. Comparison of the effects of oat bran and low-fiber wheat on serum lipoprotein levels and blood pressure. *N Engl J Med*. 1990;322:147–152. doi:10.1056/NEJM199001183220302; Brody JE. Small study challenges role of oat bran in reducing cholesterol. *New York Times*. Jan 18, 1990; Humble CG. Oats and cholesterol: the prospects for prevention of heart disease. *Am J Public Health*. 1991;81:159–160. doi:10.2105/ajph.81.2.159
7. Samuels A. Quaker funds studies on oat bran benefits. *Los Angeles Times*. Jan 31, 1990; Nestle M. *Unsavory Truth: How the food industry skews the science of what we eat*. Basic Books; 2018; Ripsin CM, et al. Oat products and lipid lowering: a meta-analysis. *JAMA*. 1992;267:3317–3325.
8. Food labeling: health claims; oats and coronary heart disease. *Fed Regist*. 1996;61(3):296–337.
9. Food labeling: health claims; soluble fiber from whole oats and risk of coronary heart disease: final rule. *Fed Regist*. 1997;62(15):3583–3601.
10. Pollack J. Ordinary people star in new fall Quaker effort. *Advertising Age*. Aug 17, 1998; Quaker Oats. Advertisement: "Eating oatmeal is good for your heart. Meet the proof." *New York Times Magazine*. Sep 27, 1998:68; Quaker Oats Co. advertisement: "30-day dietary intervention program to help lower cholesterol." *J Am Diet Assoc*. 1999;99:290.
11. Bloomberg News. Oat foods can tout benefits to heart: cereal, bread firms planning ad push after FDA ruling. *San Francisco Examiner*. Jan 22, 1997; Paul GL, et al. The Quaker Oats health claim: a case study. *J Nutraceut Funct Med Foods*. 1999;1(4):5–32. doi:10.1300/J133v01n04_02
12. Johnston L, et al. Cholesterol-lowering benefits of a whole grain oat ready-to-eat cereal. *Nutr Clinical Care*. 1998;1:6–12.
13. Schardt D. Hook, line, and Cheerios: when labels and ads don't quite add up. *Nutr Action Healthletter*. 2005;32(8).
14. National Advertising Division. NAD reviews advertising for General Mills' Cheerios. Better Business Bureau; Jul 2, 2007.
15. See: Nestle M. The FDA is going after health claims? At last! *Food Politics*. May 13, 2009; McCarthy K. FDA sinks Cheerios health claims; calls cereal an "unapproved drug." *Consumer Reports News*. May 13, 2009.
16. Edgar (Mr Consumer). Cheerios helps lower cholesterol 4%; no, make that 10%. Do I hear 20%? Mouse Print. Jun 15, 2009; Maki KC, et al. Whole-grain ready-to-eat oat cereal, as part of a dietary program for weight loss, reduces low-density lipoprotein cholesterol in adults with overweight and obesity more than a dietary program including low-fiber control foods. *J Am Diet Assoc*. 2010;110(2):205–214. doi:10.1016/j.jada.2009.10.037
17. NCL applauds FDA for warning General Mills for misbranding Cheerios. National Consumers League. May 13, 2009; Consumer group sues General

Mills for deceptive claims on Cheerios. National Consumers League. Sep 10, 2009; National Consumers League v. Gen. Mills Inc. *V/lex*. Jan 15, 2010.
18. Hanson CV, et al. Psyllium. *Corn Agronomy*. Jun 1, 1992; General Mills, Inc. The benefits of Benefit cereal. General Mills wants you to know. *New York Times*. Sep 12, 1989.
19. F.D.A. questions use of grain in 3 cereals. *New York Times*. Oct 1, 1989.
20. Burros M. Psyllium in cereal: unknown territory. *New York Times*. Sep 6, 1989; General Mills dropping Benefit cereal. UPI Archives. Jan 4, 1990; Shapiro E. Getting the most out of byproducts. *New York Times*. May 23, 1990.
21. Baker N. Kellogg's says it will not make health claims about products. UPI Archives. Aug 30, 1989; Burros M. Flirting with health claim, Kellogg announces a cereal. *New York Times*. Aug. 31, 1989.
22. Specter M. FDA warns 2 cereal makers about health claims on labels. *Washington Post*. Sep 29, 1989.
23. Lantner R, et al. Anaphylaxis following ingestion of a psyllium-containing cereal. *JAMA*. 1990;264:2534–2536; Burros M. Eating well; the food police keep busy with health claims. *New York Times*. Feb 27, 1991.
24. Meier B. Kellogg files slander suit. *New York Times*. Apr 3, 1991.
25. Food labeling: health claims; soluble fiber from certain foods and coronary heart disease. *Fed Regist*. 1998;63:8103–8121.
26. Pollack J. Kellogg's new ensemble features an old ingredient. *Advertising Age*. Nov 9, 1998:90; Pollack J. Kellogg takes light approach for Ensemble. *Advertising Age*. Apr 19, 1999:3,86; Thompson S. Kellogg loses appetite for Ensemble products. *Advertising Age*. Nov 8, 1999:1,125.
27. Food labeling: health claims; soluble dietary fiber from certain foods and coronary heart disease. *Fed Regist*. 2003;68(144):44207–44209.
28. Heavey S. Some whole oats foods can carry "low fat" claim: FDA. Reuters. Aug 9, 2007.
29. 21 CFR § 101.62. Food labeling; specific requirements for nutrient content claims.
30. Food labeling: health claims; soluble fiber from certain foods and risk of coronary heart disease. *Fed Regist*. 2008;73(85):23947–23953;Letter to Stephen Gardner, director of litigation CSPI from Jenner & Block LLP. RE: Quaker Oatmeal.
31. CSPI. Quaker agrees to tone down exaggerated health claims on oatmeal. Apr 17, 2007.

Chapter 9. Nutrient Content and Structure/Function Claims

1. FDA. *Guidance for Industry: A food labeling guide*. Jan 2013.
2. Hoyland A, et al. A systematic review of the effect of breakfast on the cognitive performance of children and adolescents. *Nutr Res Rev*. 2009;22(2):220–243. doi:10.1017/S0954422409990175

3. Zorn E. Reading "Change of Subject" will improve your awareness of current events by 70 percent. *Chicago Tribune*. Jan 31, 2008.
4. FTC. In the matter of Kellogg Company, a corporation. Docket NO. C-4262. Jul 27, 2009.
5. FTC. Kellogg settles FTC charges that ads for frosted Mini-Wheats were false. Apr 20, 2009; FTC. FTC approves final consent order in matter concerning Kellogg Company. Jul 31, 2009; FTC. Kellogg Company, in the Matter of: Case timeline. Jun 3, 2010.
6. Starling S. Kellogg to pay millions in kids' attention class action settlement. *NutraIngredients-USA*. Nov 22, 2010; Nieburg O. Kellogg settlement on attention cereal claims rejected. *NutraIngredients-USA*. Jul 16, 2012; LaFreniere M. Kellogg's Frosted Mini-Wheats class action settlement checks mailed. Top Class Actions. Apr 18, 2016.
7. Rogers M. A lot of hoopla over plain old calcium. CNN Money. May 26, 1986.
8. Bishai D, Nalubola R. The history of food fortification in the United States: Its relevance for current fortification efforts in developing countries. *EDCC*. 2002;51(1):37–53. doi:10.1086/345361; FDA. Food labeling: requirements for nutrient content claims, health claims, and statements of nutritional support for dietary supplements. *Fed Regist*. 1997;62(184):49859–49868.
9 FDA. Food labeling: health claims: calcium and osteoporosis, and calcium, vitamin D, and osteoporosis: final rule. *Fed Regist*. 2008;73(189).
10. Kellogg Company. Kellogg Company's vitamin D petition accepted by FDA. *PR Newswire*. Jan 9, 2023.
11. FDA. Food additives permitted for direct addition to food for human consumption; vitamin D. Jan 5, 2023; General Mills. Extra, extra! Read all about it: General Mills doubles vitamin D in Big G cereals. Jul 19, 2023.
12. Doering C. PepsiCo's Life launches multigrain cereal aimed at family wellness. *Food Dive*. Apr 7, 2025.
13. Herrera D. Letter to David Mackay, Kellogg Company. Oct 27, 2009.
14. Horovitz B. Kellogg pulls immunity claim from Rice Krispies. *USA Today*. Nov 4, 2009.
15. FTC. In the matter of Kellogg Company, a corporation. Docket NO. C-4262. Jul 27, 2009; FTC. FTC investigation of ad claims that Rice Krispies benefits children's immunity leads to stronger order against Kellogg. Jun 3, 2010; FTC. In the Matter of Kellogg, a corporation. Order to show cause and order modifying order. Docket No. C-4262. May 28, 2010; Hensley S. Kellogg slapped again for exaggerated health claims. NPR. Jun 4, 2010.
16. Chan S. Kellogg to restrict ads to settle U.S. inquiry into health claims cereal. *New York Times*. Jun 3, 2010.
17. See note 12.

18. Sleep Aids—Worldwide | Statista Market Forecast. Statista. National Heart, Lung, and Blood Institute. What are sleep deprivation and deficiency? Mar 24, 2022; Hyslop G. Post launches the first-ever cereal designed to promote sleep. *Food Navigator-USA*. Feb 3, 2023.
19. Agency for Healthcare Research and Quality (AHRQ). *Melatonin for Treatment of Sleep Disorders*. Evidence Report/Technology Assessment: No. 108. AHRQ 05-E002-1. 2004; Ferracioli-Oda E, et al. Meta-analysis: melatonin for the treatment of primary sleep disorders. *PLoS One*. 2013;8(5):e63773. doi:10.1371/journal.pone.0063773
20. National Center for Complementary and Integrative Health. Melatonin: what you need to know. NIH. May 2024.
21. Loria K. Does melatonin really help you sleep? *Consumer Reports*. Mar 12, 2024.
22. Doering C. Post moves from breakfast to nighttime with new sleep-promoting cereal. *Food Dive*. Feb 23, 2023.

Chapter 10. Widgets: Nutrition at a Glance

1. PepsiCo debuts Smart Spot symbol. *Nutraceuticals World*. Sep 1, 2004; Unilever U.S. unveils "Choices" program. *Nutraceuticals World*. Dec 1, 2006; Kraft Foods flagging items as "Sensible Solutions." *Progressive Grocer*. Apr 20. 2007; Nestle M, Ludwig D. Front-of-package food labels: public health or propaganda. *JAMA*. 2010;303(8):771–772. doi:10.1001/jama.2010.179
2. Armstrong K. *Stumped at the Supermarket: Making sense of nutrition rating programs*. National Policy & Legal Analysis Network to Prevent Childhood Obesity; 2010; Smith L. FSA backs "traffic light" food labelling scheme. *Guardian*. Mar 9, 2006.
3. Lupton J, et al. The Smart Choices front-of-package nutrition labeling program: rationale and development of the nutrition criteria. *Am J Clin Nutr*. 2010;91(4):1078S–1089S. doi:10.3945/ajcn.2010.28450B
4. Neuman W. For your health: Froot Loops. *New York Times*. Sep 4, 2009.
5. Artificial success. *Economist*. Sep 26, 2009.
6. Ruiz R. Smart Choices foods: dumb as they look? *Forbes*. Sep 17, 2009.
7. Nestle M. Kellogg's asks for a Froot Loops correction. More on Smart (?) Choices. *Food Politics*. Sep 5, 2009.
8. Nestle M. Smart Choices: 44% sugar calories! *Food Politics*. Aug 24, 2009; Nestle M. You don't like Smart Choices? Act now! *Food Politics*. Sep 16, 2009.
9. Nestle M. Update on not-so-Smart Choice labels. *Food Politics*. Sep 23, 2009.
10. Kennedy's letter: Nestle M. The Not-So-Smart Choices story continues. . . . *Food Politics*. Sep 26, 2009.
11. Neuman W. Connecticut to scrutinize food labels. *New York Times*. Oct 14, 2009; Neuman W. F.D.A. to clarify standards for the front of food labels.

New York Times. Oct 20, 2009; Smart Choices Program postpones active operations. Smart Choices Program. Oct 23, 2009; Nestle M. Smart Choices suspended! May it rest in peace. *Food Politics*. Oct 23, 2009.

12. Smart Choices Program postpones active operations. Smart Choices Program. Oct 23, 2009; Nestle M. Industry abandons Smart Choices! *Food Politics*. Oct 30, 2009; Dean's controversial food-labeling program suspends operations. *Tufts Daily*. Undated.
13. Laskawy T. Big Food's "Smart Choices" label raises eyebrows at the FDA. *Grist*. Sep 8, 2009.
14. Neuman W. F.D.A. to clarify standards for the front of food labels. *New York Times*. Oct 20, 2009.
15. IOM. *Examination of Front-of-Package Nutrition Rating Systems and Symbols: Phase 1 report*. National Academies Press; 2010; Neuman W. Group seeks food label that highlights harmful nutrients. *New York Times*. Oct 13, 2010.
16. Grocery Manufacturers Association. GMA and FMI announce "Facts Up Front" as theme for front-of-pack labeling program consumer education campaign. *PR Newswire*. Sep 22, 2011.
17. IOM. *Front-of-Package Nutrition Rating Systems and Symbols: Promoting healthier choices*. National Academies Press; 2011.
18. Grocery Manufacturers Association. Statement in response to the Institute of Medicine's Committee on Examination of Front-of-Package Nutrition Rating Systems and Symbols Report. Oct 20, 2011.
19. FDA. Letter of enforcement discretion to GMA/FMI re "Facts Up Front." Dec 13, 2011; FDA. *Foods and Veterinary Medicine Program Strategic Plan 2012–2016*. Apr 2012.
20. Evich HB, Parti T. Food industry to launch media blitz. Politico. Mar 1, 2014.
21. Consumer Brands Association. New research shows strong consumer preference for the Facts Up Front label on food and beverage products. Jul 14, 2025.
22. Watson E. CSPI: "Facts Up Front" is a joke that should be roundly ignored by the FDA. *Food Navigator-USA*. Mar 3, 2014.
23. Fang L. Fruity Pebbles and Lucky Charms threaten to block "healthy" food labeling guidelines in court. The Intercept. Mar 1, 2023; General Mills, Kellogg, Post Consumer Brands. RE: Docket No. FDA-2016-D-2335 for food labeling: nutrient content claims; definition of term "healthy." Feb 16, 2023.
24. Liévano W. Video: *FDA: Frosted Flakes Healthier Than an Avocado. Wall Street J.* May 11, 2016.
25. Watson E. FDA tells KIND it can use term "healthy" on pack: "Our regulations on nutrient content claims are due for a re-evaluation." *Food Navigator-USA*. Mar 18, 2017; FDA. FDA to redefine "healthy" claim for food label-

ing. Sep 27, 2016; FDA. *Guidance for Industry: Use of the term "healthy" in the labeling of human food products.* Sep 2016; Tin A. FDA to develop new "healthy" logo this year—here's what consumers could see and which foods could qualify. CBS News. Feb 27, 2024.

26. FDA. FDA proposes to update definition for "healthy" claim on food labels. Nov 28, 2022.
27. FDA. Food labeling: nutrient content claims; definition of term "healthy": proposed rule. Sep 29, 2022; Onque R. These 7 cereals do not qualify as "healthy" according to the FDA's new criteria. CNBC. Oct 11, 2022.
28. FDA. Food labeling: nutrient content claims; definition of term "healthy." *Fed Regist.* 2024;89–248:106064; FDA. Appendix G Healthy Symbols figure. FDA-2021-N-0336-0003. May 7, 2021.
29. *Biden-Harris Administration National Strategy on Hunger, Nutrition, and Health.* White House; Sep 2022.
30. Reagan-Udall Foundation. Front-of-package nutrition labeling. Nov 16, 2023.
31. FDA. Front-of-package nutrition labeling. Jul 8, 2024.
32. CSPI. Citizen petition for the U.S. Food and Drug Administration to adopt a mandatory, nutrient-specific, interpretive front-of-package nutrition labeling system for all packaged foods sold in the United States. Aug 5, 2022; FDA. Front-of-package nutrition labeling. Jul 8, 2024; Lurie P. Front-of-package nutrition labels advance to White House. CSPI. Nov 22, 2024; FDA. FDA issues proposed rule on front-of-package nutrition labeling. Jan 14, 2025; FDA. Food labeling: nutrient content claims; definition of term "healthy." *Fed Regist.* 2025;90–8249.
33. Grummon AH, et al. Nutrition info and other front-of-package labels and simulated food and beverage purchases: A randomized clinical trial. *JAMA Netw Open.* 2025;8(10):e2537389. doi:10.1001/jamanetworkopen.2025.37389

Chapter 11. Diet Claims: Fads and Fantasy

1. Kumar A. Global weight loss and diet management market size, share, trends & growth analysis report—segmented by diet . . . industry forecast from 2024 to 2032. Market Data Forecast. Jun 2024.
2. Newman AA. Pitching a product, without showing it. *New York Times.* Jan 5, 2010; Mattes RD. Ready-to-eat cereal used as a meal replacement promotes weight loss in humans. *J Am Coll Nutr.* 2002;21(6):570–577. doi:10.1080/07315724.2002.10719257
3. Zemel MB, et al. Calcium and dairy acceleration of weight and fat loss during energy restriction in obese adults. *Obes Res.* 2004;12(4):582–590; Zemel MB, et al. Dairy augmentation of total and central fat loss in obese subjects. *Int J Obes.* 2005;29:391–397.

4. Thompson S. Dairy scientist decides to milk his research for all it's worth. *Advertising Age*. Jun 20, 2005.
5. Sanders LM, et al. The relationship of ready-to-eat cereal intake and body weight in adults: a systematic review of observational studies and controlled trials. *Adv Nutr.* 2023;14(4):671–684. doi:10.1016/j.advnut.2023.05.001. Funder: General Mills' Bell Institute.
6. Culliney K. Special K US annual sales slump 9.7%. *Bakery&Snacks*. Aug 28, 2014; Kellogg. Q4 2014 results—earnings call transcript. Seeking Alpha. Feb 12, 2015.
7. Mayo Clinic Staff. South Beach Diet. Mayo Clinic. Jun 9, 2023.
8. Diet firms hope to knock out low-carb craze. NBC News. Dec 31, 2004; Kraft to launch South Beach Diet brand foods. NBC News. Jan 7, 2005.
9. Associated Press. Nutrisystem buys South Beach Diet for $15 million, plans relaunch. *Seattle Times*. Dec 18, 2015; U.S. News & World Report recognizes Nutrisystem and South Beach Diet in annual best diet rankings. *PR Newswire*. Jan 2, 2020.
10. FDA. Gluten-free labeling of foods. Mar 7, 2022.
11. Parzanese I, et al. Celiac disease: from pathophysiology to treatment. *World J Gastrointest Pathophysiol.* 2017;8(2):27–38. doi:10.4291/wjgp.v8.i2.27; Abel EK. *Gluten Free for Life*. NYU Press; 2025.
12. Choung RS, et al. Less hidden celiac disease but increased gluten avoidance without a diagnosis in the United States: findings from the National Health and Nutrition Examination Surveys from 2009 to 2014. *Mayo Clin Proc.* 2016;S0025-6196(16)30634-6. doi:10.1016/j.mayocp.2016.10.012; Statista. Gluten-free foods market in the U.S.—statistics & facts. Dec 18, 2023.
13. General Mills Foodservice. Gluten-free cereal: how we did it. Undated; FDA. Questions and answers on the gluten-free food labeling final rule. Jun 30, 2022.
14. Thompson T. Gluten-Free Cheerios: updated position statement. Gluten-Free Watchdog. Sep 1, 2015; FDA. FDA investigates complaints associated with Cheerios labeled gluten free: General Mills voluntarily recalls affected lots. Oct 2015; Wong V. "Not Safe for Celiacs"—Gluten-free Cheerios are still drawing complaints. BuzzFeed News. Jul 6, 2017; Watson E. And now the lawsuits—General Mills sued over recalled gluten-free Cheerios. *Food Navigator-USA*. Nov 3, 2015.
15. FDA. Gluten and food labeling. Jun 2018; Fritz RD, Chen Y. Oat consumption by celiac disease patients: outcomes range from harmful to beneficial, depending on the purity of the oats. *Ann Gastroenterol Dig Dis.* 2019;2(1): 003–005; Ireland N. "Gluten-free" label to be removed from Cheerios in Canada. CBC News. Oct 25, 2017.
16. Thompson T. Gluten Free Watchdog's updated position statement on Cheerios. Gluten Free Watchdog. Mar 8, 2021; Thompson T. Brief history of

oats & Gluten Free Watchdog's evolving opinion. Gluten Free Watchdog. Apr 10, 2023.

17. Consumer Lab. Rolled oats and steel-cut oats review. Dec 9, 2024.
18. Kellogg. Satisfy every "food mood" with all new flavors from Kellogg's Special K. *PR Newswire*. Dec 7, 2022.
19. Ludwig DS. The ketogenic diet: evidence for optimism but high-quality research needed. *J Nutr*. 2020;150(6):1354–1359. doi:10.1093/jn/nxz308; Gardner CD, et al. Effect of a ketogenic diet versus Mediterranean diet on glycated hemoglobin in individuals with prediabetes and type 2 diabetes mellitus. *Am J Clin Nutr*. 2022;116(3):640–652. doi:10.1093/ajcn/nqac154; Teicholz N, et al. Myths and facts regarding low-carbohydrate diets. *Nutrients* 2025;17:1047. doi:10.3390/nu17061047
20. Schueller G. We surveyed people on the keto diet. Here's what they say. US News & World Report. Aug 6, 2020.
21. Ting R, et al. Ketogenic diet for weight loss. *Can Fam Physician*. 2018 Dec;64(12):906; Global keto diet trends. Bolst Global. 2025.
22. Schouten R. General Mills unveils 16 new cereals. *Food Business News*. Dec 9, 2020.
23. Halmos EP, et al. Diets that differ in their FODMAP content alter the colonic luminal microenvironment. *Gut*. 2015;64(1):93–100. doi:10.1136/gutjnl-2014-307264; Irritable bowel syndrome (IBS). Cleveland Clinic. Nov 16, 2023.
24. Halmos EP, et al. A diet low in FODMAPs reduces symptoms of irritable bowel syndrome. *Gastroenterology*. 2014;146:67–75.e5. doi:10.1053/j.gastro.2013.09.046

Chapter 12. "Green" Claims: Natural, Organic, and Non-GMO

1. Hauter W. *Foodopoly: The battle over the future of food and farming in America*. New Press; 2012; Belasco W. *Appetite for Change: How the counterculture took on the food industry*. 2nd ed. Cornell University Press; 2014.
2. This history is discussed in FDA. Proposed rule: use of the term "natural" in the labeling of human food products; request for information and comments. *Fed Regist*. 2015;80–218:69905.
3. "Natural" will remain undefined, says FDA. *FoodNavigator-USA*. Jan 4, 2008.
4. Natural Products Association. Re: FR Doc. 2010-25000; Proposed, Revised Green Guides, 16 CFR Part 260, Project No. P954501; Request for comment. Dec 10, 2010.
5. Negowetti N. A national "natural" standard for food labelling. *Maine Law Review*. 2013;65(2):581.
6. Strom S. Kellogg agrees to alter labeling on Kashi line. *New York Times*. May 8, 2014.

7. ABC News. Kashi cereal's "natural" claims stir anger. Apr 29, 2012.
8. Astiana v. Kashi Company. Case No. 3:11-cv01967-H-BGS (S.D. Cal.); Eggnatz v. Kashi Company, Case No. 12-21678 (S.D. Fla).
9. Gorman S. Some Kashi products to lose that "all natural" label. *Huffington Post.* May 9, 2014; Watson E. Kashi agrees to pay up to $3.99m to settle "all-natural" lawsuit. *Food Navigator-USA.* Jun 14, 2015; Schroeder E. Kellogg settles suit over Kashi "all natural" claims. *Food Business News.* May 9, 2014.
10. See note #2 and FDA. Use of the term natural on food labeling. Oct 22, 2018.
11. Smith H. "Natural" claims: A thing of the past? *Food Industry Executive.* Feb 15, 2018.
12. Kellogg. *Kellogg Company Annual Report.* 2006.
13. USDA. Organic foods production act of 1990. Public Law 109-97. Nov 10, 2005.
14. Consumer Reports' guide to food labels. *Consumer Reports.* Undated.
15. Smith-Spangler C, et al. Are organic foods safer and healthier than conventional alternatives? *Ann Intern Med.* 2012;157(5):348–366. doi:10.7326/0003-4819-157-5-201209040-00007; Vigar V, et al. A systematic review of organic versus conventional food consumption: is there a measurable benefit on human health? *Nutrients.* 2020;12(1):7. doi:10.3390/nu12010007; Rahman A, et al. A comprehensive analysis of organic food: evaluating nutritional value and impact on human health. *Foods.* 2024;13(2):208. doi:10.3390/foods13020208
16. Lempert P. Will Kellogg's new attempt to support organic farming confuse shoppers even more? *Forbes.* May 17, 2016; Kashi® Launches Kashi by Kids, its first line of organic foods made for kids, by kids. *PR Newswire.* Aug 9, 2018.
17. Halloran A. General Mills is transitioning 53 square miles of South Dakota farmland to certified organic. *The Counter.* Mar 19, 2018; Skorbiansky S, et al. Rising consumer demand reshapes landscape for U.S. organic farmers. *Amber Waves.* Nov 14, 2023.
18. Organic Cereals Market Size, Share, Trends, Forecast Report, 2028. Business Research Insights; Dec 9, 2024; Organic Trade Association. Conscious consumption: younger generations fueling growth in the organic industry. Jun 18, 2024.
19. Non-genetically tweaked Cheerios a marketing boost. NBC News. Jan 4, 2014. For the fake box, see: Nestle M. Some musings on non-GMO Cheerios to start the week. *Food Politics.* Mar 24, 2014.
20. USDA/ARS. List of bioengineered foods. 2025; USDA/ERS. Recent trends in GE adoption. Jan 4, 2025.
21. USDA/ERS. Sugar and sweeteners background. Jan 7, 2025; Horovitz B. Cheerios drops genetically modified ingredients. *USA Today.* Jan 2, 2014.

22. Wunderlich S, Gatto KA. Consumer perception of genetically modified organisms and sources of information. *Adv Nutr.* 2015;6(6):842–851. doi:10.3945/an.115.008870; FDA. Programs on food from new plant varieties. Dec 16, 2024; ConAgra Foods. GMO facts. Conagrabrands.com.
23. Nestle M. *Safe Food: The Politics of Food Safety.* Rev. ed. University of California Press; 2010.
24. Non-GMO Project. Non-GMO Project program rules and procedures. Mar 31, 2023; Philpott T. Researchers: GM crops are killing monarch butterflies, after all. *Mother Jones.* Mar 12, 2012.
25. Suozzo A. The Non GMO Project, fiscal year ending June 2023. ProPublica. May 15, 2024; Roseboro K. Report: nearly half of consumers avoid GMOs. *Organic & Non-GMO Report.* Jul 7, 2018.
26. Non-GMO Project. Non-GMO Project product finder.
27. Daily R. The butterfly effect: Non-GMO Project Verified outgrow similar self-reported claims. *Food Navigator-USA.* Nov 14, 2024.
28. IARC. *IARC Monographs Volume 112: Evaluation of five organophosphate insecticides and herbicides.* WHO; Mar 20, 2015; Environmental Working Group. Roundup for breakfast, part 2: in new tests, weed killer found in all kids' cereals sampled. Oct 24, 2018; Lacey A. Going, going, gone? EWG finds glyphosate levels drop in oat-based products. EWG. Apr 21, 2023.
29. Lustin L, et al. Big win for General Mills as Eleventh Circuit Court affirms dismissal of contaminated Cheerios class action. JD Supra. May 28, 2020.
30. Organic Consumers Association. Tell General Mills to reject GMO wheat! 2024; Honeycutt Z. Shocking test results of glyphosate in breakfast cereals: Are big box brands corrupting organic? Moms Across America. Jul 7, 2025.

Chapter 13. Marketing to Kids: It's GR-R-REAT!

1. Cortini M, et al. How power is pester power? A mix-method study. *TPM.* 2021;28(1):37–46. doi:10.4473/TPM28.1.3; Zhao S, et al. Nutritional content of ready-to-eat breakfast cereals marketed to children. *JAMA Netw Open.* 2025;8(5):e2511699. doi:10.1001/jamanetworkopen.2025.11699
2. Enter Kellogg's stick up for breakfast contest. Kellogg Advertisement. 1980.
3. WK Kellogg Co. Tony's journey. Kellogg's Frosted Flakes. 2025.
4. McPherson M. *Cartoons and Cereal: A history of Saturday morning cartoons.* Independently published; 2025. Gannon M. Cereal mascots earn sales with eye contact. NBC News. Apr 4, 2014; Culliney K. General Mills slams Cornell cereal study: it is "absurd" pseudo science. *Bakery&Snacks.* Apr 9, 2014.
5. Vaala S, Ritter M. Child-oriented marketing on cereal packaging: Associations with sugar content and manufacturer pledge. *J Nutr Educ Behav.*

2020;52(3):215–223. doi:10.1016/j.jneb.2020.01.005; Schwartz M, et al. Examining the breakfast cereals marketed to kids. *J Am Diet Assoc.* 2008;108(4):702–705. doi:10.1016/j.jada.2008.01.003; Lapierre M, et al. Influence of licensed spokescharacters and health cues on children's ratings of cereal taste. *Arch Pediatr Adolescl Med.* 2011;165(3):229–234. doi:10.1001/archpediatrics.2010.300

6. Lou M. "Baby Shark" is being turned into a cereal, doo doo doo doo doo doo. CNN. Jul 29, 2019; Infectious kids' song, "Baby Shark" hits the Billboard Hot 100. NPR. Jan 10, 2019; Pinkfong. *Baby Shark Dance.* YouTube. June 17, 2016.
7. Romano A. Baby Shark (doo doo do doo do doo) explained. Vox. Mar 21, 2019; Chambers G. Baby Shark song on YouTube: What is the dance? And where did it come from? *The Standard.* Sep 6, 2018.
8. Martinez E. When were toys first added to cereal boxes and why did they stop? *TastingTable.* Apr 7, 2023.
9. US Consumer Products Safety Commission. General Mills stops sale of Cheerios with "powerball" premium. Sep 24, 1987; US Consumer Products Safety Commission. Kellogg's voluntarily recalls two toy premiums. Dec 28, 1988.
10. Korkis J. The origins of Cap'n Crunch. Cartoon Research. Dec 4, 2020; Quaker Oats. Cap'n Crunch cereal (1963–1973) commercials. YouTube; Kellogg. 7 Froot Loops commercials from 7 different decades (1963–present). YouTube; Kunkel D. Children and host-selling television commercials. *Comm Res.* 1988;15(1):71–92.
11. Beales H. Advertising to kids and the FTC: A regulatory retrospective that advises the present. FTC. Mar 2, 2004.
12. Pertschuk M. *Revolt Against Regulation: The rise and pause of the consumer movement.* University of California Press; 1982; Pertschuk M. *Giant Killers.* WW Norton; 1987; Sulzberger AO. F.T.C. staff urges end to child-ad study. *New York Times.* Apr 3, 1981.
13. Granville K. A legislative showdown for children's TV: television: backers of limiting ad time on children's TV take hope from Bush's aim to be "the education president." *Los Angeles Times.* Jun 21, 1990; Children's Television Act of 1990, Pub. L. No. 101-437, 104 Stat. 996-1000, codified at 47 U.S.C. §§ 303a, 303b, 394. The Senate Report on the CTA cited the Federal Communications Commission's 1984 decisions as precipitating factors in the enactment of the CTA.
14. CDC NCHS. Prevalence of overweight among children and adolescents: United States, 1999–2002. Nov 15, 2015; Rosenblatt R. Surgeon General takes stern stance on obesity. *Los Angeles Times.* Dec 14, 2001; HHS. The Surgeon General's call to action to prevent and decrease overweight and obesity. 2001.

15. Institute of Medicine. *Food Marketing to Children and Youth: Threat or opportunity?* National Academies Press; 2006.
16. Kolish E, Peeler CL. *Changing the Landscape of Food & Beverage Advertising: The children's food & beverage advertising initiative in action.* Council of Better Business Bureaus; July 2008; Better Business Bureau. *CFBAI Category-Specific Uniform Nutrition Criteria.* 2nd ed. BBB National Programs; Jan 1, 2020.
17. Interagency Working Group on Food Marketed to Children. Preliminary proposed nutrition principles to guide industry self-regulatory efforts. *Fed Regist.* 2011;76–65:20634–20647; Kellogg Company comments on the Interagency Working Group on Food Marketing to Children Preliminary Proposed Nutrition Principles to Guide Industry Self-Regulatory Efforts Request for Comment. FTC, Project No. P094513. Jul 14, 2011.
18. Burros M. Childhood obesity war a food fight? Politico. Oct 12, 2011.
19. Nestle M. Congress caves in again. Delays IWG recommendations. *Food Politics.* Dec 17, 2011.
20. Gillam C. Advertising sugary cereals to children needs regulation, report says. The New Lede. Jan 20, 2025.
21. Jensen M, et al. Are U.S. food and beverage companies now advertising healthy products to children on television? An evaluation of improvements in industry self-regulation, 2017–2021. *Int J Behav Nutr Phys Act.* 2023;20:118. doi:10.1186/s12966-023-01517-y; Harris JL, et al. Encouraging big food to do the right thing for children's health: a case study on using research to improve marketing of sugary cereals. *Crit Public Health.* 2015;25(3):320–333. doi:10.1080/09581596.2014.957655; Harris JL, et al. Children's cereal purchases by U.S. households: associations with child versus adult TV ad exposure. *Am J Prev Med.* 2025;68(3):598–606. doi:10.1016/j.amepre.2024.11.022
22. Powell L, et al. Trends in children's exposure to food and beverage advertising on television. *JAMA.* 2024 Aug 22;7(8):e2429671. doi:10.1001/jamanetworkopen.2024.29671

Chapter 14. Targeting Adults and Families

1. Packaged Facts. Ain't that sweet: kids, millennials and Gen Z consumers favor cereal with more sugar. *PR Newswire.* Jun 15, 2020; Beckett L. "Whatever Froots your Loops": Kellogg launches new millennial focused ad campaign. *Food Dive.* Jun 16, 2017; Commisso D. Top cereal insights for National Cereal Day. Civic Science. Mar 7, 2023.
2. King J. 5 key stats on baby boomers: a look at shopping, search, and spending. EMarketer. Jul 5, 2024; Severson K. Cereal, a taste for nostalgia looks to find its next chapter. *New York Times.* Feb 22, 2016; Zhang M. Why a bowl of cereal is a one-way ticket to '90s nostalgia. *Saveur.* Nov 2, 2022.

3. Topper A. Retro packaging from General Mills attempts to boost returns. Mintel. May 15, 2014.
4. Schouten R. General Mills brings back classic cereal recipes. *Food Business News*. Sep 11, 2020.
5. Review: General Mills ultimate taste comeback (Cookie Crips and Cocoa Puffs). *Cerealously*. Oct 10, 2020.
6. General Mills. *General Mills Annual Report 2010*; Wiener-Bronner D. Millennials abandoned cereal: General Mills is betting that kids and older people will bring it back. CNN Business. Jul 20, 2019.
7. Kellogg Company. Boomers are searching for answers on how to stay healthy for an active retirement. *PR Newswire*. Aug 28, 2013.
8. Vespa J. The graying of America: More older adults than kids by 2035. US Census Bureau. Mar 13, 2018; Battle P. Kellogg sounds alarm on unexpected shift in consumer behavior. The Street. May 7, 2025.
9. The ads, from the *Saturday Evening Post*, Oct 31, 1914, are reproduced in Fox ER. Common threads: using women's suffrage to sell soup and cereal. *Saturday Evening Post*. Oct 29, 2024.
10. Redman R. WK Kellogg seeks better performance from Special K. *Food Business News*. Nov 11, 2019; WK Kellogg Co. Molly Baz makes history as first pregnant woman on a cereal box. *PR Newswire*. Jun 4, 2024.
11. Reese's Puffs: Puffs unleashed: the art of a breakfast revolution. Mobile Marketing Association. 2014.
12. Post Consumer Brands. Pebbles cereal teams up with Susan Alexandra for a berry sweet collection. *PR Newswire*. Feb 28, 2024; Oster D. Berry Pebbles cereal collabs were not for the kids. *Marketing CPG Weekly*. Mar 11, 2024.
13. D'Ambrogio S, et al. How celebrity status and gaze direction in ads drive visual attention to shape consumer decisions. *Psychol Mark*. 2023;40(4):723–734.
14. Hauari G. Travis and Jason Kelce team up with General Mills to create Kelce Mix Cereal: here's what it is. *USA Today*. Jul 19, 2024; Devo J. General Mills teams with Kelce brothers for Cereal Training Camp. *MarketingDive*. Aug 26, 2024; Johnson B. General Mills marketing boss on reaching consumers in an era of advertising overload. *MN Star Tribune*. Oct 15, 2024.
15. General Mills. REESE'S PUFFS cereal teams up with All-Star Angel Reese to release limited edition cereal and teases upcoming fashion collab. Sep 17, 2024; Callahan K. ESPN platforms deliver unprecedented viewership success during NCAA Division I women's basketball season. ESPN Press Room US. Apr 10, 2024; Dorisca S. Angel Reese's former agents said she wouldn't make more than $2k in NIL deals, today she's shattered those expectations. Afrotech. Nov 21, 2024.
16. Rovell D. Is Wheaties dying a slow death? CNBC. Mar 21, 2012.
17. York E. Why you won't see Michael Phelps on the Wheaties box. *Advertising Age*. Aug 28, 2008.

18. Macur J. Phelps disciplined over marijuana pipe incident. *New York Times.* Feb 5, 2009; Painter KL. Wheaties puts Michael Phelps on its cereal box for third time. *MN Star Tribune.* Aug 29, 2016.
19. General Mills. General Mills unveils limited edition collectible cereal boxes featuring Gen Z icons TOMORROW X TOGETHER. Apr 16, 2024; Walmart's exclusive TXT cereal sells out instantly. Koreaboo. Apr 30, 2024.
20. Margotin P, Guesdon J. *All the Songs: The story behind every Beatles release.* Black Dog & Leventhal; 2013; Whatley J. 10 songs by The Beatles that John Lennon hated. *Far Out.* Oct 28, 2024.
21. Kritikos C. Cereal box records sound horrible. They still look incredible. *New York Times.* Sep 15, 2025.
22. Did you cut out and save these records from the back of cereal boxes? MeTV. Sep 30, 2016; Post Raisin Bran box with Bobby Sherman record offer. Hake's Auctions. Jul 11, 2019.
23. General Mills. Honey Nut Cheerios', Buzz Bee, and Ice-T team up to encourage a Change of Heart around eating and exercise. Jan 26, 2022.
24. General Mills. REESES PUFFS teams up with iconic artist KAWS to drop two cereal boxes and AR game. Nov 8, 2012.
25. Crystal Bridges Museum of American Art. KAWS: family, Mar 15–Jul 28, 2025.
26. Schroeder E. RTE cereal makers seeking seasonal boost. *Food Business News.* Nov 30, 2022.
27. Hubbard H. General Mills' classic Monster Cereals are back with a reimagined look. NPR. Aug 11, 2022.
28. Elliott S. Consumer products dress up to cash in on the Christmas spirit. *New York Times.* Dec 16, 1994.
29. Newman AA. A campaign to push Chex as an easy party snack for the holidays. *New York Times.* Dec 9, 2009; Severson K. A short history of cereal. *New York Times.* Feb 22, 2016; The history of (Chex) Party Mixes. *Quaint Cooking.* Dec 2, 2022.
30. Kellogg Company. PSA from the North Pole! Santa wants Kellogg's Rice Krispies Treats this year, not cookies. *PR Newswire.* Nov 15, 2022.
31. Meyer Z. Peeps fans, your dreams have come true. There's now Peeps cereal. *USA Today.* Jan 17, 2019.

Chapter 15. Cereal for All: Targeting Diversity, Equity, and Inclusion

1. Bruce S, Crawford B. *Cerealizing America: The Unsweetened Story of American Breakfast Cereal.* Faber & Faber; 1995.
2. Anti-Black imagery. Jim Crow Museum, Ferris State University. 2024; Fazio M. Cream of Wheat to drop Black chef from packaging, company says. *New York Times.* Sep 27, 2020.

3. Crockett D. Marketing blackness: How advertisers use race to sell products. *J Consumer Culture*. 2008;8(2):245–268. Crockett attributes the quote to Omi M, Winant H. *Racial Formation in the United States: From the 1960s to the 1980s*. Routledge; 1986; Cramer M. After Aunt Jemima, reviews underway for Uncle Ben, Mrs. Butterworth and Cream of Wheat. *New York Times*. Jun 17, 2020.
4. Chui M, et al. A $300 billion opportunity: serving the emerging Black American consumer. *McKinsey Quarterly*. Aug 6, 2021; The state of Black consumers. McKinsey & Company. Feb 24. 2024.
5. Thompson S. Why McDonald's, Coke and General Mills made African-Americans their lead consumer. *Forbes*. Jul 17, 2018.
6. In plain sight: The Black consumer opportunity. *Advertising Age*. Apr 23, 2012.
7. Kindy D. How Wheaties became the "breakfast of champions." *Smithsonian Magazine*. Jul 26, 2021; General Mills. Record-holders since 1926. 2025; General Mills. Wheaties continues 100th anniversary celebration with Michael Jordan. Dec 13, 2021.
8. Barnhill A, et al. The racialized marketing of unhealthy foods and beverages: perspectives and potential remedies. *J Law Med Ethics*. 2022;50(1):52–59. doi:10.1017/jme.2022.8; Harris JL. Targeted food marketing to Black and Hispanic consumers: the tobacco playbook. *Am J Public Health*. 2020;110(3)271–272. doi:10.2105/AJPH.2019.305518; Harris JL, et al. *Cereal FACTS 2012: A spoonful of progress in a bowl full of unhealthy marketing to children*. Yale Rudd Center; 2012.
9. Kang A. The untold truth of Urkel-O's. *Mashed*. Feb 2, 2023.
10. The tweet is reproduced in Hyslop G. Kellogg accused of "teaching racism" over insensitive Corn Pops design. *Bakery&Snacks*. Oct 27, 2017. Also see Snider M. Kellogg's to replace racially insensitive Corn Pops boxes following Twitter call out. *USA Today*. Oct 26, 2017.
11. Schmidt S. Kellogg's apologizes for lone brown corn pop on cereal box. *Washington Post*. Oct 26, 2017.
12. The video is available at Noah T. Trevor answers the age old question: is this Corn Pops box racist? *The Daily Show*. Oct 27, 2017.
13. African American cereal. *Breakfast Bowl*. Feb 13, 2008; Glanton D. Museum a chef's special. *Chicago Tribune*. Mar 10, 2008.
14. Lewis P. This Black owned cereal company is making "Cereal for the culture." *Huffington Post*. Feb 21, 2021.
15. Beaumont-Thomas B. "Diabolical actions": Snoop Dogg and Master P sue Walmart in breakfast cereal spat. *Guardian*. Feb 7, 2024.
16. US Census Bureau. New estimates highlight differences in growth between the U.S. Hispanic and Non-Hispanic populations. Census.gov. Jun 27, 2024.
17. Statista. Buying power of Hispanic consumers in the United States from

1990 to 2021, with a forecast to 2026. Mar 5, 2024; Hispanic consumers drive 16% of total US CPG growth. *Prepared Foods*. Nov 8, 2024.

18. Steinberg, D. A bowl of ole. *New York Times*. Mar 13, 1994.
19. Heneghen C. Post spices up its marketing plans with Hispanic agency of record. *Food Dive*. Oct 26, 2016; Post Consumer Brands continues to make Latino market a priority by naming LatinaWorks as Hispanic agency of record. *PR Newswire*. Oct 24, 2016.
20. Flores A. A taste of nostalgia: Kellogg's Choco Zucaritas. Spanglish Baby. Nov 26, 2012.
21. HMC honors Kellogg's with the 2022 Marketer of the Year Award: only award to honor excellence in Hispanic marketing. Hispanic Marketing Council. Jan 31, 2022; WK Kellogg Co. New Hispanic cereal campaign demonstrates importance of authentic content creation. *PR Newswire*. Jun 30, 2022.
22. Moritz L. Kellogg's tries bilingual again. *Breakfast Bowl*. Jul 13, 2016.
23. Kellogg offers insights on capturing the attention of multicultural consumers. *Candy&Snack Today*. Jun 27, 2023.
24. GLAAD. GLAAD leads millions in support against bullying for Spirit Day. Oct 20, 2016; Superville D. First Lady vows to fight cyberbullying, despite skeptics. PBS News. Mar 20, 2018.
25. GLAAD. Kellogg's and GLAAD launch special edition "All Together" cereal for Spirit Day. Oct 18, 2018.
26. Kellogg. Kellogg Company partners with GLAAD for Spirit Day launching new 2019 edition "All Together" cereal. *PR Newswire*. Oct 17, 2019.
27. Kellogg. Kellogg Company's latest collaboration with GLAAD unwraps why "Boxes are for cereal, not for people." *PR Newswire*. May 20, 2021.
28. Sweeney E. Kellogg mixes cereal brands "All Together" for GLAAD partnership. *MarketingDive*. Oct 19, 2018.
29. Gooding-Williams P. Kellogg's breakfast recipe for LGBT indoctrination. *Daily Compass*. May 15, 2021.
30. Shabad R. Ex-Trump aide Stephen Miller's legal group files complaint against Kellogg's "woke" programs. NBC News. Aug 10, 2023; The letter: America First Legal to Kellogg Company. Potential waste of the Kellogg Company's corporate assets and breach of fiduciary duty due to systemic violations of civil rights laws. Aug 9, 2023.

Chapter 16. Marketing Philanthropy: Do Good, Feel Good

1. Leffingwell B. 7 benefits of corporate philanthropy. *Austin Chamber*. May 31, 2023; Low AP, Hacker G. *Selfish Giving: How the soda industry uses philanthropy to sweeten its profits*. CSPI. 2013.
2. Kelley L. The dark side of Box Tops for Education. *The Atlantic*. Apr 16, 2021.

3. General Mills. John Legend and Box Tops for Education champion legendary teachers by supporting schools in need this back-to-school season. Jul 16, 2024.
4. Moran AJ, et al. A school-based brand marketing program's adherence to federal nutrition criteria. *Am J Prev Med.* 2017;53(5):710–713. doi:10.1016/j.amepre.2017.06.017; Dewey C. A popular school fundraiser is just "junk-food marketing to kids," experts say. *Washington Post.* Jan 17, 2018.
5. See note 4 (Dewey).
6. DeLonge M, Stillerman KP. *Champions of Breakfast: How cereal makers can help save our soil, support farmers, and take a bite out of climate change.* Union of Concerned Scientists; Jul 2019; General Mills. Regenerative agriculture: keeping our planet healthy. Undated.
7. Stein-Bachinger K, et al. To what extent does organic farming promote species richness and abundance in temperate climates? A review. *Org Agr.* 2021;11:1–12. doi:10.1007/s13165-020-00279-2; Casey C. How Cheerios works to stay relevant across generations. *Food Dive.* Aug 10, 2023.
8. Nature Conservancy. Cause marketing: how we partner with Cascadian Farm. Jan 11, 2021; General Mills. Cascadian Farm commits $750,000 to The Nature Conservancy to rebuild wildlife habitat and restore groundwater on farmland in the Sacramento Valley. Feb 3, 2021; Lappé (@annalappe) posted on X (Twitter): "I love when food companies move toward #organic & #regenerative farming but had to laugh: 25M sq ft is 68% of Central Park. Good start Cascadian Farms +@nature_org, but let's #gobigger."
9. Backhaus O, Faber S. Beware misleading "regenerative" soil claims on non-organic foods. Environmental Working Group. May 12, 2022; Regenerative certifications & verifications. Kiss the Ground. 2025; Roseboro K. Can certification programs prevent greenwashing of regenerative claims? *Organic and Non-GMO Report.* Nov 18, 2024.
10. Bruns N. How Cascadian Farm got its start. General Mills. Apr 20, 2022; Laverty KJ. Case study: Cascadian Farm a.k.a. General Mills. Global Business Center, University of Washington. Sep 2004.
11. Somervail J. Nature's Path vows to save the turtles with SEE Turtles partnership for World Sea Turtle Day. Nature's Path. Jun 16, 2020.
12. General Mills. *General Mills 2024 Global Responsibility Report.* 2024.
13. Vega T. Taking photos of breakfast and giving meals to children. *New York Times.* Mar 7, 2011.
14. Newman A. Tied together in aisle 5: Country acts and a cause. *New York Times.* Mar 29, 2012.
15. Post Consumer Brands. Fight hunger, spark change. Here's how. *PR Newswire.* May 9, 2019; Walmart, Sam's Club and Feeding America partner again to fight hunger. Spark change in the movement to end hunger. *PR Newswire.* Apr 1, 2024.

16. General Mills. General Mills Big G Cereals advocate for affordable, accessible breakfast for all kids. Oct 17, 2022.
17. General Mills. Using the power of the cereal bowl to help end childhood hunger. Mar 23, 2023.
18. Kellogg Company donation to No Kid Hungry can help provide up to 2.5M breakfasts to kids in need. *PR Newswire*. May 7, 2022; Fisher A. *Big Hunger: The unholy alliance between corporate America and anti-hunger groups.* MIT Press; 2017; Move For Hunger shatters Guinness World Records title. Move For Hunger. Oct 16, 2023; Coleman L. Fighting hunger! Students collect donated cereal boxes for local food pantries. WFMY News. Mar 6, 2024.

Chapter 17. Cereal Goes International

1. Freedonia Focus Reports. Global breakfast cereals. Sep 2019.
2. Renub Research. Top breakfast cereals companies in 2025. May 16, 2025; Sims G T. Corn Flakes clash shows the glitches in European Union. *New York Times*. Nov 1, 2005.
3. Bach D, et al. Kellogg: localizing foreign entry mode. IMD Research & Knowledge. Aug 2021; Dolan K. *Breakfast Cereal: A global history*. Reaktion Books; 2023.
4. Kellogg divests Russian operations to local snack maker Chernogolovka. Reuters. Dec 22, 2022; Circana. OmniMarket Total Store View. 52-weeks ending Dec 1, 2024; S&P Global. Kellogg Company ratings affirmed on the spin-off of North American cereal business; outlook remains negative. Sep 29, 2023.
5. Schultz EJ. Cereal marketers race for global bowl domination. *Advertising Age*. Aug 20, 2012.
6. Mote. Kellogg's failure and counterattack in the Indian market. *Food Talks*. Feb 27, 2025; Laghate G. Kellogg's India sets sights on doubling household reach. Mint. Dec. 27, 2023.
7. Sridhar D. The UK and EU cracked down on food dyes long ago—MAGA is way behind the curve. *Guardian*. Apr 30, 2025.
8. Health Canada. List of permitted food colours. Dec 12, 2023.
9. EFSA. Scientific opinion on the re-evaluation of erythrosine (E 127) as a food additive. Jan 27, 2011; EFSA. Food colours. Jan 18, 2024; Six food colors must carry warning labels in EU. *Food Engineering*. Aug 12, 2010.
10. Hari V. General Mills has been put on notice: remove dyes from Lucky Charms, Cinnamon Toast Crunch and Trix in America! *Food Babe*. Nov 2024.
11. McCann D, et al. Food additives and hyperactive behaviour in 3-year-old and 8/9-year-old children in the community: a randomised, double-blinded, placebo-controlled trial. *Lancet*. 2007;370(9598):1560–1567. doi:10.1016/

S0140-6736(07)61306-3; EFSA. EFSA evaluates Southampton study on food additives and child behaviour. Mar 14, 2008; Meikle J. EU plans warning labels on artificial colors. *Guardian*. Aug 10, 2008.

12. International Agency for Research on Cancer. The Nutri-Score: a science-based front-of-pack nutrition label. WHO. Sep 2021.
13. Chazelas E, et al. Nutri-Score and ultra-processing: two different, complementary, non-contradictory dimensions. *Nutr Hosp*. 2021;38(1):201–206. doi:10.20960/nh.03483; Scientific Committee of the Nutri-Score. Update of the Nutri-Score algorithm. Jun 29, 2022.
14. Deschasaux-Tanguy M, et al. Nutritional quality of diet characterized by the Nutri-Score profiling system and cardiovascular disease risk: a prospective study in 7 European countries. *Lancet Reg Health Eur*. 2024 Sep 10;46:101006. doi:10.1016/j.lanepe.2024.101006; Julia C, et al. Ten years of Nutri-Score front-of-pack nutrition labeling in Europe. *Nat Food*. 2025;6(3):239–243. doi:10.1038/s43016-025-01141-y
15. Southey F. Should extra virgin olive oil receive Nutri-Score "A"? *Food Navigator-Europe*. Jul 12, 2024; Ford A. Europe's biggest dietary problem? Lobbyists, says Nutri-Score creator. Politico. Dec 20, 2024; Calvert E. Food label ambush: How intense industry lobbying halted EU plans. *BEUC*. Oct 9, 2023; Besancon S, et al. A study is 21 times more likely to find unfavourable results about the nutrition label Nutri-Score if the authors declare a conflict of interest or the study is funded by the food industry. *BMJ Glob Health*. 2023 May;8(5):e011720. doi:10.1136/bmjgh-2023-011720; Garde A, et al. Unpacking front-of-pack nutrition labelling research: when the food industry produces "science" as part of its lobbying strategies. *World Nutr*. 2024;15(3):63–65. doi:10.26596/wn.202415363-65
16. Wax E, Leali G. Italy claims it's winning the war against French food labels. Politico. Jan 3, 2022; Robinson N. Nutri-score abandoned by European Commission. *Food Navigator-Europe*. Mar 4, 2025.
17. Global Food Research Program. Front-of-package labeling. Mar 2025.
18. Corvalán C, et al. Structural responses to the obesity and non-communicable diseases epidemic: update on the Chilean Law of Food Labelling and Advertising. *Obes Rev*. 2019;20(3):367–374. doi:10.1111/obr.12802
19. Campbell M. Chile: front-of-package warning labels and food marketing. *J Law Med Ethics*. 2022;50:298–303. doi:0.1017/jme.2022.55; Jacobs A. In sweeping war on obesity, Chile slays Tony the Tiger. *New York Times*. Feb 7, 2018.
20. Florko N. Kellogg's is going to war over Mexico's nutrition label rules. A similar fight is coming to the U.S. STAT News. Aug 21, 2023.
21. Korpar L. Mexican agents raid 75 outlets to seize 380,000 boxes of Kellogg's cereal. *Newsweek*. Jan 14, 2022.
22. Taillie LS, et al. Changes in food purchases after the Chilean policies on food

labelling, marketing, and sales in schools: a before and after study. *Lancet Planet Health*. 2021;5(8):e526-e533. doi:10.1016/S2542-5196(21)00172-8; Obesity Evidence Hub. Nutritional warning labels. Cancer Council Victoria. 2025.

23. Popkin BM, Ng SW. The nutrition transition to a stage of high obesity and noncommunicable disease prevalence dominated by ultra-processed foods is not inevitable. *Obes Rev*. 2022;23(1):e13366. doi:10.1111/obr.13366

Conclusion

1. Creswell J, Hirsch L. Have Americans lost their appetites? Maybe for iconic brands. *New York Times*. Jul 31, 2025; GlobalData. Lower Q1 sales, tariff outlooks sees WK Kellogg cut forecasts. Yahoo!Finance. May 7, 2025.
2. Thomas L, Dummett B. Ferrero strikes roughly $3 billion deal for maker of Froot Loops, Frosted Flakes. *Wall Street J*. Jul 10, 2025; WGB Staff. Kellogg divests Keebler cookies, related business to Ferrero. *Supermarket News*. Mar 31, 2019; Hyslop G. General Mills, WK Kellogg & Ferrero spark a fresh fight for the breakfast bowl. *Food Navigator-USA*. Nov 18, 2025.
3. Chee FY, Van Overstraeten B. Mars' $36 billion Kellanova deal gets US antitrust approval as EU opens investigation. Reuters. June 25, 2025; Mars. Mars receives final regulatory approval and moves to close acquisition of Kellanova. Dec 8, 2025.
4. General Mills flags $70 million charge in current quarter from restructuring efforts. Reuters. May 27, 2025; Redman R. Post to shut two cereal plants as category declines. *Food Business News*. Apr 10, 2025; Gelski J. After recall, Quaker decides to close plant. *Food Business News*. Apr 10, 2024.
5. Johnson B. In the land of cereal, Minnesota's breakfast upstarts offer substitute for Lucky Charms, Froot Loops. *MN Star Tribune*. May 27, 2025; Rosen A. Influence vs. evidence: the science supporting seed oils. Johns Hopkins Bloomberg School of Public Health. Jun 6, 2025.
6. Make America Healthy Again. *The MAHA Report: Make Our Children Healthy Again: Assessment*. May 2025; Kennedy E, Dwyer J. The 1969 White House Conference on Food, Nutrition and Health: 50 years later. *Curr Dev Nutr*. 2020 May 15;4(6):nzaa082. doi:10.1093/cdn/nzaa082; White House Task Force on Childhood Obesity. *Report to the President: Solving the problem of childhood obesity within a generation*. May 20, 2010; Michelle Obama's hypocritical war on junk food. Fox News. May 13, 2010; Brown M. Michelle Obama was vilified by the right. Then came MAHA. Politico. Jun 14, 2025.
7. WK Kellogg Co. Creating joy and connection since 1906. 2024.

CEREALS: A SELECTED BIBLIOGRAPHY

Bruce S. *Cereal Box Bonanza: The 1950's Identification and Values.* Collector Books; 1995. A how-to guide for cereal box collectors, with lavish color illustrations of boxes, toys, and advertising from the decade when cereals went from boring to exciting.

Bruce S, Crawford B. *Cerealizing America: The Unsweetened Story of American Breakfast Cereal.* Faber & Faber; 1995. A history of the origins of breakfast cereal, with special emphasis on the "breakfast revolutionaries" responsible for its development, and on the marketing of specific brands.

Dolan K. *Breakfast Cereal: A Global History.* Reaktion Books; 2023. An illustrated discussion of hot and cold cereals, their marketing, and their role in culture.

Fast RB, Caldwell EF, eds. *Breakfast Cereals and How They Are Made.* American Association of Cereal Chemists; 1990. Multiple experts detail historic manufacturing techniques—equipment, flavor additions, fortification, packaging, and quality assurance—for ready-to-eat breakfast cereals.

Franklin G. *Raisin Bran and Other Cereal Wars: 30 Years of Lobbying for the Most Famous Tiger in the World.* Universe; 2014. A former Kellogg lobbyist's account of how he worked to defeat regulatory limits on sugar and marketing to children.

Gitlin M, Ellis T. *The Great American Cereal Book: How Breakfast Got Its Crunch.* Abrams Image; 2012. A catalog of every cereal box the authors could find from 1892 on, identified by decade.

Hollis T. *Part of a Complete Breakfast: Cereal Characters of the Baby Boom Era.* University Press of Florida; 2012. A well-researched "baby boomer" history of the use of characters to sell breakfast cereals.

Johnson IJ. *The History and Manufacture of Breakfast Cereals*. Chicago: The Cereal Institute; 1951. A remarkably informative industry pamphlet designed for teachers.

Markel H. *The Kelloggs: The Battling Brothers of Battle Creek*. Vintage; 2017. A superbly researched history of the competition between the Kellogg brothers over credit, ownership, and marketing.

INDEX

CALIFORNIA STUDIES IN FOOD AND CULTURE

Darra Goldstein, Editor

1. *Dangerous Tastes: The Story of Spices*, by Andrew Dalby
2. *Eating Right in the Renaissance*, by Ken Albala
3. *Food Politics: How the Food Industry Influences Nutrition and Health*, by Marion Nestle
4. *Camembert: A National Myth*, by Pierre Boisard
5. *Safe Food: The Politics of Food Safety*, by Marion Nestle
6. *Eating Apes*, by Dale Peterson
7. *Revolution at the Table: The Transformation of the American Diet*, by Harvey Levenstein
8. *Paradox of Plenty: A Social History of Eating in Modern America*, by Harvey Levenstein
9. *Encarnación's Kitchen: Mexican Recipes from Nineteenth-Century California: Selections from Encarnación Pinedo's* El cocinero español, by Encarnación Pinedo, edited and translated by Dan Strehl, with an essay by Victor Valle
10. *Zinfandel: A History of a Grape and Its Wine*, by Charles L. Sullivan, with a foreword by Paul Draper
11. *Tsukiji: The Fish Market at the Center of the World*, by Theodore C. Bestor
12. *Born Again Bodies: Flesh and Spirit in American Christianity*, by R. Marie Griffith
13. *Our Overweight Children: What Parents, Schools, and Communities Can Do to Control the Fatness Epidemic*, by Sharron Dalton

14. *The Art of Cooking: The First Modern Cookery Book*, by the Eminent Maestro Martino of Como, edited and with an introduction by Luigi Ballerini, translated and annotated by Jeremy Parzen, and with fifty modernized recipes by Stefania Barzini
15. *The Queen of Fats: Why Omega-3s Were Removed from the Western Diet and What We Can Do to Replace Them*, by Susan Allport
16. *Meals to Come: A History of the Future of Food*, by Warren Belasco
17. *The Spice Route: A History*, by John Keay
18. *Medieval Cuisine of the Islamic World: A Concise History with 174 Recipes*, by Lilia Zaouali, translated by M. B. DeBevoise, with a foreword by Charles Perry
19. *Arranging the Meal: A History of Table Service in France*, by Jean-Louis Flandrin, translated by Julie E. Johnson, with Sylvie and Antonio Roder; with a foreword to the English-language edition by Beatrice Fink
20. *The Taste of Place: A Cultural Journey into Terroir*, by Amy B. Trubek
21. *Food: The History of Taste*, edited by Paul Freedman
22. *M. F. K. Fisher among the Pots and Pans: Celebrating Her Kitchens*, by Joan Reardon, with a foreword by Amanda Hesser
23. *Cooking: The Quintessential Art*, by Hervé This and Pierre Gagnaire, translated by M. B. DeBevoise
24. *Perfection Salad: Women and Cooking at the Turn of the Century*, by Laura Shapiro
25. *Of Sugar and Snow: A History of Ice Cream Making*, by Jeri Quinzio
26. *Encyclopedia of Pasta*, by Oretta Zanini De Vita, translated by Maureen B. Fant, with a foreword by Carol Field
27. *Tastes and Temptations: Food and Art in Renaissance Italy*, by John Varriano
28. *Free for All: Fixing School Food in America*, by Janet Poppendieck
29. *Breaking Bread: Recipes and Stories from Immigrant Kitchens*, by Lynne Christy Anderson, with a foreword by Corby Kummer
30. *Culinary Ephemera: An Illustrated History*, by William Woys Weaver
31. *Eating Mud Crabs in Kandahar: Stories of Food during Wartime by the World's Leading Correspondents*, edited by Matt McAllester
32. *Weighing In: Obesity, Food Justice, and the Limits of Capitalism*, by Julie Guthman

33. *Why Calories Count: From Science to Politics*, by Marion Nestle and Malden Nesheim
34. *Curried Cultures: Globalization, Food, and South Asia*, edited by Krishnendu Ray and Tulasi Srinivas
35. *The Cookbook Library: Four Centuries of the Cooks, Writers, and Recipes That Made the Modern Cookbook*, by Anne Willan, with Mark Cherniavsky and Kyri Claflin
36. *Coffee Life in Japan*, by Merry White
37. *American Tuna: The Rise and Fall of an Improbable Food*, by Andrew F. Smith
38. *A Feast of Weeds: A Literary Guide to Foraging and Cooking Wild Edible Plants*, by Luigi Ballerini, translated by Gianpiero W. Doebler, with recipes by Ada De Santis and illustrations by Giuliano Della Casa
39. *The Philosophy of Food*, by David M. Kaplan
40. *Beyond Hummus and Falafel: Social and Political Aspects of Palestinian Food in Israel*, by Liora Gvion, translated by David Wesley and Elana Wesley
41. *The Life of Cheese: Crafting Food and Value in America*, by Heather Paxson
42. *Popes, Peasants, and Shepherds: Recipes and Lore from Rome and Lazio*, by Oretta Zanini De Vita, translated by Maureen B. Fant, foreword by Ernesto Di Renzo
43. *Cuisine and Empire: Cooking in World History*, by Rachel Laudan
44. *Inside the California Food Revolution: Thirty Years That Changed Our Culinary Consciousness*, by Joyce Goldstein, with Dore Brown
45. *Cumin, Camels, and Caravans: A Spice Odyssey*, by Gary Paul Nabhan
46. *Balancing on a Planet: The Future of Food and Agriculture*, by David A. Cleveland
47. *The Darjeeling Distinction: Labor and Justice on Fair-Trade Tea Plantations in India*, by Sarah Besky
48. *How the Other Half Ate: A History of Working-Class Meals at the Turn of the Century*, by Katherine Leonard Turner
49. *The Untold History of Ramen: How Political Crisis in Japan Spawned a Global Food Craze*, by George Solt
50. *Word of Mouth: What We Talk About When We Talk About Food*, by Priscilla Parkhurst Ferguson

51. *Inventing Baby Food: Taste, Health, and the Industrialization of the American Diet*, by Amy Bentley
52. *Secrets from the Greek Kitchen: Cooking, Skill, and Everyday Life on an Aegean Island*, by David E. Sutton
53. *Breadlines Knee-Deep in Wheat: Food Assistance in the Great Depression*, by Janet Poppendieck
54. *Tasting French Terroir: The History of an Idea*, by Thomas Parker
55. *Becoming Salmon: Aquaculture and the Domestication of a Fish*, by Marianne Elisabeth Lien
56. *Divided Spirits: Tequila, Mezcal, and the Politics of Production*, by Sarah Bowen
57. *The Weight of Obesity: Hunger and Global Health in Postwar Guatemala*, by Emily Yates-Doerr
58. *Dangerous Digestion: The Politics of American Dietary Advice*, by E. Melanie DuPuis
59. *A Taste of Power: Food and American Identities*, by Katharina Vester
60. *More Than Just Food: Food Justice and Community Change*, by Garrett M. Broad
61. *Hoptopia: A World of Agriculture and Beer in Oregon's Willamette Valley*, by Peter A. Kopp
62. *A Geography of Digestion: Biotechnology and the Kellogg Cereal Enterprise*, by Nicholas Bauch
63. *Bitter and Sweet: Food, Meaning, and Modernity in Rural China*, by Ellen Oxfeld
64. *A History of Cookbooks: From Kitchen to Page over Seven Centuries*, by Henry Notaker
65. *Reinventing the Wheel: Milk, Microbes, and the Fight for Real Cheese*, by Bronwen Percival and Francis Percival
66. *Making Modern Meals: How Americans Cook Today*, by Amy B. Trubek
67. *Food and Power: A Culinary Ethnography of Israel*, by Nir Avieli
68. *Canned: The Rise and Fall of Consumer Confidence in the American Food Industry*, by Anna Zeide
69. *Meat Planet: Artificial Flesh and the Future of Food*, by Benjamin Aldes Wurgaft
70. *The Labor of Lunch: Why We Need Real Food and Real Jobs in American Public Schools*, by Jennifer E. Gaddis

71. *Feeding the Crisis: Care and Abandonment in America's Food Safety Net*, by Maggie Dickinson
72. *Sameness in Diversity: Food and Globalization in Modern America*, by Laresh Jayasanker
73. *The Fruits of Empire: Art, Food, and the Politics of Race in the Age of American Expansion*, by Shana Klein
74. *Let's Ask Marion: What You Need to Know about the Politics of Food, Nutrition, and Health*, by Marion Nestle, in conversation with Kerry Trueman
75. *The Scarcity Slot: Excavating Histories of Food Security in Ghana*, by Amanda L. Logan
76. *Gastropolitics and the Specter of Race: Stories of Capital, Culture, and Coloniality in Peru*, by María Elena García
77. *The Kingdom of Rye: A Brief History of Russian Food*, by Darra Goldstein
78. *Slow Cooked: An Unexpected Life in Food Politics*, by Marion Nestle
79. *Yerba Mate: The Drink That Shaped a Nation*, by Julia J. S. Sarreal
80. *Wonder Foods: The Science and Commerce of Nutrition*, by Lisa Haushofer
81. *Ways of Eating: Exploring Food through History and Culture*, by Benjamin A. Wurgaft and Merry I. White
82. *From Label to Table: Regulating Food in America in the Information Age*, by Xaq Frohlich
83. *Intoxicating Pleasures: The Reinvention of Wine, Beer, and Whiskey after Prohibition*, by Lisa Jacobson
84. *The Quinoa Bust: The Making and Unmaking of an Andean Miracle Crop*, by Emma McDonell
85. *On Hunger: Violence and Craving in America, from Starvation to Ozempic*, by Dana Simmons
86. *The Pierogi Problem: Cosmopolitan Appetites and the Reinvention of Polish Food*, by Fabio Parasecoli, Agata Bachórz, and Mateusz Halawa
87. *Nile Nightshade: An Egyptian Culinary History of the Tomato*, by Anny Gaul
88. *Food Justice Undone: Lessons for Building a Better Movement*, by Hanna Garth
89. *Sugar Coated: Unboxing the Hidden Forces Shaping America's Favorite Breakfast Food*, by Marion Nestle and Lisa Sutherland